ATHLETES IN APRONS

THE NUTRITION PLAYBOOK TO BREAK 100

KAREN OWOC

ACSM-CEP, ACSM/ACS-CET

Clinical Exercise Physiologist / SF Bay Area TV Health Expert

Published by BookLocker.com, Inc., Trenton, GA.

Cover and interior design by Kaneshige Design Associates

Library of Congress Cataloguing-in-Publication Data

Owoc, Karen.
    Athletes in aprons: the nutrition playbook to break 100 / by Karen Owoc.
    Includes bibliographical references and index.
    ISBN: 978-1-64719-538-0
        1. HEALTH & FITNESS / Longevity 2. COOKING / Health & Healing / Heart
3. HEALTH & FITNESS / Diet & Nutrition / Nutrition

Library of Congress Control Number: 2021924790

Printed on acid-free paper.

BookLocker.com, Inc.

2022

We don't stop playing because we grow old;
we grow old because we stop playing.

GEORGE BERNARD SHAW

THE GAME

NOTES FROM THE COACH

"Age is not how old you are, but how many years of fun you've had."

– Matt Maldre

Chronic diseases and disability were once synonymous with old age, but after over fifty years of research by the U.S. National Institutes of Health (NIH), you can prevent or at least control certain diseases through the way you live. "Normal aging" varies considerably and its rate is influenced by behavioral factors in your control, such as how well you eat, sleep, live, work, and play.

Depending on your lifestyle, your actual calendar age won't necessarily match up with your functional age (measured by how well or how poorly you look and function). For example, you may be 65 years old, but if you've avoided longevity threats like obesity, smoking, long bouts of sitting, distress, and processed, plant-less food, your functional age could be closer to 50.

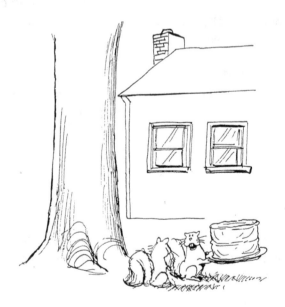

"Acorns or chocolate cake?"

Beyond Bingo

Attitudes on aging are changing. Today, people are living longer and there's been a substantial decrease in the rate of disability among older people in the last twenty years. People in their 80's (even 90's) are golfing, bowling, sailing, weightlifting, participating in Tai Chi, yoga, triathlons — and even surfing in their late 70's. The average life expectancy has changed dramatically.

80 is the New 60

According to the U.S. Census Bureau (International Database and National Vital Statistics System), the average life expectancy was:[1]

- 63.6 years in 1940
- 68.1 years in 1950
- 70.8 years in 1970
- 76.9 years in 2000 (9.3 million aged 80 years and older)
- 77.7 years in 2006
- 78.1 years in 2009
- 78.8 years in 2014
- 78.6 years in 2017

By 2030, it's estimated that individuals aged 80 years and older could grow to 19.5 million, and the "oldest-old" (aged 85 years and beyond) could grow to 10 million people.

What is "Normal Aging"?

Normal aging brings about many physiological changes. Here's what happens to some of your body systems as you age:[2]

Heart

- Your heart muscle thickens.
- The maximum pumping rate diminishes making your heart less efficient.
- The ability to extract oxygen from your blood diminishes.
- Maximal oxygen consumption during exercise declines 7.5%-10% with each decade of your life.

Blood Vessels

- Your arterial walls stiffen. Arteries transport oxygenated blood away from your heart. In order to propel blood through stiff, less elastic arteries, your heart must work harder to exert more force.

- Your capillary walls become more fragile and prone to rupture, and tissues supporting these vessels weaken. Capillaries are tiny, extremely narrow blood vessels.

Brain

- The arteries in your brain and those traveling to your brain (the carotid arteries of your neck), stiffen due to atherosclerosis (a.k.a. hardening of the arteries).

- Connections between your neurons (nerve cells) decrease. Neurons are one of the major players in healthy brain function.

- Individual nerve cell function declines. According to recent studies, the adult nervous system is capable of producing new neurons, but the exact conditions necessary for this to take place are yet to be determined.

- Brain volume diminishes (that is, your brain shrinks in size) at about 5% per decade after age 40. The rate of decline increases with age after age 70.

Kidneys

- The number of nephrons (your filtering units) decreases, so your kidneys can't filter waste material from your blood as efficiently.

- Efficiency at removing waste from your blood (filtering ability) also diminishes because the blood vessels to and within your kidneys become stiff and hard.

- The amount of tissue in your kidneys decreases.

- More than 1 in 7 (15% of Americans or 37 million people) has this disease and 9 in 10 don't know their kidneys are starting to fail.[3, 4]

Bladder

- Your muscles atrophy (that is, they waste away) and weaken, which affect your bladder control and result in incontinence.

- Elastic tissue stiffens, and your bladder's "stretchability" diminishes, so total bladder capacity declines.

Coach Karen says

The Western-style "meat-sweet diet" (high in sugar, salt, fat, and red meat) is a major risk factor for impaired kidney function.[5]

Lungs

- The vital capacity of your lungs decreases by about 40% between the ages of 20 and 70. (Vital capacity is the maximum amount of air you can expel from your lungs after first filling them up to their maximum capacity and then expiring to their maximum extent.)

Vision

- At age 40 and older, focusing on objects that are close becomes difficult.
- At age 50 and older, the susceptibility to glare increases, and your ability to see in low light becomes increasingly difficult.
- At age 70 and older, the ability to distinguish fine details diminishes.

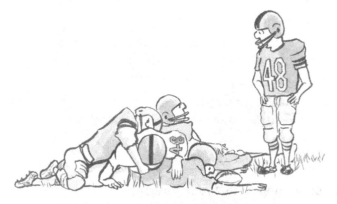

"Let me know if you see a contact lens."

Bones

- Your bone density diminishes. Although bone mineral loss is continually replaced, at around age 35, replacement cannot keep up with the loss. Bone loss accelerates in menopause.

Body Fat

- Percentage of your body fat increases until middle age, stabilizes until late life, then typically declines along with body weight.
- The cushion of fat just beneath your skin redistributes to deeper organs.

Muscles

- Between ages 30 to 70, you become less lean without exercise. Men lose an average of 23% of their lean body mass (muscle), and women lose about 22%.

Immune System

- The ability of your lymphocytes, specifically T-cells, to renew and function efficiently diminishes. T-cells attack cells that have been infected or damaged and also produce chemicals, which direct how your immune system responds.
- Your thymus gland, where T-cells develop, shrinks in size.

Hearing

- Hearing higher frequencies becomes difficult.
- Understanding speech becomes difficult, especially where there is background noise — even with good hearing thresholds. The rate of hearing loss is greater in men than in women.
- Many studies have found an association between hearing loss and cognitive decline. Hearing loss puts you at a greater risk of developing dementia because some parts of the brain (the auditory areas) shrink.

*The human body is the only machine
that breaks down when not used.*

THOMAS CURETON

PLAY 1 — GET IN THE GAME

What Makes You an Athlete...Yes, *You!*

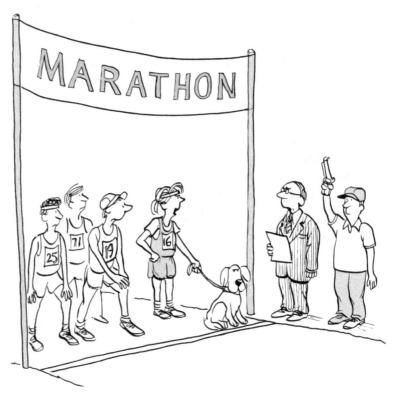

"Can't take my dog? I don't even know HOW
to run without my dog."

Y ou train. You put in the effort. You have goals to achieve. But do you reverently reserve the designation of "athlete" for the top 1% who gets paid to play? Or wears a team uniform? Or breaks a new record? If so, join those who share a mindset that's ingrained in our sports culture. But athletes are much more than that. Athletes aren't defined by dollars and cents, the number they wear, or where they finish.

The term "athlete" is loaded with these stereotypes and defined differently depending on who you ask. Let's hear what the following gents have to say...

- **Merriam-Webster:**

  "A person who is trained in or good at sports, games, or exercises that require physical skill and strength."

- **Urban Dictionary:**

  "An individual who participates in sports. Characterized by dedication, focus, intelligence, and work ethic."

- **Legendary University of Oregon track and field coach and Nike co-founder Bill Bowerman:**

  "If you have a body, you are an athlete."

Not sure if what you do counts as a sport? Let's refer to good ol' Merriam-Webster again who not only defines sport as a competitive physical game, but defines it as: "a physical activity (such as hunting, fishing, running, swimming, etc.) that is done for enjoyment".

There you go. Contrary to popular belief, the athletes' club is not so exclusive, but in fact, all-inclusive. Whether you're a retired jock, weekend warrior, back-of-the-packer, cardiac patient, or cancer survivor, you have what it takes. Everyone has the capacity to be an athlete. Being revered as an athlete doesn't hinge on your performance; it's grounded in your perseverance. True athletes focus on commitment, crave being better than yesterday, and strive to finish. So now that you're clear on what makes you an athlete...step up to the plate, embrace the identity, and read on!

PLAY 2 — FREE AGENTS

Understanding Free Radicals And Why You Age

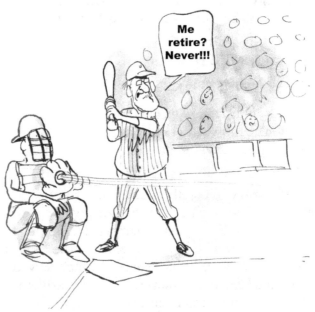

Y ou reminisce longingly of your athletic prowess and the glory days when you moved like a gazelle on the court. What happened to the strength, speed, and stamina that you flaunted back in the day? Sadly, you chalk it up to two words that make even the most macho of men want to whimper. It's called old age. Ouch. No, *double* ouch.

So why do you age? As you enter your 50's, 60's, 70's and beyond, you may think you're entering the inevitable end — call it the 'back nine of life' — but once you understand what causes you to age, you can self-correct. Aging is evidence of the minute, cumulative effects of "free radical damage" that affect your cells and the tissues in your skin, heart, blood vessels, brain, lungs, tendons, and joints.

The Energizer Bunny Within

You're pumped up, full of energy, and head out to set a new personal best. Ever wonder how your body gets energized? Well, simply put, it comes down to the oxygen you breathe and your mitochondria ("my-toh-KON-dree-ah"). Mitochondria are the "power plants" of your cells. They're called power plants because they break down or "burn" glucose from the food you eat to release energy. If you eat crummy food, don't expect to produce energy that keeps you going and going and going and going...

Fill 'Er Up With ATP

The energy molecules that your power plants produce have to be in a form that your cells can use, which is in a *chemical* form called ATP. Think of ATP (adenosine triphosphate) as your own personal high-octane fuel. Without a constant supply of ATP, your body won't work — e.g., your heart won't beat, your muscles won't contract, you won't heal, you won't absorb nutrients.

A single human cell contains thousands of these power plants. The number of mitochondria in a cell depends on your cells' energy needs. For example, your active heart, brain, liver, kidneys, and beefy muscles have thousands of mitochondria, while less active cells have a lot fewer.

Oxygen + Iron = Energy

Your power plants need oxygen to produce ATP. They get oxygen from proteins in your red blood cells (hemoglobin) and inside your heart and muscles (myoglobin), which function as "oxygen storage units". When you take a breath, the oxygen you inhale travels through your bloodstream in these storage units until they reach your power plants.

But to make these oxygen storage units, your body needs iron, so a healthy diet is critical for you to produce ATP. That's why doctors routinely order blood tests that check iron, red blood cell, hemoglobin, and myoglobin levels if their patients complain of fatigue and generalized weakness.

How Oxygen Goes Free and Goes Rogue

In the process of turning air and food into energy, an oxygen molecule may break apart into two single atoms with unpaired electrons. These atoms are aptly named "oxygen free radicals" or "free radicals" for short. Electrons (like snow skis and golf shoes) like to be in pairs. When unpaired, the chaos begins! These single atoms are highly charged and scavenge the body seeking out electrons to complete its pair.

Coach Karen says

Your power plants need high-quality food and oxygen to generate limitless energy and endurance.

Coach Karen says

Red blood cells don't contain any mitochondria. That's because they get their energy from glucose (sugar).

Coach Karen says

An oxygen molecule is composed of two oxygen atoms that are bonded together (O_2).

The Radical Chain Reaction

A free radical is unstable while scavenging to find a sidekick for its unpaired electron. The scavenger looks for the nearest target and steals an electron from another molecule. Then that molecule becomes unpaired and scavenges the body to seek out other electrons, so they can become a pair. It's the classic domino effect. During this electron stealing spree (called oxidation), parts of the cell, such as DNA, proteins, and cell membranes, are damaged. The damage builds up until eventually, the cell is so damaged, it can't function and survive. The cell may die.

How Cell Damage Translates to Disease

If the cell damage is in your eyes, you could have macular degeneration or cataracts. If it's in your blood vessels, you could have clogged arteries or high blood pressure. If it's in your heart, you could have a heart attack or stroke. If it's in your cartilage, you could have arthritis. If it's in your kidneys, you could develop chronic kidney disease. If it's in your brain, you could have memory loss or develop full-blown Alzheimer's or Parkinson's disease. Get the picture?

Sometimes damaged molecules don't die, and DNA is damaged — a major culprit in tumor initiation and progression. All cancers begin when one or more genes in the DNA of a particular cell mutate, which makes a normal cell go horribly awry.

To summarize, oxygen free radicals are highly reactive, unstable particles that eventually damage healthy cells of any type. Free radicals speed up cell death and cause you to "rust" from the inside out. The imbalance between free radicals and your body's defense team (the **anti**-oxidants) is what's known as *oxidative stress*.

How Mitochondria Are Damaged and Lost

Cells that require a lot of energy to function, such as your eyes, brain, and heart, have more mitochondria. If you're healthy, you have the right amount of these power plants in a given cell but become chronically ill, and you may only have half that amount. How many mitochondria you have and how well they're functioning determines your level of energy. Damage to your mitochondria not only impairs energy production, it also increases production of toxic free radicals. So if you want to keep playing your sport and more importantly, if you want to continue to thrive, you have to take care of your mitochondria.

How do mitochondria get damaged? Well, first, aging is a factor. As you age, you lose mitochondria, and they just don't work as well

Coach Karen says

Free radicals are natural waste products from various chemical processes in the cell that can build up and do bodily harm.

anymore. But remember, you have control over how well and how fast you age. There's increasing evidence that supports the link between preventable environmental factors and disease.[1] Besides aging, here are the top five offenders that can reduce your mitochondria number and their ability to function:

1. **Heavy metals (non-essential)** — Mercury and arsenic are two of the most toxic pollutants.[2]

2. **Medications**

3. **Parasites**

4. **Viruses**

5. **Severe oxidative stress** — Heavy metals, medications, parasites, and viruses are all causes of significant oxidative stress. Severe oxidative stress is also caused by lifestyle influences, such as:

   - **Air pollutants**
   - **Chemicals** — e.g., chemical cleaners, chlorine, deodorizers, nail polish, synthetic fragrances
   - **Chronic stress**
   - **Cigarette smoke**
   - **Excessive alcohol consumption**
   - **Exercising too much or too little**
   - **Exposure to fungal toxins** — e.g., environmental molds in bathrooms and basements
   - **High blood sugar levels**
   - **Lack of sleep**
   - **Pesticides**
   - **Plastics and phthalates**
   - **Pro-inflammatory foods** — e.g., food that's fried, charred, over-processed, overcooked, over-sugared, over-salted, and high in saturated fat
   - **Radiation exposure** — e.g, from excessive sunlight to X-rays
   - **Unhealthy microbiome** (gut bacteria imbalance)

Coach Karen says

Avoid these pro-inflammatory foods that damage your mitochondria:

- Fried
- Charred
- Over-processed
- Over-cooked
- Over-sugared
- Over-salted
- High in saturated fat

MITOCHONDRIAL MENACES (MEDICATIONS)

Medications have now emerged as a major cause of mitochondrial damage.[3] The medications documented to damage mitochondria include:

- **Analgesic (for pain) and anti-inflammatory** — e.g., aspirin, acetaminophen (Tylenol®), naproxen (Aleve®, Naprosyn®)

- **Anesthetics** — e.g., lidocaine (Xylocaine®), propofol (Diprivan®)

- **Angina medications** — e.g., amiodarone (Cordarone®)

- **Antiarrhythmic medications** (regulates heartbeat) — e.g., amiodarone (Cordarone®)

- **Antibiotics** — e.g., tetracycline, antimycin A

- **Antidepressants** — e.g., citalopram (Cipramil®), fluoxetine (Prozac®, Symbyax®)

- **Antipsychotics**

- **Anxiety medications** — e.g., alprazolam (Xanax®), diazepam (Valium®)

- **Barbiturates**

- **Cholesterol medications** — includes statins, e.g., atorvastatin (Lipitor®), simvastatin (Zocor®), lovastatin (Mevacor®), colestipol (Colestid®)

- **Diabetes medications** — e.g., Metformin (Glucophage®, Fortamet®)

- **Mood stabilizers** — e.g., lithium

- **Others,** such as medications for alcoholism, cancer

Damage to Disease

Damage to mitochondria is now understood to be associated with a wide range of common diseases, disorders, and conditions, such as:[4]

- **Alzheimer's disease, a.k.a. type 3 diabetes** (progressive death of brain cells resulting in brain atrophy, or shrinkage, caused by cellular changes, such as chronic inflammation and the abnormal buildup of plaque in the arteries of the brain and between brain cells) — Per recent estimates, Alzheimer's disease is now the third leading cause of death in the U.S. after cardiovascular disease.[1]

- **Ataxia** (degeneration of the brain causing loss of muscle control, speech, and balance)
- **Atherosclerosis** (hardening and loss of elasticity within the arteries due to plaque buildup in the arterial wall)
- **Cardiomyopathy** (disease of the heart muscle that makes it harder for the heart to pump blood to the rest of the body and can eventually lead to heart failure)
- **Chronic fatigue syndrome**
- **Dementia**
- **Diabetes, type 2** (inability to process food as energy)
- **Fibromyalgia**
- **Hepatitis C**
- **Macular degeneration** (central vision loss caused by the buildup of plaque in the macula, a part of the retina, and subsequent atrophy and death of photoreceptors and retinal cells in the eyes)
- **Migraine headaches**
- **Neuropathic pain**
- **Parkinson's disease** — Parkinson's is an example of a disease where the mitochondria are ultimately destroyed and brain cells slowly die.
- **Liver cirrhosis** (death of liver cells)
- **Retinitis pigmentosa** (degenerative eye disease causing vision loss)
- **Schizophrenia**
- **Strokes**
- **Transient ischemic attacks (TIA)**

The Anti-Aging Antidotes

Free radicals also contribute to the visible signs of *external* premature aging. Yes, those sporty crinkles around your eyes and freckles on your face. You can blame them on oxidative stress too. What do your wrinkles say about your lifestyle?

Most free radicals can be repaired and passivated with reasonable efficiency via antioxidants. But when antioxidants are outnumbered, they can't keep up with high levels of free radicals that have accumulated in your cells. If cell death outpaces building new well-functioning cells, disease wins.

PLAY 2 — FREE AGENTS | 13

You may already be experiencing signs and symptoms of aging and oxidative stress. How quickly do you heal? Do skin wounds take weeks or months to close and heal? Is your hair turning gray? Is it harder to see close objects and read small print? Do you have headaches or muscle and joint pain? Are you tired and fatigued? Is your memory as sharp as it used to be?

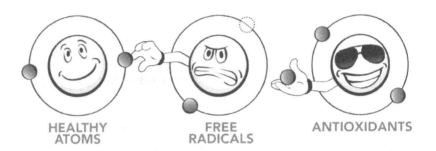

HEALTHY ATOMS   FREE RADICALS   ANTIOXIDANTS

Antioxidants stop the degenerative chain reaction of free radicals. They donate an electron to a free radical, so the radical no longer has an unpaired electron and is no longer a scavenging threat. Antioxidants can donate an electron without becoming a free radical themselves. Your body produces some antioxidants on its own, but not a sufficient amount. The solution? Acquire them through the food you eat. Thousands of antioxidants reside in the colorful roots, seeds, leaves, and flesh of plants (more on pg. 38).

PLAY 3 — THE BENCHWARMERS

Foods To Ditch

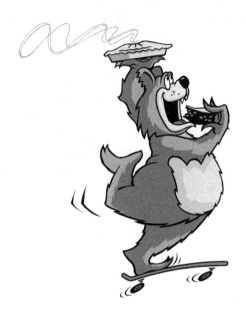

I f you've ever moaned, "Ugh. It's tough growing old," you're likely in pain or you simply can't move like you used to do. Swinging, running, throwing, and even bending over are now HARD. Walking, for that matter, can be a stretch. But all is not lost. You can control how well you feel and how fast you age. Let's start with why sugar makes your once limber body, brain, and arteries *old*.

DITCH: Sugar

Blame Aging on Sugar. Eating too much sugar not only adds empty calories to your diet and inches to your curves, it overcharges your system. One of the key suspects of cell deterioration (aging) is your own blasts of circulating blood sugar (glucose). These glucose molecules cling to proteins in a process called "glycation", and a chain of chemical reactions takes place in your body.

In the end, proteins clump together, known as "crosslinked" proteins, which accumulate over time and disrupt the normal functioning of your cells. This is why diabetes — a disease caused by prolonged elevated levels of sugar in the blood — is considered an "accelerated model of aging".

Why You Get Stiff

These "crosslinks", also known as advanced glycation end products (AGEs) or glycotoxins, seem to stiffen tissues. A stiff body is an aging body, and the most vulnerable proteins to crosslinking are **collagen** and **elastin**. Collagen is one of the most common and longest living protein molecules in the human body. Skin care companies spend billions of dollars trying to replicate, package, and sell it as their revolutionary secret to erasing wrinkles.

Collagen not only provides structure, support, and elasticity to your skin, but to other tissues as well. It's in your muscles (including the heart), blood vessels, bones, joints, tendons, ligaments, organs, skin, intestinal lining, corneas, teeth, and other connective tissues. Think of collagen as the "glue" that holds your parts together. In addition to AGEs, the following factors promote the breakdown of collagen and result in skin laxity and wrinkling:

- Cigarette smoke
- Hormone loss (estrogen levels decline after menopause)
- Pesticides
- Pollution
- Sun exposure, radiation
- Other sources of free radicals

The skin is the largest organ of the human body and one of the most revealing places where aging occurs. The condition of your skin is a good reflection of what's happening on the inside. Do you notice a lot of wrinkles or is your skin loose and fragile like crepe paper? When skin ages, it loses its suppleness, elasticity, and rebound.

When your skin becomes less flexible, expect your internal tissues like your lungs, arteries, and tendons to correspondingly stiffen too. When your arteries are stiff, they lose their contractility, and are limited in their ability to expand and contract. When that happens, your vessels lose their power to squeeze large volumes of blood through them.

Coach Karen says

Eating a diet high in added sugar and refined carbohydrates results in a stiff, aging, less functional body.

HOW WELL DO YOU REBOUND?

Elasticity (the ability to stretch and rebound) diminishes as AGEs accumulate. Fibrous connective tissue, or elastic tissue, loses specialized cells called elastin fibers. In your prime, these fibers could be stretched, but returned to their original length instantaneously.

Take the following "Skin Rebound Test" to measure your skin's elasticity:

1. Gently take a pinch of skin between your thumb and forefinger (on the back of your hand).

2. Raise it 1/4" above the surface into a little ridge, hold for 5 seconds, then let go.

If the ridge completely flattens out in **less than 2 seconds or in nothing flat**, then your skin is very elastic and youthful; **2 seconds or more**, then your skin is probably that of someone in their 50's or 60's; **6-7 seconds**, then your skin is probably that of someone in their 70's.

Age-Related Diseases Linked to AGEs

Stiff tissues can contribute to the development of inflammation and the progression of age-related diseases, such as:

Coach Karen says

When you reduce the number of AGEs circulating in your body, you reduce your risk of the age-related lifestyle diseases.

- **Atherosclerosis** (hardening of the arteries) — AGEs trap "bad" cholesterol in the inner walls of blood vessels, which develop into hardened plaque. It's now known that coronary arteries start developing plaque as early as age 15.[1] Atherosclerosis is a chronic, slow, progressive disease, so without dramatic game changers, the disease will progress.

- **Cancer cell metastasis** (when cancer cells spread to a different body part from where it started)

- **Cataracts** (clouding of the lens of the eye due to proteins clumping together)

- **Diabetes (type 2) and insulin resistance** — Studies show 65% of those with type 2 diabetes will go on to develop Alzheimer's.

- **Nephropathy** (reduced kidney function)

- **Neurodegenerative disease** (such as Alzheimer's) — Studies suggest Alzheimer's is a form of diabetes that occurs in the brain.

Researchers refer to Alzheimer's as **"type 3 diabetes"** or **"brain diabetes"** because brain cells don't respond to insulin, which lead to impairments.[2]

· **Sarcopenia** (loss of skeletal muscle due to aging)

Anti-AGEing Defense Team

Your body fights glycation with immune cells that have special AGE receptors. (Relate this to your golf ball finder that locates your errant golf balls.) When AGEs are detected, your immune cells surround the AGEs, attack them, and break them down. Once the crosslinked proteins are 'unlinked', they make their way into your bloodstream, travel to your kidneys, and race to the nearest exit via your pee.

But whoa! Not so fast. You're not out of the sand trap just yet. As you age, your kidneys become less functional, and your immune cells become less active. When you tack on more years, it's more difficult for your natural defense system to win the battle against the AGEs, and you become even more susceptible to serious diseases. It's no coincidence that everything starts breaking down as you get older, and you're constantly calling on your doctor about one ailment or another. Being vigilant about controlling the production of AGEs is the key to crossing the 100-year mark.

DITCH: Collagen Supplements

The Perfect Counterpunch to AGEing? Supplements are not regulated by the FDA, so anyone can claim their wonder pill contains what (and does what) they say it does. Ingestible collagen, in the form of supplement powders and pills, are being touted as the answer to reversing aging. But even if you swallowed collagen supplements by the fistful, they won't end up as collagen somewhere else. Here's why...

Once swallowed, collagen molecules are dismantled into 'chains of amino acids' by your potent digestive juices (pepsin in your stomach). These new chains scurry down to your small intestine where they're broken apart and become very small individual amino acids that run amuck. Imagine how American footballers line up in formation and at hearing the quarterback shout "Hut! Hut! Hut!", everyone scatters and starts running at each other. Same as these 'free' amino acids. After breaking loose, they reassemble in different ways to become different proteins like enzymes, antibodies, or hormones. At that point, they're absorbed and make their way into the bloodstream.

With that said, your body is absorbing the smaller fragments of what was once a whole intact collagen molecule. Currently, no randomized controlled trials and published clinical studies on ingestible collagen have been proven to have any effects on your skin or body. Better to focus on eating more protein-rich foods (like beans, chia seeds, lentils, quinoa, soy milk, soy nuts, tempeh, tofu) that help your body make its own collagen. This process requires vitamin C, so eat plenty of citrus fruits, bell peppers, tomatoes, broccoli, strawberries, and greens — in other words, plants!

DITCH: Bone Broth

The Lowdown on Bones In addition to collagen supplements, bone broth has become a trendy anti-aging soup du jour. It's true that simmering animal bones and animal parts slowly for long periods of time in water (a minimum of 4 hours and up to 48 hours) leach collagen into the broth. That's how our forefathers made glue. But bones are known to store heavy metals, in particular, lead.

Food scientists found high levels of lead in bone broth made from organic chickens (with the most lead coming from the skin and cartilage).[3] Other studies found bone broth to be a poor source of calcium and magnesium too.[4] Bone broth belongs in the penalty box. Drink vegetable broth instead, and make a rich plant-iful soup.

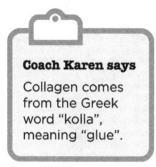

Coach Karen says

Collagen comes from the Greek word "kolla", meaning "glue".

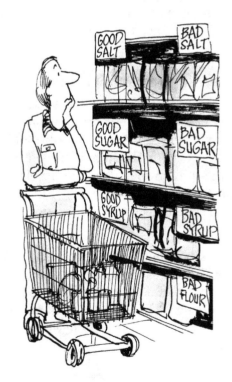

Coach Karen says

Plaque is a sticky substance made up of cholesterol, fat, calcium, fibrin (a blood clotting agent), and metabolic waste.

DITCH: Sodium

Blame Your Aging on Salt Too You may think you've dodged a bullet if you have normal blood pressure, and yet you freely eat salty food. You're one of the lucky ones in that respect, but here's the bad news. Excess dietary sodium damages the inner lining of your blood vessels, called the endothelium. Like sugar, elevated sodium levels cause your arteries to stiffen.[5]

Stiff blood vessels make it hard for your heart to pump blood throughout your body. After a while, your heart wears out, and you end up with heart failure. When your arteries are hit with a constant barrage of bullets — sodium, stress hormones, high blood sugar, high insulin levels, and high LDL cholesterol (the bad guys) — your arteries become a breeding ground for chronic inflammation and plaque build-up. In addition to compromising your blood vessels and heart, sodium can damage and impede blood flow to other target organs, such as your kidneys and brain.

Can One Salty Meal Be All That Bad?

You're pretty good about staying within your sodium limits on most days of the week, but perhaps you have a heavily salted meal every once in a while. "What's the harm in that?" you ask. *Lots*. A high-salt meal can significantly impair blood flow within 30 to 60 minutes after eating it.[6]

DITCH: Foods Cooked at High Temperatures

Coach Karen says

AGEs are not only formed in your body, you ingest them as well. Remember, what you eat becomes a part of you.

Playing With Fire and AGEs You take pride in manning a raging hot fire and huge slabs of meat. In your mind, it's a sacred ritual, a 'Rite of Passage', and evidence that you can cook. But modern-day diets are now linked to high levels of AGEs due to their high percentage of heat-processed food. In addition to sugar, high levels of inflammatory AGEs are formed when products are cooked at high temperatures, including being pasteurized, dried, roasted, broiled, seared, smoked, fried, or grilled.

Researchers found a link between heat-processed foods and AGEs by comparing different types of cooking methods.[7] Animal-derived foods, which are high in protein and fat, are generally rich in AGEs and form AGEs during cooking. On the other hand, fruits, vegetables, peas, beans, and whole grains, contain relatively few AGEs and maintain low levels of AGEs even after cooking.

DITCH: Flour-y Grain Foods

Worst Offenders Bread, breakfast cereals, baked goods, pasta, and packaged snacks. Did you ever make paper-mâché paste in elementary school? It's made with one part flour and one part water, then mixed until it becomes a thick glue-like consistency. Once it dries, the craft project is very hard and stiff. Hmmm...do you ever feel "bloated" or "gassy" after eating flour-based foods?

From Intact to Flour-y

When a grain is "intact", you can actually see the grain. An intact grain (more on pg. 102) hasn't been stripped of any of its layers nor has it been pulverized into flour. An intact grain doesn't have much effect on your blood sugar, like flour, because it literally moves right on through to your gut intact. Your good gut bacteria then feast on all the fiber. To keep your microbiome ("my-kroh-BYE-ohm") healthy, **step up your grain game**.

When a grain, such as wheat, is ground into a fine flour, its effect on your blood sugar changes, that is, it causes it to rise. Grinding grains (both whole and refined) into flour increases the grain's surface area — just like when you roll a rolling pin over a clump of dough and flatten it like a pancake. The increased surface area exposes it to more digestive enzymes, which causes the starch to quickly convert into glucose. If this excess energy isn't used, then it has to be stored.

Prolonged levels of blood sugar surging through your arteries cause more cell deterioration (AGEs) and more fat to be stored, especially around your middle. Do you eat a lot of flour-y foods...bread, brownies, bagels, rolls, energy bars, cereal, chips, crackers, pretzels, cake, cookies, muffins, pie, pasta, potstickers, pancakes, waffles, or pizza? Now, look down. Has your belly become a long-term parking lot for fat? Or how about your liver (pg. 187-189)?

Better Defenders Legume and nut flours don't have the same effect on your blood sugar as grain flours.[10] They're low in carbohydrates, high in fiber and protein, and contain healthy fat that won't stir up a sugar attack. Just be mindful of what you *add* to them (like oil and sweeteners). Use ground flaxseed and/or almond, chickpea, hazelnut, soy, and walnut flours instead of grain flours. *The exception...*oat flour. Oats are grains, but oat flour contains more soluble fiber than any other grain and more healthy fats, which causes a slower rise in blood sugar.

Coach Karen says

Microbiome is where microorganisms, including trillions of both good and bad bacteria in your digestive tract live, a.k.a. gut microbiota. Think of your large intestine as one large 'garden' of bacteria that protects, strengthens, and nourishes you.

Coach Karen says

Sub out wheat flour with legume flour. Ground up pulses (beans, peas, chickpeas, and lentils) don't spike blood sugar like white and whole wheat flours.[8, 9]

Flour Rankings

Flours with the lowest glycemic index (cause a slower and smaller rise in blood sugar levels.[10]

#1 - Walnut (lowest)

#2 - Almond

#3 - Ground flaxseed

#4 - Hazelnut

#5 - Soy

#6 - Chickpea, Oat (tied)

Coach Karen says

Always carry your own personal "First Aid Kit" with you (i.e., some freeze-dried berries) because you never know when you might need to blunt a sugar spike.

When Pasta Is a Protein

Protein pastas are made with legume flour from black beans, chickpeas, edamame, and soybeans, not wheat or rice flour. They're often a lower carb, high-protein, and high-fiber product vs a starchy one. Many companies are producing these pastas now, but read the nutrition facts. Be sure they still meet the 5-to-1 ratio of carbs to fiber (pg. 100). Some of them contain starch additives, which increase the carbs and not the fiber.

DIG IN: Berries

Blunt Blood Sugar Spikes Researchers studied eating grain flours (white and rye bread) with a combination of berries and found the berries suppressed blood sugar and insulin spikes typically caused by these flour-y grain foods.[11] So if you can't refuse an occasional starchy, flour-y meal (like a plate of Nonna's homemade raviolis at Christmas), be sure to eat a handful of berries with it.

HOW "RESISTANCE" FOSTERS FATNESS

When the sugar in your blood climbs too high and lingers, it promotes inflammation, and your cells become more resistant to insulin. First, a short lesson on insulin, a hormone produced by your pancreas. Think of insulin as the 'key' that opens the door to your cells and allows blood sugar to get in where the sugar can be used as energy. Sugar can't get into your cells without the key to unlock the cell door. When your blood sugar spikes, your pancreas spews out more insulin 'keys'.

Insulin Resistance Over time, the locks on the cell doors eventually wear out, and the keys won't open the cell doors anymore. This is called insulin resistance, which causes your blood sugar and insulin levels to remain high. Your pancreas, which takes orders from your brain, keeps spewing insulin because it continues to get the signal that your blood sugar is high. Eventually your pancreas poops out and stops producing insulin. Then, inevitably you have to inject insulin to survive.

Selective Resistance Insulin tells your cells when and where to store the energy — either in your fat or as glycogen. While your cells can become resistant to taking up insulin, they are not

(continued on next page)

(continued from previous page)

resistant to taking up fat. That is, your cells are selectively resistant.[12] Continue eating those donuts that spike your blood sugar and insulin levels, and you'll blow up those fat cells. The fat will likely land in one of the most dangerous parking spots too — deep within the belly where it surrounds vital organs.

Leptin Resistance And there's more! High blood sugar and insulin resistance interfere with leptin, the satiety hormone that's produced by your fat cells. The leptin system keeps you from starving and overeating. This hormone is released into the bloodstream from your fat cells and circulates to the brain. Fat cells produce leptin in proportion to the size of the fat cell.

So in theory, a person who is overweight should have their own built-in appetite regulator. BUT...sometimes the leptin signaling stops working, which means your brain isn't getting the leptin signal. Even if leptin is being released from the fat cells at full throttle, the brain thinks the body is starving.

As a result, you're not satisfied even after eating a meal. In fact, you want more! Sound familiar? And if that isn't bad enough, since your brain thinks you're starving, it tells your metabolism to slow down to preserve energy. **To summarize, think of high blood sugar, insulin resistance, and leptin resistance as the leading drivers behind gaining fat and having a tough time losing it.**[13]

Coach Karen says

Glycogen is a stored 'package' of glucose in liver and muscle cells.

Coach Karen says

Leptin's job is to tell your brain you've had enough to eat and that you have plenty of energy stored.

DIG IN: Probiotics, Prebiotics, and Polyphenols

Foods That Feed Your Immune System An aging immune system is associated with chronic inflammation, which increases the risk of almost all conditions associated with *old age*. The key to your longevity lies in your gut. That's because 70% of your immune system is located in your digestive tract. In other words, your gut wall houses 70% of the cells that make up your immune system.[14] A healthy gut promotes a healthy immune system, and is effective at battling day-to-day assaults. Keeping it healthy is a proactive way to fight off infections faster and better. Refined foods, sugar, salt, and AGEs all negatively affect your gut microbiome.[15]

Coach Karen says

Gut bugs need probiotics (live bacteria) and prebiotics (fiber). Feed them well to fend off inflammation and infections.

Coach Karen says

Not all fermented foods contain active cultures. Heat inactivates the organisms, so heat-treated fermented foods, like baked bread and canned sauerkraut, do not have probiotic activity. Also, beer and wine remove the live organisms (yeasts that allow fermentation).

Many inflammatory diseases (e.g., cardiovascular disease, type 2 diabetes, chronic lung disease, dementia, cancer, allergies, arthritis, chronic fatigue, obesity, depression, and gastrointestinal disorders), are linked to a "malfunctioning gut", that is, it's housing too many of the *bad* bacteria. Certain foods build up good bacteria in your gut, which in turn, support a healthy gut and immune system. These foods include probiotics, prebiotics, and polyphenols — the 3 P's.

Probiotics (Live Bacteria)

Probiotic foods contain live bacterial cultures that help your gut bacteria stay in balance or in "equilibrium". That is, the good bacteria are able to keep the bad bacteria (like E. coli) from multiplying and going out of control. Probiotics include:

- **Cultured milk products**, such as yogurt and kefir that contain live and active cultures like S. Thermophilus, L. Bulgaricus, L. Acidophilus, Bifidobacteria.
- **Fermented plant foods**, such as kimchi, kombucha, raw (not pasteurized) sauerkraut, miso, tempeh

Prebiotics (Fiber)

Prebiotics boost the growth of friendly bacteria in the gut. Think fiber! Foods most beneficial to the microbiome are those that contain dietary fibers — the parts of the plant that your body can't digest or absorb. Instead, the fiber passes relatively intact through your stomach, small intestine, large intestine (colon), and out the back door.

Here are some prebiotic foods to get you started:

- Intact whole grains (particularly barley, oats, wheat)
- Apples, bananas (unripe), berries, citrus fruits, grapes
- Onions, garlic, leeks, shallots
- Artichokes, asparagus, broccoli, cabbage. cauliflower, mushrooms (especially shiitake), seaweed
- Beans, soybeans (including tofu, edamame), chickpeas, lentils, peas
- Beets, burdock root, carrots, sunchokes, jicama, konjac, yams
- Nuts (particularly almonds, pistachio nuts, walnuts), flaxseeds

Polyphenols (Antioxidants)

Polyphenols ("pah-lee-FEE-naalz") are beneficial compounds in many plant foods. They're packed with antioxidants, decrease inflammation, and increase the growth of friendly gut bacteria. They include:

- Fruits, vegetables, lignans
- Herbs, spices
- Green tea, matcha, red wine
- Cocoa powder, unsweetened (100% cacao)

THINGS THAT HARM THE GOOD BUGS

Diet, antibiotics, and toxins affect the composition of your microbiome. Your gut relies on just the right balance of bacteria diversity and abundance to prevent inflammation and infection. When the bad bugs outnumber the good ones, the unhealthy imbalance affects the rate of health decline.[16] The following things can cause bad gut bacteria to damage the friendly gut bugs:

1. **Eating the same thing day after day.** A microbiome that is rich in diverse gut bacteria increases your chances of recovering from harmful opponents. Eat a wide variety of COLORS to promote the growth of many different types of bacteria. Your microbiome can be altered after just a few days of eating a wide variety of whole foods.[17]

2. **Using antibiotics.** Antibiotics can't tell the difference between good and bad bacteria, and eliminate both of them.[18]

3. **Eating unfriendly gut foods.** These foods destroy and starve healthy bacteria and promote the growth of damaging bacteria. Processed foods, high-fat foods, meat, fried foods, sugar, salt, and alcohol can all harm the delicate balance and ecosystem of your gut microbiome.

4. **Lack of regular physical activity.**[19]

5. **Cigarette smoking.**[20]

6. **Not getting enough sleep.**[21]

7. **Too much stress.**[22]

Coach Karen says
Think of your gut as a large vegetable garden, the probiotics as the seeds, and the prebiotics and polyphenols as the fertilizer to help the seeds flourish.

Coach Karen says
If you've been sick, lack energy, or abused your body, you can restore your gut microbiome with a healthy and diverse diet, some exercise, and more relaxation.

 TRY THESE REAL FOOD RECIPES!

Mango Berry Freeze pg. 246
PB & Peach Toast pg. 238

PLAY 4 — FIRED UP MEANS AGING UP

Chronic Inflammation

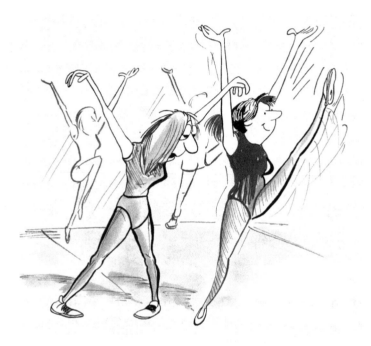

"I thought this was supposed to energize me."

Are you wondering if it's time to hang up your cleats? Do you feel like you've aged out of your sport? Well, chronic inflammation might be the *silent* culprit behind your perpetual slump...but all is not lost. If you know what's curtailing your athleticism, then you can fix it.

Chronic inflammation is different from the more familiar "acute inflammation". Acute inflammation is actually a healthy response to injury and infection. If you've ever sprained your ankle or received a nasty bug bite, the affected area likely became swollen, warm, painful, and red. That's because immune cells and key nutrients are attacking the area as a line of defense. This is an acute inflammatory response — and it's actually a good thing.

On the other hand, chronic inflammation is happening *inside* your body and is something you can't see. It's imperceptible and dangerous. Studies have shown a correlation between heart disease and elevated levels of C-reactive protein (CRP), a protein in your blood that signals inflammation.[1] A high-sensitivity CRP test (hs-CRP) indicates inflammation in your blood vessels. It's not a test for cardiovascular disease, but it's the strongest and most significant predictor of your risk for future cardiovascular events.[2]

"Inflamm-aging"

Chronic inflammation is the cause of most chronic diseases and may progress quietly to end-organ damage. Inflammation threats your health and longevity and is considered a major player to diseases, such as:

- **Asthma**
- **Atherosclerosis** (hardening of arteries caused by plaque buildup)
- **Chronic kidney disease**
- **Depression**
- **Diabetes**
- **Macular degeneration** (a common form of age-related blindness)
- **Neurodegenerative disorders** — e.g., vascular dementia, Alzheimer's disease, Parkinson's disease
- **Obesity**[3]
- **Osteoporosis or 'porous bones'** (weak and brittle bones)
- **Rheumatoid arthritis**
- **Some cancers**
- **Stroke**
- **Vascular calcification** (Calcium travels through the bloodstream and can leave deposits in the heart, vessels, or valves, which can lead to tissue stiffening, plaque rupture, and heart failure.)

Risk Factors That Ignite

There are four key risk factors that promote chronic inflammation, and they're all caused by the way you live.[4] Check off any of the following lifestyle risk factors that may have snuck into your lifestyle:

☐ **Obesity**

Coach Karen says

Chronic inflammation is associated with systemic bone loss and osteoporosis. High serum levels of C-reactive protein (CRP) have been linked to lower bone mineral density in women and older adults.[19]

Coach Karen says

Plaque is a sticky substance made up of cholesterol, fat, calcium, fibrin (a blood clotting agent), and metabolic waste.

☐ **Poor diet** — high in saturated fat, trans-fat, sodium, refined carbohydrates, or refined sugar

☐ **Smoking**

☐ **Stress and sleep disorders** — Stress can often trigger sleep disorders. Both physical and emotional stress contribute to the release of pro-inflammatory proteins and increased CRP.[5]

If you checked off any of the above, you may already be suffering from a chronic inflammatory disease, or it'll likely emerge if you don't change things up soon.

The Dietary Culprits of Aging

Do you have memory lapses, body pain, skin problems, digestive issues, persistent fatigue, hearing or vision loss, weight gain, frequent infections, or any inflammatory risk factors? If so, then it's time you face your toughest opponent — YOU. It's likely you're not being fed against your will (although it might feel like it when Aunt Clara insists you eat her vintage ham and celery jello mold at Easter), but the bottom line is...**you have choices**. And the foods you choose will either heal you or kill you.

Coach Karen says

Remember, what you eat becomes a part of you.

Researchers have identified certain foods as significant contributors to chronic inflammation. If you eat any of the following foods every day, your body is in a constant state of alarm, and the incessant inflammatory response is taking its toll. In addition to being a highly inflammatory food, the (*) foods also contain high levels of advanced glycation end products (AGEs).

1. **Alcohol** (more than one round) — e.g., beer, wine, or hard liquor

2. **Artificial colorants** — Food dyes are derived from petroleum and common in everyday foods, e.g., breakfast cereals, candy, chewing gum, jello, ice cream, sodas, sports drinks, vitamins, yogurt.

3. **Artificial sweeteners** — e.g., "diet" or "zero calorie" drinks, "no-sugar-added" products

4. **Fast food** — Fast foods are particularly aging due to the chemical toxins found in plastic food and beverage packaging and phosphates.

5. **Flour** (the kinds made from grains) — e.g, wheat flour, rice flour

6. **Fried foods*** — e.g, blooming onions, chips, fish and chips, French fries, fried chicken, wontons

7. **High fat meats, particularly red*** — e.g., beef/pork ribs, prime rib

8. **Phosphates** — Phosphate is hidden in common foods and beverages.

9. **Processed meats*** — e.g, bacon, chorizo, cold cuts, corned beef, hot dogs, pepperoni, pastrami, salami, sausage

10. **Refined carbohydrates** — e.g., white flour products, such as white bread, bagels, breakfast cereals, crackers, flour tortillas, pasta, pretzels, pizza crust

11. **Saturated fats*** — e.g., beef fat, butter, cheese, cream, ice cream, lard, red meat, tropical oils

12. **Sugar** — e.g., cakes, candy, coffee drinks, cookies, pastries, snack bars, soda

13. **Trans fats/hydrogenated oils*** — e.g., canned frosting, fried fast foods, non-dairy coffee creamers, shortening, and baked goods including biscuits, cakes, cookies, crackers, doughnuts, frozen pizzas (dough), pie crusts, stick margarines and other spreads

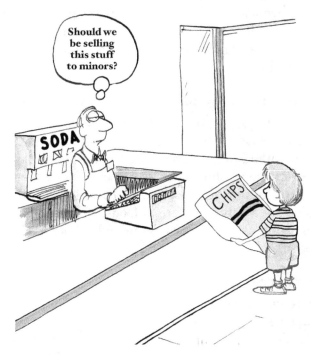

Sugar Overload

When reading food labels, what may seem like a wee bit of added sugar, realize that four grams of added sugar is equivalent to one full teaspoon. The leading sources of added sugar in the U.S. are sugar-sweetened drinks, candy, grain-based desserts like cakes and cookies, and dairy desserts like ice cream.[6] Chug a 44-ounce Super Big Gulp after a tennis match, and you're shooting a nocuous sugary tonic into your veins — 32 teaspoons (128 grams) of added sugar! You'll trigger a disastrous flash flood of glucose and insulin in your bloodstream.

Coach Karen says

Think of blood sugar like shards of glass traveling through your blood vessels. As they move through your arteries, they damage the delicate inner lining (endothelium).

Strike Three! YOU'RE OUT!

Just like there's a limit on how many times you can swing and miss when you're up at bat, there's a limit on how much sugar you should consume a day. Here are the American Heart Association recommendations for added sugar per day:

- Men — less than 9 teaspoons (36 grams)
- Women — less than 6 teaspoons (24 grams)

Let's say you polished off an entire can of soda (39 grams of added sugar) with your lunch. At this point, you may as well call it a day. Hit the showers. You just exceeded your entire day's allowance of added sugar in one sitting. A 12-oz soda contains 39 gm (9-3/4 teaspoons) of added sugar! Don't even think about putting ketchup on your fries because that has sugar in it too. To break 100, what's the recommendation for added sugar? It's less than the AHA recommendation. In other words, **zero, zilch, nada.**

Phosphates and Premature Aging

Researchers have shown that sugary sodas can cut life short, but the culprit in one particular study wasn't sugar, it was phosphates.[7] A diet high in phosphates is linked to an increased prevalence and severity of age-related diseases and conditions, such as muscle and skin atrophy (wasting away), chronic kidney disease, and vascular calcification. Phosphates are hidden in many commercial foods. Read the labels. Eating too many phosphates accelerates aging and influences your chances of breaking 100.[7]

The Double Whammy of Soda

Sodas contain two aging components — phosphoric acid (a form of phosphates) and sugar. Phosphoric acid is a clear, colorless, odorless, syrupy liquid that's added to sodas to give them their tangy taste. It also creates an acidic environment that slows mold and bacterial growth, which multiplies easily in a sugary solution.

Sodas are caustic cocktails. Consider them 'corrosives in a can', and watch them in action. To clean corroded car battery terminals, just pour a can of soda over the terminals. The phosphoric acid will bubble away all the corrosion. Try it — this actually works!

Phosphates in Disguise

Phosphates are disguised in many ways. Here are words to look for when reading food product labels:

- Aluminum phosphate
- Calcium phosphate
- Dicalcium phosphate
- Hexametaphosphate
- Monocalcium phosphate
- Phosphoric acid
- Polyphosphate
- Pyrophosphate
- Sodium phosphate
- Sodium polyphosphate
- Sodium tripolyphosphate
- Tetrasodium phosphate
- Tricalcium phosphate
- Trisodium phosphate

Coach Karen says

Phosphate is added to some commercial plant-based milks, so read the labels carefully.

Phosphate Overload and Bone Loss (Osteoporosis)

Calcium and phosphorus work together as a team to form and maintain healthy teeth and bones. These teammates need to be in sync in order to be effective. When you have too much phosphorus in your blood (a.k.a. hyperphosphatemia), your body pulls calcium from your bones, which makes them weak and brittle (osteoporosis).

The bottom line...phosphoric acid causes imbalances in the body that result in age-related, debilitating diseases that appear after many years of consuming it. Phosphate overload induces systemic inflammation, oxidative stress, vascular calcification, and higher risk of and premature death in patients with chronic kidney disease.[8] Patients with chronic kidney disease are especially at risk because their kidneys have difficulty removing phosphorus.

WHERE PHOSPHATES ARE HIDING IN YOUR FOOD

Phosphates are not only in sodas, they're in processed foods. They're used to thicken food, cure meat, help dough rise, balance pH to extend shelf life in processed foods, and emulsify/stabilize milk proteins, such as in cheese. Phosphates are added to:

- **Baking powder** (sodium acid pyrophosphate, calcium acid pyrophosphate, monocalcium phosphate, and/or sodium aluminum phosphate)
- **Bottled coffee beverages**
- **Breakfast or cereal bars**
- **Commercially baked goods and mixes** — e.g., biscuits, cake mixes, donuts, pancakes, refrigerated bakery products, waffles
- **Meat and chicken products (processed)** — e.g., bacon, chicken tenders or nuggets, deli meat, ham, sausage
- **Fast food**
- **Flavored waters**
- **Iced teas**
- **Instant puddings and sauces**
- **Mashed potato mixes**
- **Nondairy creamers**
- **Sodas and other bottled beverages**
- **Some plant-based milks** — e.g., almond, cashew, coconut, flax, hemp, oat, pea, quinoa, rice (read the labels carefully)
- **Other manufactured food** — e.g., ready-to-eat meals

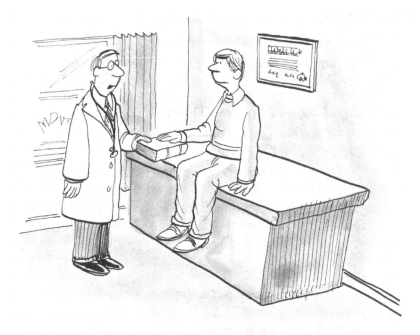

"Do you solemnly swear to listen to my advice?"

Sat Fat Facts

Saturated fats are stable fats, that is, they're not as sensitive to heat and light like other oils. That's why they're solid or waxy at room temperature, can withstand high cooking temperatures, and have a long shelf life. Even though the saturated fat in tropical oils are chemically different from the saturated fat in animals, the health organizations* recommend against consuming palm oil and other tropical oils because they also promote coronary artery disease.

*The World Health Organization; National Heart, Lung and Blood Institute; National Institute of Diabetes and Digestive and Kidney Diseases; and USDA's Agricultural Research Service

Here's how some of the saturated fats compare:

- **92% - Coconut oil** (13 gm saturated fat per tablespoon)
- **89% - Coconut milk**
- **84% - Palm kernel oil**
- **64% - Butter**
- **60% - Chocolate**
- **52% - Palm oil (a.k.a. palm fruit oil or red palm fruit oil)**
- **43% - Lard**

- **40% - Beef fat**
- **14% - Olive oil** (1.9 gm saturated fat per tablespoon)
- **10% - Avocado oil** (1.5 gm saturated fat per tablespoon)

COCONUT OIL — IS IT HEALTHY OR HYPE?

Coconut oil from the tropics has gained considerable traction over the olive oils of the Mediterranean. But remember, coconut oil may be trending on the Internet, but not necessarily in medicine. Much of the research examining the effects of coconut oil on cholesterol levels consist of short-term studies and instead, supports the long-term effects and benefits of omega-3 fatty acids.

The Jury is Out

Coconut oil is widely marketed as having many health benefits. Same goes for MCT oil, a popular supplement extracted from coconut oil. In July 2017 the American Heart Association issued an advisory recommending against using coconut oil.[9, 10] Analysis of more than 100 published research studies reaffirmed that saturated fats significantly raise LDL cholesterol (the artery cloggers). In addition, seven controlled trials showed that coconut oil raised LDL levels. Another study found that anti-inflammatory HDLs (the good guys) become pro-inflammatory in the presence of saturated fats in coconut oil.[11]

Palm Oils, Coconut Water, and Coconut Milk

Palm oils come from 'oil palm' trees, unlike coconut oil that comes from 'coconut palm' trees. Palm oil, sometimes called "red palm fruit oil" or "palm fruit oil" comes from the palm fruit — the orange flesh that surrounds the palm seed. On the other hand, palm kernel oil is extracted from the palm kernel (seed). Fat-wise, the oils are not similar.

Coconut water is the clear liquid found inside young coconuts and contains zero saturated fat. In contrast, coconut milk is thick and creamy, 89% saturated fat, and comes from the grated white meat inside of a mature coconut. Coconut oil comes from pressing the fat from the white meat.

The current American Heart Association and American College of Cardiology guidelines suggest limiting saturated fat intake to less than 5% to 6% of your total daily calories. For example, if you need about 2,000 calories a day, no more than 100 to 120 calories should come from saturated fats, which equals about 11 to 13 grams. On 1,200 calories a day, 7 to 8 grams of saturated fat is the daily limit. Here's a sampling of what sat fat in food looks like...

- 1 **burger** - Quarter Pounder® with cheese (20 gm saturated fat)
- 1/4 cup **coconut milk** (13 gm)
- 1/2 cup **ice cream** - Chunky Monkey® (10 gm)
- 3 strips of **bacon** (9 gm)
- 1 tablespoon of **butter** (7 gm)
- 1 slice **cheddar cheese** (6 gm)
- 1 ounce **dark chocolate** (5 gm)
- 1 cup **whole milk** (5 gm)
- 1 cup **2% milk** (3 gm)

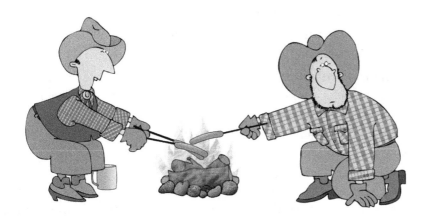

Why Meat Ain't So Neat

In addition to the phosphates in meat that cause cellular fires, meat is problematic in itself for two reasons:

1. It's high in saturated fat (containing about twice the recommended levels), which increases systemic inflammation, risk of kidney and heart disease, and risk of certain cancers.

2. It's rich in choline. The bacteria in your gut interact with this nutrient and help produce a compound called **TMAO** (trimethylamine-N-oxide).

TMAO is a newly recognized key blood biomarker linked closely to major adverse cardiovascular events (heart attack, death, and stroke).[12] It plays a role in systemic inflammation, coronary artery disease, and the dysfunction of large arteries caused by arterial stiffness.[13] Not only does red meat bump up the TMAO levels, but it also causes the kidneys to become less effective at clearing them out.[14]

New research from the Cleveland Clinic strengthens the case against a diet rich in choline. Their study provided direct evidence that showed dietary choline increased TMAO levels 10 times in two months, and the tendency for platelets to clump together, which can cause clots to form, increased proportionately as well.[15]

Coach Karen says

Vegetarians and vegans, who avoid meat products, produce little TMAO.

Coach Karen says

A heavy meal can trigger a heart attack within 26 hours. Heart attack risk jumped four times in the two hours after a large meal, known as the two-hour "hazard period".[18]

How to Lower TMAO

You can lower your TMAO and risk of major adverse cardiac events by cutting back on foods that produce high levels of TMAO and increase clot risk. These foods include:

- **Full-fat dairy products** — e.g., butter, cream cheese, whole milk
- **Processed and unprocessed animal products**[12] — particularly beef, lamb, pork, poultry, eggs[17]
- **Nutritional supplements and energy drinks** promoted for gaining muscle, weight loss, and athletic performance. Such products contain the building blocks of TMAO, namely choline, phosphatidylcholine (lecithin), and L-carnitine.[12]

The promising news is you may be able to reverse the concentrations of TMAO in your blood within a short period of time. Studies reveal that by switching from a diet rich in red meat to either a white meat or non-meat protein source, you can substantially reduce choline intake and TMAO levels *within four weeks*.[14]

Putting Out the Fire

So there you have it, the top inflammatory foods that fire up your body and cause you to age...and oh-so ungracefully. But with every food that makes you older, there's a plethora of foods that will reverse it. An anti-inflammatory diet consisting of a high intake of fiber (whole plant foods) has been shown to lower CRP levels. Doctors are learning that one of the best ways to combat chronic inflammation lies in your fridge — not your medicine cabinet.

THE PALEO EFFECT

Some researchers found that people that followed the Paleo Diet for over a year had twice the amount of TMAO in their blood. They attribute this to a diet rich in animal-based protein and low in dietary fiber due to an exclusion of whole grains and legumes.[14]

Proponents of the Paleolithic or "Paleo" Diet, (a.k.a. Caveman, Hunter-Gatherer, or Stone Age Diet) think humans should stick to eating foods that our caveman ancestors ate two million years ago. They believe the human body hasn't adapted to a modern diet and eating like a caveman will promote good health.

The diet includes animal-based protein, nuts, seeds, and limited fruit and vegetables — i.e., foods that could be obtained by hunting and gathering. Since farming did not exist during this period, the diet excludes whole grains, legumes, refined white cane sugar, and dairy.

Per a meta-analysis of 19 studies, elevated levels of TMAO increase the risk of death by 63%, and increase the risk of a major adverse cardiovascular event by 62%.[12] Even if you aren't "officially" following the Paleo diet, but eat a diet heavy in animal-based protein and few whole grains and legumes, you're vulnerable to the same negative Paleo Diet health effects.

Coach Karen says

TMAO is associated with brain aging and cognitive impairment.[20] What's bad for your heart is also bad for your brain.

 TRY THESE REAL FOOD RECIPES!

Raspberry Lime Gazpacho pg. 261
Summer Fruit Bruschetta pg. 235

PLAY 5 — YOUR DEFENSIVE LINE

How Colorful Is Your Food?

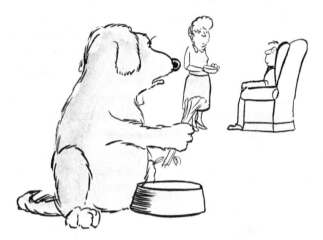

"Tell me this isn't celery."

A good defensive line is a game-altering weapon. Imagine running out onto the football field to face the biggest, baddest team in the league. You get out to the field only to realize your entire defensive line has decided to sit out the second half. Panic sets in. With no reinforcements to help fend off your opponent, your body is now hugely vulnerable.

That's pretty much the scenario when you don't eat enough phyto-chemicals. Phyto-what, you say? "Phyto" (FY-toe) is the Greek word for plant. Phyto + chemicals = phytochemicals (also called phytonutrients). These naturally occurring biochemicals impart the plant's color, flavor, smell, and texture and many act as antioxidants. In the phytochemical world, *color matters*. The colors are the antioxidants!

Phytochemicals aren't essential for you to stay alive like vitamins and minerals, but are thought to be your armor against the day-to-day cellular assaults from free radicals. They incapacitate cell-damaging free radicals, and the colors provide a rough guide to the type and amount of phytochemicals in your food. As a general rule, the deeper the color, the more powerful the antioxidants.

Don't get too cross-eyed with all the scientific names. Just know that there are six major and diverse families of phytochemicals. Within each of these families are colorful plant groups and within each group, there are sub-groups of pigments. In other words, plants contain a boatload of phytochemicals. Nutrition researchers at UC Davis estimate that there are more than 10,000.[1] By eating a lot of plants, you have the potential to eradicate a lot of free radicals. Here are the All-Stars of antioxidants...

Your Colorful Defensive Line (Phytochemical Pigments)

1. RED

- Red-Pink
- Red

2. ORANGE

- Orange / Dark Green
- Yellow-Orange

3. GREEN

- Yellow-Green and Leafy Greens
- Green

4. WHITE

- White / Green
- White / Tan
- White

5. BLUE

- Blue / Purple / Black

6. BROWN

- Brown
- Reddish-Brown

Add Color to Your Years

New experimental studies continue to emerge that demonstrate the multiple human health effects of phytochemicals. These potent plant compounds can:

- Slow the aging process.

- Keep you able, active, and alert.

- Provide special nutrients or specific antioxidants that have a direct link to cancer prevention.

- Prevent chronic inflammation.

- Protect against chronic and age-related diseases, such as heart disease, stroke, high blood pressure, diabetes, cataracts, macular degeneration, and bone loss.

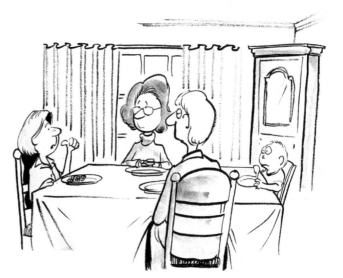

"I'll save the peas for later, when
I can properly enjoy them in my room."

Pass the Colors Please

Fill up on a vibrant plate of fruits, vegetables, grains, beans, peas, teas, herbs, spices, nuts, and seeds. Now let's go color by color with examples of each one...

1. RED

RED-PINK

Phytochemicals — **lycopene** *(carotenoid)*

Benefits — bone, brain, eye, and heart health; cancer prevention (breast, prostate); immune support

Fruits — papaya; pink grapefruit; pink grapefruit juice; pink guava; watermelon

Vegetables — tomatoes, raw and especially cooked tomatoes; tomato products, e.g., tomato juice, tomato paste, tomato puree, tomato sauce, tomato soup, tomato juice

Legumes — kidney beans; red beans

RED

Phytochemicals — **anthocyanin, quercetin** *(polyphenols)*, **beta-carotene** *(carotenoid)*, **capsaicin** *(capsaicinoid)*, **ellagic acid** *(aromatic acid)*

Benefits — blood vessel health; cancer prevention; immune support; inflammation reduction

Fruits — cherries; cranberries; red apple skin; red currants; red pitaya (a.k.a. dragon fruit, strawberry pear); pomegranate (very high); raspberries; strawberries

Vegetables — chili peppers; sweet red bell peppers

 TRY THESE RED RECIPES!

Pomegranate Balsamic Vinaigrette pg. 250
Watermelon Ice pg. 247

2. ORANGE

ORANGE / DARK GREEN

Phytochemicals — **alpha-carotene, beta-carotene** *(carotenoids)*

Benefits — bone, eyes, heart, and skin health; cancer prevention; immune support; inflammation reduction; vision preservation (cataracts, macular degeneration)

Fruits — apricots; cantaloupe; mango; papaya; peach; persimmon

Vegetables — acorn squash; broccoli; butternut squash; carrots; collard greens; kabocha squash (Japanese pumpkin); kale; pumpkin; spinach; sweet orange bell peppers; sweet potato; winter squash; yellow squash; sweet potato, tatsoi

YELLOW-ORANGE

Phytochemicals — **beta-cryptoxanthin** *(carotenoid)*, **hesperidin** *(polyphenol)*

Benefits — bone, eye, and skin health; immune function; vision preservation

Fruits — apricot; guava; kumquat; lemon; mango; nectarine; orange; papaya; peach; persimmon; pineapple; starfruit; tangelo; tangerine; yellow apple; yellow pear

Vegetables — sweet orange/yellow bell peppers; yellow corn

 TRY THESE ORANGE RECIPES!

Mango Salsa pg. 233
Tropical Berry Quinoa Salad with Zesty Citrus Dressing pg. 252

Coach Karen says

The ORANGEs are classified as "precursors" of vitamin A, a.k.a. provitamin A. That means, once ingested, the body converts provitamin A to an active form of vitamin A (essential for immune function and bone, eye, and skin health). "Preformed" vitamin A is found in animal products, fortified foods, and vitamin supplements.

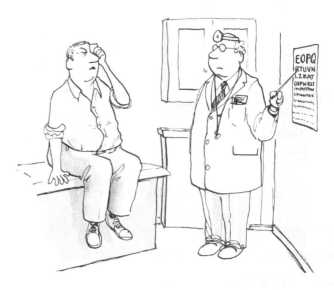

"Can I buy a vowel, Pat?"

3. GREEN

YELLOW-GREEN and LEAFY GREENS

Green plants may contain more yellow pigment (lutein) than it appears. That's because chlorophyll, nature's green pigment that colors fruits and vegetables green, often masks the yellow color.

Phytochemicals — **lutein**, **zeaxanthin** *(carotenoids)*

Benefits — heart health; cancer prevention; vision preservation (cataracts and macular degeneration)

Fruits — avocado; green pears; honeydew melon; kiwi; mango; yellow pears

Vegetables — arugula; artichokes; asparagus; basil; beet leaves; broccoli; Brussels sprouts; celery; cilantro; collard greens; cucumber; dill; edamame; green peas; green bell peppers; kale; mustard greens; parsley; Romaine lettuce; snap peas; spinach; Swiss chard; turnip greens; yellow bell peppers; yellow corn; zucchini

Nuts — pistachio nut (green skin around the nut)

GREEN

These sulfur-containing compounds are responsible for the pungent aroma and bitter flavor of cruciferous vegetables.

Phytochemicals — **sulforaphane** *(isothiocyanate)*, **indole-3-carbinol** *(indole)*

Benefits — heart health; cancer prevention

Vegetables (Cruciferous) — arugula (rocket); bok choy; broccoli; Brussels sprouts; cabbage; cauliflower; collard greens; Chinese cabbage; horseradish; kale; kohlrabi (turnip cabbage); mustard greens; rutabaga; savoy cabbage; tatsoi; turnips; turnip greens; wasabi (Japanese horseradish); watercress

 TRY THESE GREEN RECIPES!

Cilantro Lime Farro pg. 279
Wild Salmon or Tofu Tacos with Citrus Salsa pg. 274
Wilted Power Greens pg. 286

ARUGULA, CILANTRO, AND OTHER HEART-BRAIN PROTECTORS

When it comes to preventing strokes and memory loss, arugula and cilantro (a.k.a. coriander, Chinese parsley) are powerful protectors. These GREENs contain high levels of compounds called nitrates, which provide a natural way to treat high blood pressure and reduce risk of a stroke or heart attack. In scientific studies, nitrates have been shown to widen (dilate) blood vessels, which lowers blood pressure.

A study revealed that cerebral blood flow was 20% lower in patients with Alzheimer's disease compared to those without dementia.[2] Research has also shown that nitrates increase blood flow to areas of the brain involved in executive functioning.[3] For a healthy heart and brain, eat at least two cups of dark green leafy veggies per day.

Of foods containing high levels of nitrates (over 1,000 mg per kg), here's how a few popular greens size up:

1. Arugula = 4,800 mg nitrate/kg
2. Cilantro = 2,468
3. Butter leaf lettuce = 1,978
4. Spring mix = 1,878
5. Basil = 1,827
6. Beet greens = 1,770
7. Red/green leaf lettuce = 1,628
8. Swiss chard = 1,510
9. Dill = 1,123
10. Romaine = 1,097

Coach Karen says

Allicin is garlic's defense molecule. When the garlic plant is crushed, attacked, or injured, it produces allicin, which is toxic to insects and microorganisms.[2]

4. WHITE

WHITE / GREEN

Phytochemicals — allyl sulfides (*organosulfides*), particularly **allicin**[4]

Benefits — blood vessel and heart health; cancer prevention

Allium Vegetables — chives; garlic; leeks; onions; scallions; shallots

WHITE / TAN

Phytochemicals — **lignans** *(polyphenols)* and various groups of substances

Benefits — bone and heart health; cancer prevention; healthy cell growth

Fruits — banana; brown-skinned pears; dates, fresh and dried; figs; white nectarine; white peach

Vegetables — black-eyed peas; garlic; ginger; Jerusalem artichoke; jicama; leeks; mushrooms; parsnips; rutabaga; shallots; white cauliflower; white corn; white onion; white-fleshed potatoes

Legumes — butter beans; cannellini beans; garbanzo beans (chickpeas); Great Northern beans; navy beans (pea beans); peanuts

Nuts — almonds; Brazil nuts; cashews; hazelnuts (filberts); macadamias; pecans; pistachios; walnuts

Seeds — amaranth; chia seeds; flaxseeds; hemp seeds; pumpkin seeds; sesame seeds; quinoa; 100% cacao

Grains — barley; brown rice; farro; millet; oats; popcorn

WHITE

Phytochemicals — **isoflavones**, particularly **daidzein** and **genistein** *(polyphenols)*, **saponins** *(triterpenoid)*

Benefits — blood vessel, bone, and heart health; cancer prevention; inflammation reduction

Legumes — edamame; soybeans; soy nuts; soy products, e.g., miso, soy milk, tempeh, tofu

 TRY THESE WHITE RECIPES!

Cocoa Almond Milkshake pg. 243
Tofu Lettuce Wraps pg. 273
Vanilla Bean 'Nice Cream' pg. 298

Coach Karen says

Upgrade your lifestyle. Get regular exercise, and eat real food.

5. BLUE

BLUE / PURPLE / BLACK

Phytochemicals — anthocyanins, ellagic acid, resvervatrol (polyphenols)

Benefits — blood vessel, brain, eye, and heart health; cancer and diabetes prevention; inflammation reduction; vision preservation

Fruits — blackberries; black currants; black grapes; blueberries; boysenberries; elderberries; figs, Black Mission*; Concord grapes; Concord grape juice; plums; pomegranate (very high); prunes; purple grapes; purple passion fruit; raisins; red-skinned pears; red grapes; red wine

Black figs are significantly higher in phytonutrients compared to the yellow, brown, or purple varieties.

Vegetables — beets; eggplant, especially the skin; purple asparagus; purple basil; purple cabbage; purple carrots; purple kohlrabi; purple potatoes; purple sweet bell pepper; purple sweet potato; radicchio; radishes; red onions; red potatoes

Beans, Grains, Seeds — black beans; black popcorn; black rice; red rice; wild rice; black sesame seeds

Herbs — hibiscus tea

 TRY THESE BLUE RECIPES!

Black Rice Bento Bowl with Mellow Lime Dressing pg. 258
Pear and Blueberry Crumble pg. 295

6. BROWN

BROWN

Phytochemicals — flavonoids, particularly **epicatechin, catechin,** and **procyanidin** *(polyphenols)*

Benefits — blood vessel, brain, heart, and skin health; cancer and diabetes prevention

Fruits and Beans — cocoa (non-alkalized)

REDDISH-BROWN

Phytochemicals — **flavonoids, lignans, phenolic acid** *(polyphenols)*, **beta-carotene** *(carotenoid)*

Benefits — brain, eye, heart, and skin health; cancer and diabetes prevention

Fruits — dates

Coach Karen says

Dates have the highest concentration of polyphenols among the dried fruits.[5]

DATE "SUGAR" — THE WHOLESOME SWEETENER

Dates have the best nutrient score of any fresh fruit and the highest concentration of polyphenols of any dried fruit. The reason? They grow in deserts, and the harsh environment promotes the formation of polyphenols in order to provide protection from oxidative stress to the palm's fruit.[5, 6]

Dates are a good source of fiber, BROWNs, and vitamins and minerals, including iron, potassium, B vitamins, copper, manganese, and magnesium. Date sugar can be substituted for other sweeteners in recipes. It's similar in color and texture to brown sugar. Date Lady contains two grams of sugar per teaspoon. (Cane sugar, honey, coconut sugar, agave contain two to three times more sugar at four to six grams of sugar per teaspoon.) Date sugar will not dissolve, so it's not something you'd add to sweeten up your coffee. For your morning brew, you'd want to use date syrup instead.

 TRY THESE BROWN RECIPES!

Chocolate Hummus pg. 232
Razzberry Chocolate Pudding pg. 296

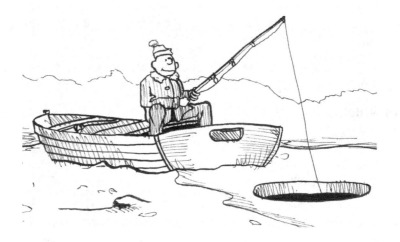

The Freezer Is Your Friend

Fruits and veggies can be purchased fresh or frozen. Seasonal produce is picked when ripe and "flash frozen" (frozen quickly at an extremely low temperature), so nutrients are at their peak when you eat them. Unlike fresh, they aren't subject to sitting on a truck, driving long distances, then sitting in a supermarket warehouse for sometimes months before making an appearance in the produce section. They're also not subject to sitting in your fridge for a week before finally ending up on your plate.

When you keep your freezer stocked with frozen produce (everything from peaches to beets and peas), you'll always have a variety of nutrient-dense COLORS on deck that are ready to eat. They're lifesavers when you're off the Active List and can't get out to play, much less shop for groceries.

Befriend Freeze-Dried Too

Freeze-dried fruits and vegetables — not to be confused with *dehydrated* — are a healthy alternative to fresh and frozen. They maintain a low profile in your golf bag, gym bag, and backpack without crowding out your other sports essentials. You'll always have plenty of shelf-stable COLORS at your fingertips without the bulk.

Several studies show that the antioxidant-rich phytochemicals found in freeze-dried fruits were almost as high as fresh — with the exception of vitamin C, which is prone to breaking down more than in fresh or frozen fruits.[7, 8, 9] So stock up on bulk bags of freeze-dried berries, beets, persimmons, corn, carrots, peas, and the like for the fiber and phytos. You can eat them as is, or toss them in your salads, pancakes, hot oatmeal, cereals, smoothies, soups, or stews. Grind some freeze-dried berries into a powder, and add them to yogurt and baked goods like cookies, muffins, and quick breads.

Dehydrated vs Freeze-Dried — They're NOT the Same Thing

Freeze-dried foods are first frozen to around 40 degrees below zero in a "freeze dryer" (vacuum chamber). Once the moisture is frozen, the food is slightly warmed to transform the ice into a vanishing vapor. You can eat your freeze-dried produce in their "crunchy" form, or you can rehydrate them to regain their original water-rich state. In contrast, dehydration applies high evaporating heat (95°F to 155°F) for several hours to remove the moisture, which can strip much of its food value and produce those dreadful AGEs.

Coach Karen says

Anti-aging starts with COLOR-ful food. As a general rule, the more vibrant and intense the COLOR, the more powerful the antioxidants.

PLAY 6 — RAW VS COOKED

Which Is the Winner?

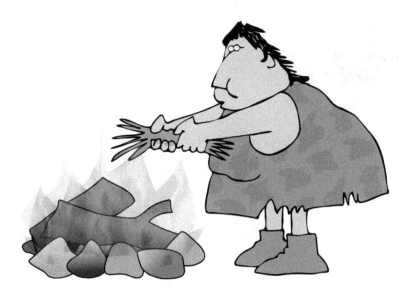

Congratulations! You decided to start eating more COLORS, but you wonder...is it healthier to eat your vegetables raw or cooked? You may have heard from some people (perhaps the "raw foodists") who say cooking destroys valuable vitamins, minerals, and enzymes. So now you're not sure if you should eat your tomatoes off the vine or simmered in a sauce.

Let's take a lesson from your prehistoric relatives who discovered that cooking has a purpose. After eating a diet of tough roots and raw meats and having to pound everything with a rock to tenderize it, cooking became a vital part of human adaptation. You see, cooking breaks down the insoluble fiber, which softens your food and makes them edible.

Get Rich on Lycopene

As it turns out, raw vegetables are not always healthier than cooked. According to a study, people that followed a strict raw food diet had low levels of lycopene (the REDs) in their blood. Lycopene is found largely in tomatoes and in other rosy fruits, such as watermelon, pink grapefruit, and papaya. Cooking lycopene-rich vegetables actually increases their lycopene content due to the heat and the water loss.

Heat breaks down a plant's thick cell walls. This releases some of the nutrients that are bound to these surfaces and makes the REDs, ORANGEs, and GREENs *(the carotenoids)* more available and more easily absorbed. Also, raw tomatoes are water-rich (95% water by weight), but when they're cooked, such as in tomato paste, their water evaporates, which increases total lycopene concentration.

Eat 10K a Day

Lycopene has the ability to attack free radicals, reduce inflammation, lower cholesterol, improve immune function, help lower the risk of prostate and other cancers, and possibly prevent strokes, particularly ischemic strokes. Researchers suggest getting 10,000 micrograms (µg) of lycopene a day — from food.[1,2] Well, how much is *that*? Keep reading...

Cooked tomato-based products top the list of lycopene-rich foods and give you the biggest bang for your buck.[3] There's no evidence of lycopene toxicity by getting it from food, so don't worry about eating too many of these REDs. A 4-oz mug of tomato juice or a homemade Virgin Mary (not Bloody please) with breakfast or lunch will do the job. You can also get your 10K a day by consuming 2/3 cup minestrone soup, 1/2 cup tomato juice, 1/3 cup spaghetti sauce, 3 tablespoons tomato purée, 2-2/3 medium raw tomatoes, 23 cherry tomatoes, 1-1/2 cups watermelon, or 1-1/4 cups guava.

Coach Karen says

Ischemic strokes are caused by plaque buildup or clots that block blood flow to the brain.

Here's how the lycopene-rich REDs compare:[4]

FOOD	LYCOPENE
Tomato soup, canned (condensed), low sodium	**26,426 mcg** per 1 cup
Tomato and vegetable juice, low sodium	**23,377 mcg** per 1 cup
Tomato juice, canned, no salt	**21,960 mcg** per 1 cup
Tomato paste	**18,984 mcg** per 1/4 cup
Vegetable juice cocktail, low sodium	**18,082 mcg** per 1 cup
Tomato sauce, canned, no salt	**17, 022 mcg** per 1/2 cup
Spaghetti sauce, low sodium	**16,211 mcg** per 1/2 cup
Minestrone soup, canned, reduced sodium	**15,580 mcg** per 1 cup

FOOD	LYCOPENE
Tomato purée, canned, no salt	**13,597 mcg** per 1/4 cup
Tomatoes, canned, stewed	**10,424 mcg** per 1 cup
Pink guavas, raw	**8,587 mcg** per 1 cup
Watermelon, raw	**6,979 mcg** per 1 cup
Salsa, ready-to-serve	**6,728 mcg** per 1/4 cup
Tomato, raw, chopped	**6,082 mcg** per 1 cup
Tomato, raw, cherry	**5,244 mcg** per 12
Pink grapefruit, sections	**3,264 mcg** per 1 cup
Chili with beans, canned	**2,737 mcg** per 1 cup
Papayas, raw, 1" pieces	**2,651 mcg** per 1 cup
Tomato catsup, low sodium	**2,051 mcg** per tablespoon
Cocktail sauce	**2,026 mcg** per 2 tablespoons
Pink grapefruit, half	**1,745 mcg** per 1/2 fruit
Baked beans, canned, vegetarian	**1,298 mcg** per 1 cup

Coach Karen says

Age can affect lycopene absorption, so as you celebrate more birthdays, eat more lycopene-rich foods.

Hold the Salt, Add the Fat

Lycopene is fat soluble and better absorbed if eaten with fat.[5] Add some hemp seeds to your marinara sauce, or pair an avocado salad with your tomato soup to better absorb the REDs. And just for the record, a fatty burger and fries will increase the formation of free radicals and AGEs, so eating lycopene with *that kind* of fat would be like getting slapped with a 15-yard penalty. That is, you'll be traveling even farther away from your goal! Remember, you're trying to grow younger, not older. Also, for the same reason, choose no-salt cooked tomato products to bypass the aging effects of sodium.

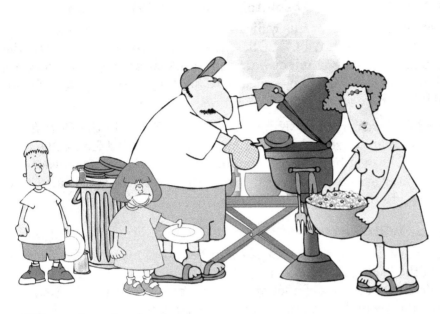

Healthier When Cooked

Cooking increases the antioxidant levels in some vegetables, so cook them up.[6] More GREENs (indole), are available when cruciferous vegetables, such as broccoli, cauliflower, cabbage, and Brussels sprouts, are cooked. More ORANGEs are released when cooked, particularly in broccoli, carrots, and zucchini as well as asparagus, cabbage, mushrooms, peppers, and spinach.[7]

Healthier When Raw...Huh?

After just saying broccoli is healthier cooked, now it's healthier raw? Yep. Cooking not only increases the antioxidant levels in some vegetables, cooking also decreases them.[8] Broccoli, for example, contains an enzyme called myrosinase ("my-ROH-sin-ayze"), but extreme heat destroys this enzyme, which is necessary to form one of the cancer-fighting GREENs (sulforaphane). So eat your broccoli raw — or steam it for no more than four minutes. Cooking certain vegetables, such as beets and cabbage, causes a significant loss of COLORS.

The Bottom Line...

Totally confused? Remember, plants contain a multitude of phytochemicals, so eaten cooked, you may get more of some, while you may get more of others when eaten raw. To keep it simple, just be sure your training table includes a combination of both raw and cooked vegetables. When it comes down to it, just do as Mom always told you to do. Eat your vegetables.

All Vegetables Are Absolutely Unhealthy When Fried

Deep fried foods form free radicals due to the oils being heated at high temperatures. All COLORS are used up just trying to battle the oxidizing hot oil. You might want to rethink those deep-fried zucchini sticks — not only are they sponges for fat, they're void of phytochemicals.

Fried foods are a "Silent Killer". A study published in the *British Medical Journal* revealed a link between eating fried food and earlier death.[9] Those at highest risk of dying from all causes, cardiovascular, and cancer ate fried food daily. Next in line were those who ate fried food one to three times a week.

Foods With the Most AGEs

AGEs are not only formed inside your body, you ingest AGEs directly from the foods you eat, a.k.a. "dietary AGEs". That's because the modern diet consists of a lot of heat-processed food and, like you, animals (abound with protein and fat) form lots of AGEs in their bodies. So if you eat cooked meat, you're assaulted twice — by the dietary AGEs and by the AGEs formed when you cook it.

High levels of AGEs are known to contribute to oxidative stress and inflammation, which are linked to the recent epidemics of cardiovascular disease and diabetes. In a study supported by the National Institute on Aging (NIA), researchers analyzed 549 foods and their AGE content. Foods with the highest AGE levels were **beef** and **cheeses** followed by **poultry**, **pork**, **fish**, and **eggs**.

If you shiver with excitement when you hear the words, "Hot dogs here!" at the ballpark, the NIA analysis might flatten your frankfurter. Of the 549 foods tested, a broiled beef hot dog was one of the foods highest in AGEs. And one up from the deadly dog was...BACON. Yes, those smoky, salted pork strips contain over eight times more AGEs than the dog.[10]

- **Beef** — The meat group contains the highest levels of AGEs. Although fats contain more AGEs per gram, meats are served up in larger portions than fats, so meats will likely contribute more to the overall intake of AGEs.

- **Cheeses** — High-fat and aged cheeses, particularly Parmesan, full-fat American, and Greek feta, contain more AGEs than lower-fat cheeses (e.g., reduced-fat mozzarella, 2% milk cheddar, and cottage cheese). Although cooking drives the formation of AGEs in foods, even uncooked, animal-based foods, such as cheeses, can

Coach Karen says

Tofu is quite high in AGEs if cooked or broiled at high temperatures, but it is still lower than most meats.

contain large amounts of AGEs. This is likely due to pasteurization and the aging process.

- **Lamb** — Lamb ranked relatively low in AGEs compared to other meats even when broiled at high heat (450°F) for 30 minutes.

- **High-fat spreads**, including butter, cream cheese, margarine, and mayonnaise, are among the foods highest in AGEs, followed by **oils** and **nuts**, *except* pistachios. Butter and certain types of oils are AGE-rich, even when uncooked.

Carbs Have the Least AGEs Unless...

Carbohydrates contain lower amounts of AGEs compared to meat and fat groups. This may be because these foods often contain more water, antioxidants, and vitamins, which may reduce the formation of AGEs. **Grains**, **legumes**, **breads**, **fruits**, and **vegetables** contain the least AGEs *unless* prepared with added fats. For example, French fries from the Golden Arches has 90 times more AGEs than a boiled potato.

In the carbohydrate group, dry-heat processed foods, such as crackers, chips, and cookies, have the highest AGE levels per gram of food. This is likely due to the addition of ingredients, such as butter, oil, cheese, eggs, and nuts. The dry-heat processing substantially accelerates AGE formation. Even though the amount of AGEs in snack-type foods is far below those present in meats, they're a health hazard if you graze on several snacks during the day, or eat them as a fast meal.

Best Age-Defying Tactics and Cooking Methods

You can significantly reduce your intake of AGEs and how fast you age by changing what you eat and the way you cook. Here's how...

- **Eat less dense foods.** Think of dense foods as being higher in calories per forkful, e.g., solid fats, fatty meats, and full-fat dairy products. Even "lean" red meats and poultry contain high levels of AGEs.

- **Eat more water-rich foods.** These are foods that naturally contain higher percentages of water or absorb a lot of water from being soaked in and/or cooked in water, e.g., legumes, whole grains, fruits, vegetables, and fish.

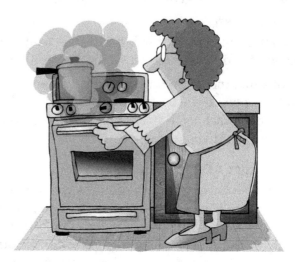

- **Avoid high heat (greater than 300°F).** To reduce the formation of AGEs, it's better to cook foods over medium heat for an extra minute or two rather than at a high temperature in less time. This is when patience pays off.

- **Avoid processed foods.** Processed foods are generally high in fat and salt and cooked at high temperatures.

- **Avoid dry heat, e.g., roasting, grilling, broiling, and barbecuing.** Researchers found a link between heat-processed foods and AGEs.[10] Compared to uncooked food, cooking with dry heat (whether on the grill, in a skillet, or in the oven) promotes AGE formation by more than 10 to 100 times. Opt for moist cooking methods, such as poaching, steaming, stewing, and boiling.

  Browned or charred foods (e.g., charcoal-broiled or smoked foods) indicate that AGEs are present. Meats high in protein and fat are likely to form AGEs during cooking. On the flip side, carbohydrate-rich foods, like fruits, vegetables, and whole grains, maintain low AGE levels after cooking.

- **Use acidic ingredients**, such as marinades made with lemon juice, cranberry juice, or vinegar. Add herbs, spices, hot pepper flakes, and other WHITEs for added flavor, such as garlic, onions, shallots, green onions, and fresh grated ginger. Food marinated in acids form less than half the amount of AGEs during cooking compared to food not exposed to acidic solutions.[10]

NOTE: Controlling AGEs is particularly important if you have diabetes or kidney disease. People with diabetes generate more AGEs in their bodies and those with impaired kidneys have difficulty clearing them out.

The Bottom Line...

Eat more COLOR-ful plants and cook them at low temperatures with moist heat for shorter cooking times.

Beyond AGEs — When High Heat Meets Meat

Churning out picture-perfect grill marks on your steaks is not only a sign of being an expert grillmaster, it's a sign of something else. According to lab studies, when you cook muscle at high temperatures (whether it's beef, pork, poultry, or fish), two potentially cancer-causing chemicals are formed — HCAs and PAHs. So watch out if you're sharing the bar-b with some carnivores and their slabs of meat.

- **Heterocyclic amines (HCAs)** — HCAs form when cooking muscle at high temperatures and particularly when the grilling produces black char marks. The proteins react to the intense heat, and lab studies have shown HCAs alter DNA, which could lead to cancer.

  According to the National Cancer Institute, well-done meat contains higher concentrations of HCAs than when cooked medium or rare. Cooking muscle above 300°F, whether grilling, pan frying, broiling, or cooking for long periods of time tend to form more HCAs.

- **Polycyclic aromatic hydrocarbons (PAHs)** — PAHs are formed when fat and juices drip off the meat and into the grill, which burn and cause flames and smoke. PAHs come back up in the smoke, and these potentially carcinogenic compounds cover and stick to the food.

Maillard Magic — Cooking Starch With High Heat

AGEs, HCAs, PAHs, now there's one more... *acrylamide*. **Acrylamide** was first detected in the food world in April 2002. Acrylamide is a chemical typically found in starchy plant-based foods that are cooked at high temperatures (a recurring theme here), e.g., fried, roasted, grilled, baked, or barbecued, but *not* boiled or steamed.

When an amino acid (asparagine) and naturally occurring sugars meet up while being blasted with dry high heat (above 248°F), a chemical reaction occurs. It's called the Maillard ("ma-LARD") reaction, a.k.a. "browning". You've probably seen this reaction take place many times.

Coach Karen says

On the stove, **low** heat corresponds to about 275°F, **medium** to 300°F, **medium high** to 330°F, and **high** to 375°F.

Coach Karen says

PAHs can be found in smoked foods as well as cigarette smoke and car exhaust fumes.

It is the Maillard magic that creates flavor and color changes. If you ever watched in wonder while your mom's soft buttery dough transformed into crispy brown cookies in the oven, that was the Maillard reaction.

Unfortunately, the product of this Maillard browning reaction is acrylamide, which has been known to cause cancer in animal studies. Acrylamide has been identified as:

- **"Probable human carcinogen"** by the International Agency for Research on Cancer (IARC)

- **"Reasonably anticipated to be a human carcinogen"** by the U.S. National Toxicology Program (NTP)

- **"Likely to be carcinogenic to humans"** by the U.S. Environmental Protection Agency (EPA)

What?! Cookies? Cancer? Acrylamide is produced mainly by deep-fat frying, baking, or roasting food rich in starch. But before you throw up your hands in exasperation, there are ways to *reduce* your exposure to acrylamide in your food. According to the FDA, here's how...

1. **Limit certain starchy foods**, such as **potato products**, especially French fries and potato chips, and **foods made with grain flour** (e.g., cookies, pastries, toast, pretzels, and ready-to-eat breakfast cereals). More reasons to clean out your stash of processed snacks.

   NOTE: Acrylamide levels vary depending on the manufacturer, the cooking time, method, and temperature of the cooking process. For example, according to Food for Life®, they evaluate all of their organic sprouted grain products (breads, tortillas, pastas, cereals, and more) for presence of acrylamide. Based on some comprehensive product testing and evaluations, Food For Life has determined that acrylamide concentrations are well below the safe harbor daily levels of 0.2 micrograms per day (established by California Office of Environmental Health Hazard Assessment).

2. **Avoid high-heat cooking**, such as frying, air frying, baking, barbecuing, and roasting. Higher cooking temperatures and longer cooking times produce more acrylamide. Reactions start at 248°F. Frying dramatically increases acrylamide formation. Air frying circulates air heated up to 400°F. Grilling temperatures vary from 200°F to 550°F. Charcoal grills can get up to 700°F. Moist heat, such as boiling and steaming, do not typically form acrylamide.

3. **Soak raw potato slices in water for 15 to 30 minutes** before roasting to reduce acrylamide formation during cooking. Keep in

mind, high temperatures and low moisture conditions produce acrylamide. (Soaked potatoes should be drained and blotted dry before cooking to prevent splattering or fires.)

4. **Cook potatoes and toast bread to a lighter color** (as opposed to dark brown), which produces less acrylamide. Brown areas tend to have more acrylamide. Very brown areas should be avoided. Don't cook starchy foods, like potatoes and root vegetables, at high temperatures for a long time. Crispy, brown roasted potatoes and hash browns contain more acrylamide than yellow, lightly golden brown ones.

5. **Don't eat scorched food.** Cut off burnt areas.

6. **Avoid storing potatoes in the refrigerator**, which can result in increased acrylamide levels during cooking. Store them in a cool, dark place, such as a closet or pantry, to prevent sprouting.

7. **Drink more hibiscus tea and green tea.** Acrylamide forms in coffee when the beans are roasted. So far, scientists haven't come up with a way to reduce the formation of acrylamide in the roasting process. In an analysis of 42 coffee samples, coffee substitutes made from roasted and ground grains and herbs had the highest concentrations of acrylamide followed by instant coffee, and then roasted coffee.[11]

8. **Avoid smoke.** Acrylamide is also found in cigarette smoke. So stop smoking if you do, and get away from those that smoke.[12] Steer clear of smoke from *any* source — including a BBQ pit.

9. **Focus on your "overall" diet and nutrient intake.**

Coach Karen says

Be sure to keep your spuds away from onions. Onions emit ethylene gas, which triggers plant cells to degrade and will speed up sprouting.

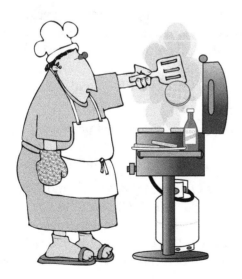

Coach Karen says

All in all, avoid frying, BBQ'ing, broiling, and roasting your food at high temperatures. Steam, stew, or poach instead.

Tips for Cancer-Safe Grilling

No need to stop firing up the grill especially since it's a fast and easy way to get a meal on the table. Besides, breaking off your summer affair with your Weber could be too traumatic. So here are some tips to healthify your grill skills.

- **Go Green** — Fruits and vegetables don't produce HCAs and non-starchy vegetables produce less acrylamide at high temperatures. Grill up some artichokes (pre-steamed), avocado halves, bell peppers, cucumbers, grapes, onions, pineapple, peaches, portobello mushrooms, Romaine lettuce, squashes, and watermelon. Use a stainless steel grilling basket, roasting pan, or outdoor griddle.

- **Cut It** — Skewer smaller cuts of vegetables (think kabobs), which will cook faster and reduce the amount of time exposed to the heat and reduce acrylamide formation.

- **Wrap It** — Don't cook your fruits and veggies with meat. The fat dripping from the meat will fall into the flames and coat your COLORS with PAHs. If you do cook them together, wrap your fresh produce in foil to protect them from the cancer-causing smoke.

- **Clean the Grill** — Clean the grill grates before grilling to remove any old char, and keep it clean throughout the grilling as well.

- **Pre-Cook It** — Pre-cook your veggies first by steaming them (e.g., in a Lékué steam case) to reduce the time they're spent exposed to high heat and flames.

- **Marinate It** — When grilling any starchy vegetables, soak them in an acidic marinade (e.g., lemon-, cranberry- or vinegar-based) to add to their water content. The moisture will minimize the production of acrylamide, and the acids will reduce the formation of AGEs. Sugary marinades/glazes and BBQ sauces that contain a lot of sugar burn easily and cause more charring.

- **Flip It Frequently** — Creating the pretty, but unhealthy, black char marks means letting the food sit on the grill to scorch. Don't grill vegetables, fruit, tofu, and bread until they're dark or charred.

- **Go for Gas** — The heat on a gas grill is more controllable, so opt for gas versus a charcoal grill. Charcoal burns hotter than gas, and you can't dial down the heat. Resist setting your grill on blow-torch mode. Light up the outside burners only. Don't light the center one, but cook your food in the center of the grill with the lid closed.

- **Use Moist Heat** — Steam, stew, or poach. Cook at lower temperatures and for shorter cooking times. These methods reduce the formation of AGEs.

- **Avoid Boiling Vegetables** — Boiling is moist heat, but totally immersing your veggies in water will increase the loss of their water-soluble vitamins. Instead, hydrate your vegetables by steaming, stewing, and poaching them. These methods are best to reduce the formation of AGEs and acrylamide.

Crank down the heat, and cook more non-starchy veggies (e.g., asparagus, red peppers, tomatoes, peaches, mangos, and pineapple). They're less inclined to form cancer-causing chemicals and are cancer-protective on their own. Get creative with cooking off the grill too, such as with a slow cooker, which cooks at low temperatures. At the low setting, it cooks at 190°F, while the high setting cooks at 300°F.

 TRY THESE REAL FOOD RECIPES!

Lemon Dill Potato Salad pg. 247
Plant-Powered Pizza pg. 269
Vegan 'Parmesan' pg. 285

PLAY 7 — STARTING LINEUP

The Fab 15 Recruits

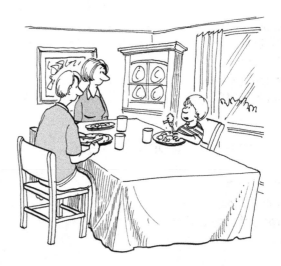

"Broccoli is biodegradable
if you want to throw mine away."

Introducing the Fab 15 brain-friendly foods! These notable recruits will put the brakes on what's aging your amazing brain. As you age, your brain's "cleanup crew" starts slacking off. Eat these foods to literally keep your head in the game. Blood vessels, whether in your heart or in your head, can accumulate plaque. Plaque hardens and narrows your arteries. Too much of it in your pipes can result in a stroke, heart attack, and/or vascular dementia.

And there's more...the blood vessels in your legs can clog up with plaque too, known as peripheral artery disease (PAD). When this happens, you can't get enough oxygen to your working muscles, resulting in pain, numbness, or a serious infection in your legs and feet. No need to say how much you need functioning, cramp-free glutes, hips, hams, quads, calves, and feet to play your sport, much less to just walk.

A plant-centered, fiber-rich training table that consists of lots of COLORS can reduce your risk of 'rusting' from the inside out. Recruit all of the following every day, and you'll slow down the aging pace:

1. **Herbs and spices** — particularly black pepper, cayenne, cinnamon, cumin, ginger, red pepper flakes, rosemary, turmeric. Herbs and spices add COLORS to your food in concentrated form.[1] Double up on herbs.

2. **Berries** — particularly acai ("AH-sy-EE") berries, blueberries, strawberries. Think of berries as your brain's natural "housekeeper". They clean out and recycle the biochemical debris that builds up in your brain and is linked to age-related memory loss and cognitive decline).[2] Berries are loaded with tiny fibrous seeds, and raspberries win the fiber race with a whopping eight grams per cup!

3. **COLOR-ful fruits** — particularly citrus, pomegranate, red grapes. Eat them fresh, dried, frozen, and freeze-dried. Enjoy fruit for dessert.

4. **Tomatoes** — particularly cooked tomatoes for their high concentration of REDs (lycopene).

5. **Dark green leafy vegetables** — particularly arugula, bok choy, kale, spinach, and other greens like beet tops, chards, fennel tops. Start your day with a salad for breakfast. Why wait for lunch to get in your first dose of leafy greens? These superstars are versatile and pack a powerful potassium punch. Eat them raw or cooked, toss them in your smoothie, sauté, soup, or sandwich.

6. **Cruciferous vegetables** — particularly broccoli, Brussels sprouts, cabbage, cauliflower, collard greens, horseradish, radishes, turnips. Save your leaves and stems. They're full of valuable nutrients. Add them to another dish, or freeze them for later to simmer in a homemade or store-bought vegetable broth.

7. **COLOR-ful vegetables** — particularly avocado, eggplant, kabocha (Japanese pumpkin), orange sweet potatoes, pumpkin, purple sweet potatoes (a.k.a. "beni imo", a staple of the centenarians in Okinawa), red beets. Stock up on frozen veggies for convenience, and don't forget canned too.

8. **Whole "intact" grains** — particularly amaranth, barley, buckwheat, bulgur, millet, steel-cut or rolled oats, wild rice.

9. **COLOR-ful legumes** — particularly beans, lentils, peas, tofu.

10. **Ground flaxseeds** — Eating these mighty seeds daily will help you break 100. Find out more in *Play 12: No. 1 Seed* on pg. 94.

Coach Karen says

Eat iron-rich plants, like spinach, soybeans, and other legumes, with foods high in vitamin C, like oranges, bell peppers, and strawberries, to absorb more iron.

Coach Karen says

Canned pumpkin works well in marinara sauces, smoothies, and muffins. Puréed beets add moistness, and boost the nutritional profile of chocolate cupcakes!

11. **Garlic** — Don't let garlic breath stop you from loading up on these pungent cloves. The science behind the stink supports their neuroprotective effects. In addition to WHITEs, a team of University of Missouri researchers discovered another antioxidant in garlic. This active compound, known as Fru-Arg (fructosyl arginine) is capable of penetrating the blood-brain barrier and offers protection against brain aging and disease. Its potent antioxidant effects may prevent and even possibly reverse age-related neurological diseases, such as Alzheimer's and Parkinson's.[3, 4]

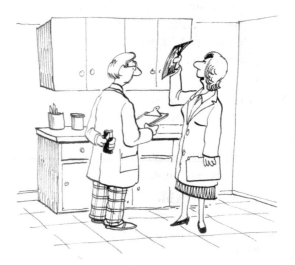

"This 'dark area' on the x-ray
looks suspiciously like chocolate."

12. **100% natural cocoa powder (non-alkalized), unsweetened** — Enjoy chocolate in its purest form. Be sure to buy cocoa in its "natural" state as it still contains the natural acids. Alkalized cocoa (a.k.a. "Dutched cocoa" or "Dutch-process cocoa") is processed with an alkaline solution to neutralize the beans' acidity, but alkalization decreases the cocoa's rich supply of BROWNs.[5]

13. **Green tea, loose leaf, freshly brewed** — Green tea undergoes much less processing than the other teas, so it contains more antioxidants and less caffeine. These hand-picked green tea leaves are high in catechins *(polyphenols)* called epigallocatechin gallate (EGCG), which are the most active and most studied of the polyphenols. Practice the whole ritual of making tea, a calming vehicle for both inner peace and good health. Warm tea = warm heart.

Sip your tea *between* meals. Green tea interferes with iron absorption and can lead to iron deficiency anemia.[6] Be sure to purchase tea leaves from Japan. Tea from China has been shown to contain high levels of lead since their tea plants are contaminated by heavy metals from excessive industrial pollution.[7]

14. **Nuts and other seeds** — particularly almonds, almond butter, hazelnuts (filberts), macadamia nuts, pecans, walnuts; and chia seeds, hemp seeds, pumpkin seeds, sesame seeds. Scatter these wherever your heart desires for a boost of healthy fat and fiber.

Coach Karen says

When brewing green tea, don't use boiling hot water. It destroys the COLORS and burns the delicate leaves. Your tea will be bitter. Heat water to 140°-180°F (based on variety).

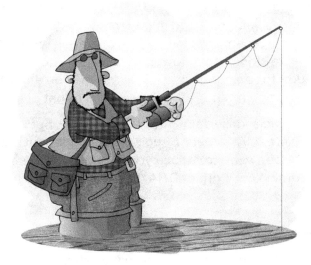

15. **SMASH, canned, fresh or frozen** — SMASH is an acronym that refers to five types of fish that you're encouraged to eat: **S**almon, **M**ackerel (Pacific Atka, Pacific or Atlantic Chub, or US/Canada Atlantic mackerel), **A**nchovies, **S**ardines, and **H**erring. SMASH have health benefits, particularly due to being rich in omega-3 fatty acids and low in mercury. SMASH range in size from the tiny anchovy to the larger salmon. The bigger the fish, such as halibut, mahi mahi, shark, swordfish, and tuna, the longer their lifespan, and the longer fish live, the more mercury they contain.

Mercury is a naturally occurring heavy metal that's released into the environment. It's a potent neurotoxin and exposure to high levels can harm the brain, heart, kidneys, liver, lungs, and immune system of people of all ages. Mercury can be passed to the fetus during pregnancy, and newborns through breastmilk. This metal is a highly toxic element. There is no known safe level of exposure, and it provides NO physiological benefit.

Coach Karen says

Avoid King and Spanish mackerel. They're high in mercury. Eat Pacific Atka, Chub, or US/Canada Atlantic mackerel instead.

Coach Karen says

Ischemic strokes occur when an artery that supplies blood to your brain is blocked by fatty buildup (plaque) or a blood clot.

Coach Karen says

EPA/DHA can prevent clotting, but **large doses** can increase risk of bleeding and hemorrhagic strokes. Eating fish 2-3X a week is not enough to increase this risk.

Coach Karen says

One tablespoon of olive oil contains 1.9 gm of saturated fat.

THE ABCs OF EPA AND DHA

EPA and DHA, the all-star omega-3 fats abundant in fish, have been shown to favorably affect some of the key factors, such as blood pressure and cholesterol, that can reduce your risk of ischemic strokes. The fish omega-3s seem to make your blood less 'sticky' and less likely to clump together. As a result, you're less likely to form clots that cause heart attacks and ischemic strokes. Eating fish as seldom as one to three times per month might significantly reduce the incidence of ischemic stroke.[8]

In various studies, levels of both EPA and DHA in the red blood cell membranes were reduced in patients with dementia. In patients with pre-dementia syndrome, the levels of EPA (but not DHA) were significantly lower. Studies point to EPA as a viable marker for dementia and low levels may be a risk factor for cognitive impairment.[9] All good reasons to get SMASH'ed!

There is no official daily value for EPA and DHA, but the American Dietetic Association suggests eating about 3.5 gm of DHA/EPA per week to reduce your risk of heart disease. SMASH contain 1.0-1.7 gm of DHA/EPA per 3-oz serving.[10]

Why Olive Oil Didn't Make the Cut

Scientific facts about olive oil get distorted, whereby this oil has been elevated to "magic bullet" status. Here are some of the reasons why olive oil didn't make the starting line-up.

- Oil is the most calorie-dense food on Earth.
- At 100% fat, oils average 120 calories per tablespoon. One-quarter cup (four tablespoons) of olive oil has more calories than each of these: a Triple Whopper® with cheese, a large order of McDonald's French fries, and two slices of a medium Domino's® pepperoni and sausage pizza.
- Oil is better than butter, but that doesn't mean it's "good" for you.
- Olive oil is 14% saturated fat. Two tablespoons of olive oil contains nearly 4 gm of saturated fat. On 2,000 calories per day, that's one-third of your total daily limit of sat fat, while on 1,200 calories per day, it's one-half.
- Oil is nutrient-poor.

- The functionally independent centenarians of Okinawa, Japan (one of the world's longevity "hot spots") don't use olive oil. These older Okinawans solidified their diets long before the fast food invasion. What they *do* eat is a lot of fiber-rich, whole foods — lots of fruits, vegetables, intact grains, and beans. They eat little animal protein, usually seafood or lean meat.

THEN AND NOW: THE MEDITERRANEAN LIFESTYLE

Then: In the 1950s, scientists recognized the association between an eating pattern, now popularly called "The Mediterranean Diet", and low rates of heart disease. Farmers living on the isle of rural Crete, Greece were lean, but they also walked about nine miles a day (often behind a plow and a pair of oxen or donkeys), cleared their land with a single-bladed ax, washed their clothes by hand, and swam in the sea for hours to harpoon fresh fish for the day. Historically, Cretans only ate what their land produced — olives and an abundance of fruits and vegetables, herbs and spices, coarse whole-grain breads, pulses (beans, lentils, and peas), wild greens, and fish. Crete farmers had the lowest rates of heart disease and cancer.

Now: Today, the people of Crete still maintain an olive oil-rich diet, but in a follow-up study, 86.1% of the farmers was overweight and/or obese. Mean weight increased by 44 pounds with an alarming increase in abdominal obesity.[11] Childhood obesity is highest in Crete and 50% of its children are overweight. Rates of heart disease and its risk factors have increased significantly.[12]

How could this happen if olive oil is the secret to heart health? Well, the modern-day islanders traded in their traditional staples for more meat, cheese, and T.V.[13] Daily intake of organic whole foods decreased, as well as the amount of physical activity. The message? Olive oil in and of itself is NOT the key to living longer and disease-free.[14]

 TRY THESE REAL FOOD RECIPES!

Raspberry Pecan Salad with Raspberry Champagne Vinaigrette pg. 251
Slow-Baked Miso Maple Salmon pg. 272

PLAY 8 — ONE-ON-ONE DRILLS

Salt Assaults

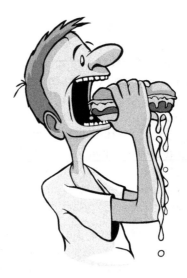

Y ou may think you're one of the lucky ones because you can eat unlimited bags of chips and other troves of salt, and it doesn't affect your blood pressure. But even if you don't have hypertension, excess sodium can adversely affect other target organs. If you want to stop aging, stop buying processed food and grinding salt over everything you eat. If you're a salt junkie, then here's what you need to know.

Coach Karen says

One teaspoon of table salt is equivalent to about 2,300 mg sodium.

According to the Centers for Disease Control and Prevention, bread is the No. 1 source of sodium in the American diet. And that doesn't include the ketchup, mustard, cheese, pickles, and cold cuts that are stacked on top of it. Nor does it include the chips you eat alongside your artfully composed hoagie. A seemingly benign large chicken breast sub from your favorite franchise can rack up 3,330 mg of sodium. Spice up that sub with some jerk mustard and add another 350 mg.

How Much Sodium

Salt is a mixture of 40% sodium and 60% chloride. A healthy, active adult needs between 200 to 500 mg of sodium per day to function normally, which is equivalent to about 1/8 to 1/4 teaspoon of refined table salt. But Americans consume seven times more sodium than what their bodies need — over 3,400 mg sodium per day (about 1-1/2 teaspoons table salt) — with most of it coming from processed food. The Institute of Medicine set the current recommended sodium limits for healthy adults, which are based on age:

- Ages 19-50: **1,500 mg*** (equivalent to 2/3 teaspoon or 3,800 mg salt)
- Ages 51-70: **1,300 mg*** (equivalent to ~1/2 teaspoon or 3,200 mg salt)
- Ages 71+: **1,200 mg*** (equivalent to 1/2 teaspoon or 2,900 mg salt)

These values may be higher for people who lose large amounts of water through sweat, such as athletes and workers exposed to extreme heat.

Coach Karen says

Refined table salt, coarse Kosher salt flakes, and large grain sea salts vary in crystal size, so the amount of sodium in one teaspoon will vary.

ALL SALTS ARE NOT CREATED EQUAL

It's true that salts vary in mineral content, which affects their color, texture, and taste, but it's a huge leap to think that salt is actually *good* for you. Any clinical health claims associated with the trace elements in Celtic or Himalayan sea salts have not been substantiated, e.g., they detoxify and mineralize the body, lower blood pressure, balance blood sugar, prevent muscle cramps, and improve bone health. These minerals aren't present in large enough quantities to have any effect. The bottom line...salt is salt and their differences vary the flavor, not the nutrition, of your food..

Coach Karen says

Your body cleanses on its own. Your liver, kidneys, and intestines are detoxifying every minute of the day.

The 1-to-1 Sodium Rule

An on-the-spot way to determine if a food product is high in sodium is to apply the 1-to-1 sodium rule, which compares sodium to calories. Simply put, if a product has 100 calories, the sodium content should hover around 100 mg. If not, put it back on the shelf.

Watch out for canned foods, especially soups. Half a cup of canned 'classic' tomato soup contains 90 calories and 480 mg sodium. That computes to a colossal 1-to-5 ratio. Worse yet, people often eat the whole can of soup in one sitting and ingest the entire 1,920 mg of sodium, not to mention five teaspoons of added sugar! M'm! M'm! Not So Good!

Coach Karen says

Use the 1:1 sodium rule to quickly determine if a food product is high in sodium. Sodium (mg) and calories should be about equal.

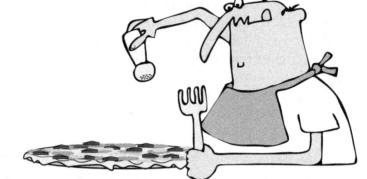

Your Blood Vessels on Sodium

Healthy blood vessels will help keep your heart and brain young and functional. Studies show elevated sodium levels can cause the inner lining of blood vessels, called the endothelium, to "malfunction".[1] The following occurs as a result:

1. **Vessels stiffen and blood flow slows.** Arteries that become less elastic lose their ability to fully contract and relax, which makes it harder for your heart to pump large volumes of blood throughout your body and brain. Eventually, the heart wears out (heart failure).

   Keep in mind that your brain is a very vascular organ. It requires a *lot* of blood to function. Every four minutes, a gallon of blood flows through your brain's rich network of blood vessels. Studies indicate a link between low blood flow to the brain combined with cardiovascular disease and the incidence of neurodegenerative diseases. When neurons don't receive oxygen and nourishment, they die. Cerebral blood flow is 20% lower in patients with Alzheimer's disease compared to those without dementia.[2]

2. **Vessels become sticky.** The inner lining of healthy blood vessels should be smooth (think slick like Teflon), but when the endothelium is assaulted with sodium, as well as blood sugar and stress hormones, it becomes inflamed and "rough" (think sandpaper or Velcro). The result? Plaque sticks to the vessel wall — a primer for forming clots.

   In addition to the plaque attack, your body breeds dangerous inflammation, especially when you're sick. Inflammation may cause plaque to crack, rupture, and dislodge from the arterial wall. In fact, inflammation is the primary reason why heart attacks are more likely to occur seven days after a confirmed flu diagnosis.[3]

Your Heart on Sodium

Researchers found that elevated sodium levels may increase the wall thickness of your heart's main pumping chamber, known as the left ventricle.[1] High blood pressure is a major risk factor for this muscle tissue enlargement, but it's also found in healthy people with normal blood pressure who consume high amounts of sodium. This thickening can lead to cardiac issues, such as:

- Arrhythmia (abnormal heart rhythm)
- Heart attack
- Sudden cardiac arrest (sudden loss of heart function)
- Heart failure (inability of the heart to pump enough blood throughout the body)

Your Kidneys on Sodium

Healthy kidneys remove extra fluid and waste from your blood. Studies show that too much sodium damages the kidneys, and the kidneys start excreting protein.[1] Other sodium-related complications include:

- **Swelling in the legs, hands, and face** — The kidneys can't eliminate excess
- **Heart failure** — Excess fluid in your bloodstream can overwork your heart, making it enlarged and weak.
- **Shortness of breath** — Fluid can build up in your lungs, making it difficult to breathe.
- **Increased blood pressure** — Blood pressure rises as sodium and fluid build up in your tissues and bloodstream.

Coach Karen says

Just like your biceps grow in size from pumping iron, your heart (a muscle) gets larger and thicker if it has to pump too hard.

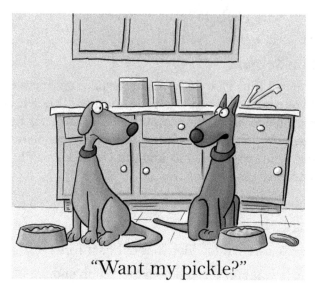

"Want my pickle?"

Your Brain on Sodium

Scientists found that eating excess salt causes the brain to overreact to stressful situations. This overreaction causes your nervous system to release chronically high levels of stress hormones and results in short-term spikes in blood pressure. This blood pressure variability used to be considered harmless by physicians as long as overall blood pressure was normal, but it's increasingly associated with a higher risk of cardiovascular death and events.[1]

But Wait! It's Not Just the Salt

Living a long and functional life today means you don't shake or utter that four-letter word...SALT. You've banished it from your favorite recipes, family table, and your cupboards. Low sodium, salt-free, reduced sodium, lightly salted, and unsalted have painfully crept their way into your vocabulary and into your pantry. But the dietary approach to managing your blood pressure involves another key mineral — potassium. Low levels of potassium in your diet may be just as much of a risk factor for high blood pressure as high levels of sodium.[4] Aim for a balance of less salt and more potassium in your daily training plan. Potassium helps to:

- Relax your blood vessel walls, leading to lower blood pressure.[5]

- Excrete excess sodium through your urine, leading to lower blood pressure.[6]

- Reduce damage to your arteries from the decrease in arterial pressure.

Coach Karen says

Potassium and sodium are the dynamic duo. They work TOGETHER. When sodium goes up, potassium goes down, and when sodium goes down, potassium goes up.

NOTE: Not only do studies suggest a link between low potassium levels and high blood pressure, but it's linked to diabetes as well. That means, higher glucose and insulin levels could indicate you're not getting enough potassium.[7]

Beyond Bananas

Eat more potassium-rich foods, such as a wide variety of fruits, vegetables, and legumes — *not just bananas*. Many people think of bananas when they think of foods high in potassium, but they're actually near the bottom of the list of high potassium foods (foods with over 400 mg potassium per serving). Aim for 4,700 mg per day.

POTASSIUM CONTENT

FOOD	POTASSIUM (mg)
Swiss chard, 1 cup	961
Potato, baked, 1 medium	941
Squash, winter, cooked, 1 cup	896
White beans, canned, drained, 1 cup	829
Potato, baked, 1 small	738
Lentils, cooked, 1 cup	731
Prune juice, canned, 1 cup	707
Prunes, dried, 1/2 cup	699
Carrot juice, canned, 1 cup	689
Edamame, 1 cup	676
Pomegranate, one 4" fruit	666
Tomato paste, 1/4 cup	664
Beet greens, cooked, 1/2 cup	654
Acorn squash, mashed, 1 cup	644
Watermelon, 1/8 of a melon	640
Black beans, 1 cup	611
Kidney beans, canned, 1 cup	607
White beans, canned, 1/2 cup	595
Butternut squash, 1 cup	582
Yogurt, nonfat, 1 cup	579
Tomato juice, canned, 1 cup	556
Tomato purée, 1/2 cup	549
Sweet potato, baked in skin, 1 medium	542
Spinach, frozen, 1 cup	540

Coach Karen says

Lower your blood pressure by eating potassium-rich foods. Did you know that a medium baked potato has 123% more potassium than a banana?

Coach Karen says

Avoid relying on potassium supplements as they can more easily result in an excessive intake of potassium.

Coach Karen says

Boiling depletes potassium. A boiled potato has almost half the potassium of a baked potato.

FOOD	POTASSIUM (mg)
Salmon, wild, cooked, 3 oz	534
Pomegranate juice, 1 cup	533
Beets, 1 cup	518
100% orange juice, 8 oz	496
Apricots, dried, 6	488
Avocado, 1/2 fruit	487
Lima beans, cooked, 1/2 cup	478
Mackerel, various types, cooked, 3 oz	474
Coconut water, plain, unsweetened, 8 oz	471
Great northern beans, canned	460
Tomato sauce, 1/2 cup	453
Soybeans, mature, cooked, 1/2 cup	443
Pink beans (light red kidney), cooked, 1/2 cup	430
Cantaloupe, cubed, 1 cup	427
Banana, 1 medium	422

Sources: National Institutes of Health; U.S. Department of Agriculture[8]; Advances in Nutrition[9]

Medications and Conditions That Affect Potassium

Most people shouldn't have any problems eating a potassium-rich diet. WARNING: If you have kidney failure or a kidney disorder, check with your doctor as to how much potassium you can consume per day. Too much potassium can be harmful when your kidneys aren't functioning at full capacity. They're less able to remove this mineral from your blood, and the potassium can accumulate to a dangerous level.

Potassium affects the way your heart muscles work and plays a role in each heartbeat. Too much potassium in your blood may cause your heart to beat irregularly, and in the worst cases, can cause a heart attack. Some blood pressure-lowering medications can *increase* potassium levels and require periodic blood and/or urine testing. These medications include:

- **Beta-blockers** — e.g., carvedilol (Coreg®); metoprolol (Toprol XL®, Lopressor®); atenolol (Tenormin®)

- **ACE inhibitors** — e.g., lisinopril (Zestril®, Prinivil®); benazepril (Lotensin®)

- **ARBs or angiotensin II receptor blockers** — e.g., valsartan (Diovan®); losartan (Cozaar®); olmesartan (Benicar®)

Some medications can *decrease* potassium levels:

- **Steroids** (e.g., prednisone), **thiazide diuretics** (e.g., hydrocholorthiazide (Microzide®, Hydrodiuril®), and **laxatives** — If you're taking a corticosteroid, such as prednisone, for osteoarthritis, you'll tend to lose potassium and retain excess sodium.

HOW BLADDERS AND BOWELS AFFECT POTASSIUM

Diuretics make the kidneys pump water and sodium into your pee, but potassium also slips through the open floodgates. Bulk-forming laxatives absorb water and electrolytes, which can cause a loss of potassium in your stool. To help offset this sodium-potassium balancing act, eat fruits and vegetables high in potassium and cut back on bread, processed foods, and restaurant food, which are some of the highest sources of daily sodium.

The Bottom Line...

- **Eat mostly "real food"**, that is, unprocessed or minimally processed food.

- **Use herbs, spices, and flavored vinegars to season food.**

- **Read nutrition labels.**

- **Go easy on condiments**, e.g., soy sauce, Worcestershire sauce, salad dressings, ketchup, seasoned salts, pickles, olives.

- **Beware of baked goods**. In addition to salt, baked goods, like bread and pastries, are made with baking soda and/or baking powder, which contain sodium. These foods aren't typically thought of as "salty" but can be significant sources of hidden sodium.

- **Speak up when dining out.** Ask to have your food prepared with less salt. Use squeezes of lemon or lime to add flavor to your food.

- **Limit the use of salt substitutes**, which contain potassium chloride, and use COLOR-ful herbs and spices instead.

- **Ditch the sports drinks, and drink water.** Gatorade® has built a brand synonymous with sports hydration, that is, replacing lost fluid, carbohydrates, and electrolytes. But unless you're engaged in prolonged, vigorous physical activity (e.g., hill climbing on a bike for an hour and a half or working out in extreme heat), water will do.

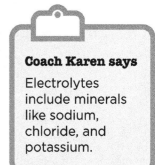

Coach Karen says

Electrolytes include minerals like sodium, chloride, and potassium.

Coach Karen says

The vast majority of people who drink sports drinks aren't athletes and aren't as physically active as they should be.

Spare yourself the refined sugar, phosphates, modified food starch, artificial colorants, artificial flavors, not to mention the extra calories. A 20-oz Gatorade Thirst Quencher contains 34 grams of sugar. That's nearly nine teaspoons of sugar! Drink one of these after every workout, and you'll be aging at an accelerated rate.

- **Eat a balanced diet consisting of fresh fruits and vegetables.** You'll get a healthy dose of heart- and brain-healthy nutrients, COLORS, and fiber.

 TRY THESE REAL FOOD RECIPES!

Cajun Spice (No Salt) pg. 276
Red Lentil Hummus (No Oil) pg. 233

PLAY 9 — THE FUNDAMENTALS

How to Play the Eating Game

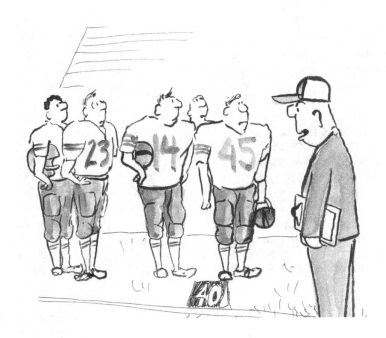

The Game Plan — Memorize These Six Plays!

1. Eat "First-String" foods 90% of the time.

2. Eat all the COLORS.

3. Eat protein with every meal, preferably plant-based protein.

4. Eat when you're hungry; don't eat when you're not.

5. Eat from The Power Plate.

6. Eat until you're 80% full. That is, you can still put away a few more bites, but stop at this point..

The Anti-Aging Training Table

First-String food = *Go for It!*
Second-String food = *Tread Lightly!*
Benchwarmers = *Out of Bounds!*

Coach Karen says

To make dried fruit more water-rich, place them in a bowl, cover with hot water, and steep for 10-15 minutes, then strain.

FIRST STRING Go for it!	SERVINGS PER DAY	TRAINING NOTES
Berries, 1/2 cup (fresh or frozen), 1/4 cup dried	1	BLUEs and REDs: Acai berries, barberries, blackberries, blueberries, cherries, Concord grapes, cranberries, goji berries, mulberries, raspberries, strawberries
Other Fruits, 1 medium-sized fruit, 1 cup cubed (fresh or frozen), 1/4 cup dried	3	Various COLORS: particularly apples, avocados, citrus, dates, pomegranate, plums (especially black plums), red grapes
Leafy Greens, 1 cup raw or 1/2 cup cooked	2	GREENs: Arugula, assorted baby greens, beet greens, collard greens, kale (black, green, red), mustard greens, sorrel, spinach, Swiss chard, turnip greens
Cruciferous Vegetables, 1/2 cup chopped, 1/4 cup Brussels or broccoli sprouts, 1 tablespoon horseradish	1	GREENs: Arugula, bok choy, broccoli, Brussels sprouts, cabbage, cauliflower, collard greens, horseradish, kale (black, green, red), radishes, turnip greens, watercress, kimchi
Other Vegetables, 1 cup raw or 1/2 cup cooked (fresh or frozen), 1/4 cup dried mushrooms; **Vegetable Juice,** 4 oz	2	Various COLORS: **Non-starchy** —artichokes, asparagus, beets, bell peppers, carrots, garlic, mushrooms, okra, onions, sea vegetables, snap peas, summer squash, zucchini **Starchy** — corn, peas, potatoes, pumpkin, sweet potatoes (orange, purple), taro, winter squash, yams
Lycopene-Rich Food*,	10,000 micrograms	REDs: Tomatoes, guava, papaya, pink grapefruit, watermelon, etc.
Beans, 1/2 cup cooked beans, split peas, tofu, tempeh; 1 cup fresh peas or sprouted lentils; 1/4 cup hummus or bean dip; 1/2 cup cooked lentil/bean pasta	3	Various COLORs: Beans, peas, lentils WHITEs (soy)**: Edamame, edamame/soy pasta, miso, soy milk, soy nuts, tempeh, tofu
Intact Grains and Pseudo-Grains, 1/2 cup cooked; **Sprouted Whole Grain Products (flourless),** 1 slice bread or tortilla, 1/2 English muffin, 1/2 cup cereal; **Popcorn,** 3 cups popped	3	WHITEs: Amaranth, barley, buckwheat, bulgur, farro, oats, rice (black, brown, red, wild), millet, popcorn, quinoa, rye, spelt, teff, whole wheat; sprouted whole grain products

FIRST STRING Go for it!	SERVINGS PER DAY	TRAINING NOTES
Flaxseeds, 1-2 tablespoons	1	Ground golden or brown
Nuts and Seeds, 1 oz (~1/4 cup) raw, unsalted; **Chia Seeds, Hemp Seeds**, 1-2 tablespoons; **Nut/Seed Butters**, 2 tablespoons	1	WHITEs: Almonds, Brazil nuts, cashews, hazelnuts, macadamias, peanuts, pecans, pepitas, pistachios, seeds (pumpkin, sesame, sunflower), walnuts
Nutritional Yeast, 2 teaspoons	1	
Turmeric, 1/4 to 1 teaspoon	1	Combine with black pepper to enhance absorption.
Herbs and Spices, 1-2 teaspoons dried or 1-2 tablespoons fresh	Eat liberally	Various COLORS: e.g., basil, bay leaves, black pepper, garlic, ginger, cayenne, chili powder, cilantro, cinnamon, cumin, curry powder, dill, paprika, parsley, rosemary, thyme
Beverages, 1 cup • **Green Tea/Matcha** • **Hibiscus Tea** • **Other Beverages**	8 cups total	No sweeteners added. Drink green tea between meals. REDs and BLUEs Water, black tea
Vinegar, 2 teaspoons with each meal[1]	3	Apple cider, balsamic, champagne, distilled white, fruit, rice, white/red wine, sherry

First-Stringers are:
- Recommended — the healthiest choices
- Naturally rich in water (fruits, vegetables, beans are "water-rich")
- High volume
- High in fiber (requires more chewing)
- Low in calories
- Low in sodium

One lycopene serving: minestrone soup (2/3 cup), tomato juice (1/2 cup), spaghetti sauce (1/3 cup), tomato purée (3 tablespoons), raw tomatoes (2-2/3 medium), cherry tomatoes (23), watermelon (1-1/2 cups), or guava (1-1/4 cups)

**One soy protein serving: edamame (1/2 cup), edamame/soy pasta (1/2 cup cooked), fortified soy milk (1 cup), soy nuts, roasted, unsalted (1/4 cup).

Coach Karen says

Don't drink straight vinegar. Sprinkle it on your salads. Rinse your mouth with water after eating anything acidic to protect your tooth enamel.

Coach Karen says

If you don't make First-String choices and hit your food goals on one day, shake it off. Just eat better the next day.

SECOND-STRING Tread lightly!	SERVINGS	TRAINING NOTES
SMASH, 3-4 oz	2 servings per week	SMASH — Salmon, mackerel, anchovies, sardines, herring
Extra virgin, cold-pressed oils*	Eat minimally	See product recommendations on pg 223.
Poultry, 3-4 oz	No more than 1-2 days per week	Organic, pasture-raised, skinless white meat
Salt Products	Not to exceed sodium limit**	Kosher salt, sea salt, low-sodium soy sauce (tamari), white miso
Alcoholic Beverages	1 or none per day	4-5 oz wine; 12 oz beer; 1-1.5 oz of 80-proof liquor. (In order of first to last place: red wine, white wine, beer, hard liquor.)

Second-Stringers are:
- Harmful to your health if consumed often. Consume occasionally and/or in small amounts.

All oils are 100% fat, calorie-dense, and about 120 calories per tablespoon. One teaspoon of oil is considered one serving of fat.

Daily sodium limit — Ages 19-50: **1,500 mg**; 51-70: **1,300 mg**; Ages 71+: **1,200 mg** (1/2 teaspoon).

BENCHWARMERS Out of Bounds!	SERVINGS	TRAINING NOTES
Animal Fats, Dairy*	0	Butter, cheese, cow's milk, cream, cream cheese, cream sauce, half-and-half, ice cream, lard, sour cream, yogurt
Tropical fats*	0	Coconut milk, coconut oil, palm kernel oil, palm oil
Trans-Fat, Hydrogenated Fat, Partially Hydrogenated Fats	0	Margarine, shortening, fried fast food, non-dairy creamer, non-dairy whipped topping, no-stir nut butter, theatre/microwave popcorn, etc.
RBD Oils (highly processed)	0	"Refined, Bleached, and/or Deodorized"
Red Meat, Processed Meat*	0	Beef, lamb, pork, veal, organ meat; Cured, dried, salted, smoked red meat, e.g., bacon, bologna, chorizo, deli meat, hot dogs, pepperoni, sausage, etc.
Eggs	See note**	Includes foods made with eggs, e.g., mayonnaise
Sweeteners	0	All refined sugars, less refined sugar ("raw"), sugar substitutes, high-fructose corn syrup; High-sugar jams, jellies, glazes

Coach Karen says

Treat meat (anything animal) as a condiment and not the main attraction.

Coach Karen says

Reduce or eliminate dairy consumption due to insulin-like growth factor 1 (IGF-1) and its link to prostate and breast cancer. Substitute with plant-based dairy.[5, 6]

BENCHWARMERS Out of Bounds!	SERVINGS	TRAINING NOTES
Sweetened Drinks, Sodas	0	
Artificial Colorants	0	Neon-green, electric orange, and the like don't count as your daily COLORs. Artificial colorants are derived from petrochemicals (or crude oil).
"Lite Salt" (salt substitutes with potassium chloride)	0	
Miscellaneous	0	Food that's fried, charred, or cooked with direct high heat. Highly salted, pickled, smoked foods.

Benchwarmers are:
- Risky for your health
- Calorie dense
- Dry
- Firm
- Fatty
- Salty
- Sugary

Saturated fats — *American Heart Association/American College of Cardiology Guidelines: Less than 5%-6% of total daily calories, e.g., on 2,000 calories a day, no more than 100-120 calories should come from saturated fats (11-13 gm). The Anti-Aging Training Table keeps saturated fats out of bounds.*

**Studies show eating 2 or more egg yolks in a 2-week period increased formation of TMAO.[2] If eaten, opt for soft/hard boiled or poached vs scrambled or fried. Based on published meta-analyses, consider avoiding eggs completely if you have had a reproductive cancer or at high risk for breast, ovarian, and prostate cancer.[3, 4]

Crank Up the Volume

Water-rich foods are high-volume foods due to all the water they contain, so they fill you up. Take the caloric density of raisins, for example. A handful (1/4 cup) of raisins is equal to one full cup of water-rich grapes. Did you know that the following foods have the same number of calories?

Coach Karen says

Remember, what you put in your mouth becomes a part of you.

Coach Karen says

Popcorn is an intact whole grain, and great source of fiber. Make your own at home to control the amount of sodium, oil, and the type of oil used, if any.

BENCHWARMERS (dry, dense, sugary, firm, fatty)	OR	FIRST STRING (high volume, high fiber, water-rich)
2 medium glazed doughnuts	or	2 pint-sized clamshells of blueberries (about 310 blueberries)
20 potato chips	or	8 cups (2 quarts) of air-popped popcorn
1 medium serving of French fries	or	4 ears of corn (6" long)
1 energy bar	or	1 pound of seedless grapes (2 1/2 cups; about 80 grapes)
1 chocolate chunk muffin	or	6 medium apples
1 scoop (1/2 cup) of mint chocolate chip ice cream	or	1 medium orange, 30 sweet cherries, and 6 baby carrots
1 bag (8 oz) potato chips	or	11 sweet potatoes

The Power Plate

Since the '60s, plates (like TV screens) have been growing in size. The standard dinner plate increased from 8-1/2" (now considered a salad plate) to 12 inches. It's no surprise that people have grown bigger along with the plates. If your plate is the size of a manhole cover, it's time to seriously downsize. Opt for a 9-inch round one.

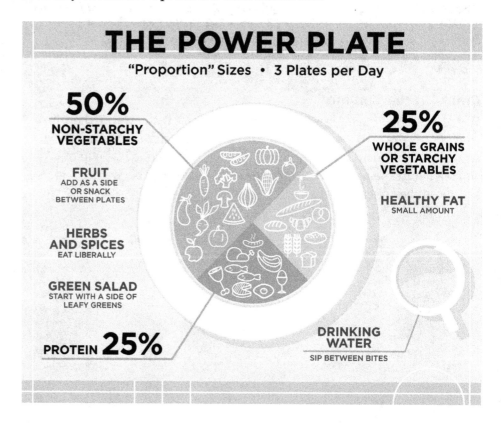

When filling your plate, focus more on *proportions* than portions. Here's how your First Stringers would look on your Power Plate:

- **50% of the plate — Non-starchy vegetables**
- **25% of the plate — Plant-based protein**, e.g., beans, lentils, peas, hummus, tofu, tempeh, edamame); **SMASH**
- **25% of the plate — Intact grains or starchy vegetables**, e.g., potatoes; sweet potatoes; sprouted whole grain breads; black, brown, or red rice; corn, popcorn; hot cereals
- **On the sidelines — Leafy green salad, fruit, and water**

Coach Karen says

To lose weight and lower blood pressure, start meals with a high-volume, low-sodium salad or soup.

A SUPERPOWER PILL?

When something good comes along, someone always tries to bottle it. Why hover over a whole platter of rabbit food when you could pop a little pill? Sorry, it doesn't work that way, and it's still better to eat your plate of plants. First, unlike drugs, supplements cannot make disease claims and are not regulated by the FDA. That means, the FDA is **not** authorized to review supplements for safety and effectiveness **before** they are sold to you. Pretty scary, isn't it?

Second, according to a Cornell University study, the health effects attributed to eating phytochemicals are primarily due to all the COLORS working synergistically with the micronutrients in the *whole plant foods*. When the individual antioxidant compounds are isolated from the food source, such as in a pill, the protective and anti-inflammatory health effects are inconsistent. The long-term safety, doses, and efficacy of consuming these compounds as dietary supplements are still in need of further study.[7]

SAMPLE POWER PLATES

Breakfast

- Steel-cut oats mixed with unsweetened soy milk, walnuts, ground flaxseed, cinnamon, and berries
- Low-sodium tomato juice

Lunch

- Meal-sized salad with dark, leafy greens, bell peppers, tomatoes, and zucchini sprinkled with hemp seeds and topped with Lemon Dill Potato Salad (pg. 247)

Dinner

- Broccoli, carrots, shiitake mushrooms, onions, and garlic stir-fry
- Baked tempeh or wild salmon
- Wild rice cooked with herbs and garlic
- Side salad with dark, leafy greens, sunflower seeds and Pomegranate Balsamic Vinaigrette (pg. 250)

Between Plates

- Navel orange + handful of cashews
- Apple slices + almond butter
- Chopped vegetables + Red Lentil Hummus (pg. 233)

Water

Drink plenty of water throughout the day.

Coach Karen says

If you're fighting to stay awake, eat a WHOLE apple. The theory? Biting into the apple and navigating around the core require dexterity and concentration, which activate brain regions and can perk you up.

Power Plate to Power Bowl

"Bowl food" has emerged as a whole new category of food that has gained popularity and doesn't seem to be going away anytime soon. It starts out with a base layer of whole grains, greens, starchy or spiralized vegetables, and is topped with other hearty components (e.g., fish, grilled tofu, Brussels sprouts), then sprinkled with garnishes, and finished with a sauce to tie it all together. Basically, it's a Power Plate in a bowl!

So once you proportion out your Power Plate, transfer it to a bowl and dig in. Eating with a fork and knife off a plate is a more formal and rigid style of eating. On the other hand, bowl food is "comfort food". You can bring a bowl closer to you, which makes the eating experience more intimate since the flavors and textures are right under your nose and close to your eyes. It's why food tastes better in a bowl. Bowls are a great way to build a meal with more vegetables, stretch proteins, repurpose leftovers, and use up odds and ends in your locker (pg. 206).

The Aging Analysis

Your diet, your lifestyle, and your positivity all have an influence on how well you age. To summarize, healthy aging is a process affected by the combination of *many* mechanisms, such as:

1. Free radicals
2. Mitochondrial damage
3. AGEs (glycotoxins)
4. Microbiome imbalance
5. Chronic inflammation
6. TMAO
7. HCAs and PAHs
8. Acrylamide

Coach Karen says

"Whole" foods are foods as nature made them — no added fat, sugar, sodium, flavorings, or other manufactured ingredients. They're processed minimally or not at all.

 TRY THESE REAL FOOD RECIPES!

Grilled Oatmeal with Fresh Fruit 'n Nuts pg. 235
Wild Salmon or Tofu Tacos with Citrus Salsa pg. 274

*The aging process can be slowed
by the substances found naturally in
whole, plant-based foods.*

Check off all the First-Stringers you eat in one day.

THE POWER PLATE PLAYERS (DAILY ROSTER)

FIRST STRING – GO FOR IT!

BERRIES
- 1/2 cup (fresh or frozen)
- 1/4 cup dried

1 DAILY SERVING
☐

OTHER FRUITS
- 1 medium fruit
- 1 cup cubed (fresh or frozen)
- 1/4 cup dried

3 DAILY SERVINGS
☐ ☐ ☐

LEAFY GREENS
- 1 cup raw
- 1/2 cup cooked

2 DAILY SERVINGS
☐ ☐

CRUCIFEROUS VEGETABLES
- 1/2 cup chopped
- 1/4 cup Brussels or broccoli sprouts
- 1 Tbsp horseradish

1 DAILY SERVING
☐

OTHER VEGETABLES
- 1/2 cup raw or cooked
- 1/4 cup dried mushrooms
- 4 oz vegetable juice

2 DAILY SERVINGS
☐ ☐

RED FRUIT OR VEGETABLE
Lycopene
Include 10K mcg, such as:
- 2/3 cup minestrone
- 4 oz. tomato juice
- 1/3 cup spaghetti sauce
- 1-1/2 cups watermelon

BEANS
- 1/2 cup cooked
- 1 cup fresh peas/ sprouted lentils
- 1/4 cup hummus or bean dip
- 1/2 cup cooked lentil/bean pasta

3 DAILY SERVINGS
☐ ☐ ☐

INTACT & SPROUTED GRAINS
- 1/2 cup cooked intact grains
- 1 slice sprouted whole grain bread
- 3 cups popped popcorn

3 DAILY SERVINGS
☐ ☐ ☐

FLAXSEEDS
- 1 to 2 Tbsp ground

1 DAILY SERVING
☐

NUTS & SEEDS
- 1 oz (about 1/4 cup)
- 2 Tbsp nut or seed butter

1 DAILY SERVING
☐

NUTRITIONAL YEAST
- 2 tsp

1 DAILY SERVING
☐

TURMERIC
- 1/4 to 1 tsp

1 DAILY SERVING
☐

HERBS & SPICES
- Eat liberally

1 DAILY SERVING
☐

BEVERAGES
- **Green Tea or Matcha**
  1 cup (1-4 servings)
  ☐ ☐ ☐ ☐

- **Hibiscus Tea**
  1 cup (1 serving)
  ☐

- **Water & Other Beverages**
  1 cup (3-6 servings)
  ☐ ☐ ☐ ☐ ☐ ☐

8 DAILY SERVINGS
☐ ☐ ☐ ☐ ☐ ☐ ☐ ☐

VINEGAR
- 2 tsp with each meal

3 DAILY SERVINGS
☐ ☐ ☐

FIRST STRINGERS ARE:
- Recommended – the healthiest choices
- Naturally rich in water ("water-rich")
- High volume
- High in fiber (requires more chewing)
- Low in calories
- Low in sodium

PLAY 10 — YOUR BEST OFFENSE

Eat More Beans!

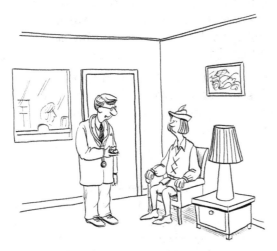

"Typically, I don't accept
magic beans for payment."

Beans, peas and lentils (a.k.a. legumes or pulses) could be the world's oldest and most perfect food. This diverse group is an excellent source of protein, dietary fiber, and complex carbohydrates. These edible seeds are nutritionally dense, inexpensive, flavorful, and extremely versatile. Firehouse chili, bean burritos, hummus, baked beans, bean dip, and split pea soup are just a few of the delish dishes that show off the mighty bean's versatility.

Since beans are high in water and fiber (averaging 7-10 grams of fiber per half cup serving), you'll feel fuller, feel fuller faster, and feel satisfied longer. Trade in your belt-busting steak for an ultra-lean, plant-based protein that's lower in calories, void of saturated fat, and superrich in COLORS *(polyphenols)*. Researchers studied 24 common beans and identified a varied mix of phytochemicals in each bean.[1] So don't get fixed on just one type of bean, mix 'em up! Eat a three-bean

Coach Karen says

Keep a container of beans in your fridge to have a handy add-on for your bowls, salads, soups, and more.

salad or chili on one day, then a black bean dip or pinto bean burrito on another.

Stop Offensive Fouls

Despite all the glowing health benefits of beans, do you have the ability to clear a room after eating them? Do they inflate you with flatulence? Fear no more! There are ways to lessen these effects, so don't deprive yourself of the nutritional superpower of beans.

1. **Soak uncooked dried beans before cooking.** Drain the beans well. By discarding the soaking water, you'll get rid of some of the potent culprits (water-soluble carbohydrates called oligosaccharides) that make it tougher for you to digest beans.

2. **Increase your bean consumption *gradually*.** This is when you need to just hunker down and eat more beans. If you do, you'll encourage the presence of the enzyme you need to digest these starches, which are great fertilizers for your good gut bacteria (prebiotics). Start with 1/4-cup increments of beans two to three times per week.

3. **Cook your beans with a large strip of dried kombu** ("KOHM-boo"), an edible Japanese sea vegetable, a.k.a. dried kelp, to reduce the gas-producing properties of beans. This "King of Seaweeds" contains enzymes that help break down the gas-producing culprits in beans. The amino acids in kombu help soften beans and make them more digestible. Eden® prepares all their cooked canned beans with kombu. See kombu (pg. 219).

4. **Add some gas-reducing dried herbs, like bay leaves or a few pinches of cumin.**

5. **Opt for plain ol' beans.** Refrain from adding sweeteners like honey, maple syrup, or brown sugar, which may cause you to bloat and expel even more wind.

Don't Be a Killer Cook

Some raw beans contain high levels of a protein called **phytohaem-agglutinin** ("fy-toh-hee-mah-GLOO-tin-in") or PHA. PHA is present in *raw or undercooked* kidney beans, white kidney beans (cannellini), and fava beans (broad beans). If consumed, the toxin can cause acute intense food poisoning within a few hours. Just eating four or five raw or improperly cooked red kidney beans can make you very sick with severe vomiting followed by diarrhea (a.k.a. red kidney bean poisoning).

Coach Karen says

The amount of gas you produce from eating beans depends on your intestinal health, the bacteria and enzymes in your gut, and the way the beans are prepared.

Coach Karen says

Cook now, freeze for 6 months. Drain cooked beans; rinse with cold water. Cool and drain completely. Transfer to freezer-safe containers. 1-3/4 cups = 1 standard-sized can.

PHA is most concentrated in raw red kidney beans. White kidney beans only contain a third of the toxin as red kidney beans, while broad beans contain just 5 to 10 percent. But the toxin is killed if you cook it long enough and at a high enough temperature.[2] Slow cookers cook at lower temperatures and won't get hot enough to kill this toxin.[4]

Research shows that PHA is destroyed when presoaked beans are boiled at 212°F for 15 minutes.[5] **DO NOT USE A SLOW COOKER** for this stage of cooking. After boiling, simmer until tender, then drain and rinse. There's no need for concern if you eat canned beans, which are processed at high temperature and pressure, so the PHA is destroyed.

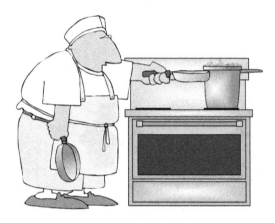

Coach Karen says

DO NOT give young children beans as toys or art objects. If ingested, they can choke and be poisoned by the PHA.

Coach Karen says

Add acidic ingredients (e.g., tomatoes, vinegar, wine) to beans AFTER they're fully cooked. The acids prevent the beans from softening.

Bean Additives

Some companies prepare their cooked beans with food additives, such as calcium chloride, which is used to harden the skins, so they don't fall apart during cooking. Some companies use calcium disodium EDTA (ethylenediaminetetraacetate) to preserve the bean's color. In beans prepared without additives, you may find broken beans and black beans may appear more reddish black than deep black. Basically, they will appear just as if you prepared them at home.

The Life of a Bean

Fresh beans are dried to extend their shelf life — but that doesn't mean they'll break 100 along with you. Beans don't go "bad", but age and exposure to air make beans *hard*. Dispose of those age-old beans in your pantry as they may never soften — no matter how long you soak and cook them!

Buy beans in small quantities from a store with good turnover. Check "sell-by" dates, and don't buy beans that have been stored in bulk bins. Once home, store your little fellas in sealed glass containers in a cool, dry place away from any light.

 TRY THESE REAL FOOD RECIPES!

BAMburgers with Chipotle Mayo pg. 263
One-Pot Mexican Quinoa pg. 268

PLAY 11 — FIXING THE CHRONIC SLICE

Slurp Up Some Souper Stuff

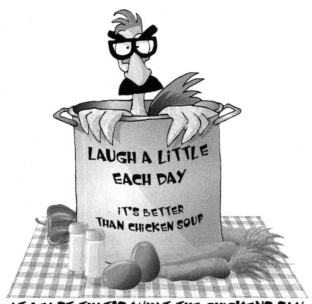

LAUGH A LITTLE
EACH DAY

IT'S BETTER
THAN CHICKEN SOUP

AT LEAST THAT'S WHAT THE CHICKENS SAY

Too many slices on the golf course are never good, but neither are too many slices of pizza, bacon, and cheesecake. Habits that keep you in your comfort zone, like emotional eating, are hard to break, but the best way to fix a chronic slice is with...*(drumroll please)*...soup! Whaaat?

Think about it. What could be more comforting than a hot bowl of homemade goodness? Soup warms you up from the inside out and tucks away a truckload of those mighty phytos. Like salad, soup is an awesome vehicle for getting in more COLORS.

Souping is genius. Where else can you clean out your fridge and end up with a soul-soothing meal? Add whole grains, beans, and your soup becomes the quintessential healthy meal. Here are some other great reasons to start souping and overcome those exasperating eating habits:

1. **Soup is water-rich.** It's not only delicious, but naturally filling, so you can feel satisfied and enjoy loads of good fuel. Several studies have shown that people eat fewer total calories on days when they eat soup.[1]

2. **Soup saves money.** The most expensive food you buy is the food you toss in the trash. Per a 2018 USDA study, higher quality diets were linked to higher levels of waste. Researchers found that 39% of the fruits and vegetables Americans buy are thrown away! This equates to about one pound of food wasted per person per day.[2]

3. **Soup is a slurpable surprise that's always in season.** No matter what time of year, DIY soup makes a nutrient-dense, one-pot wonder. Toss in frozen winter squash in the summer, fresh-from-the-garden veggies in the spring, and you'll have some of the most flavorful and nutritious real food in a single bowl.

   You can eat soup for lunch, dinner, and yes, even breakfast! In Japan, a traditional breakfast starts with a warm bowl of miso soup, which is a nice contrast from the typical Western breakfast of cold, sweet breakfast cereal from a box. Consider a healthy homemade bowl of black bean chowder instead of a breakfast burrito to jumpstart your day. Try it. Who knows. A steamy cup of soup in the A.M. may even replace that hot mug of morning Joe.

4. **Soup is convenient and the ideal go-to meal.** Don't forget to use your ultimate convenience appliance — the slow cooker. Toss in your goodies in the morning and voila! At the end of the day, you'll have a hot pot brimming with savory soup. Not only does soup often taste better the next day, it can be rewarmed and ready to eat in just minutes.

Coach Karen says

Red or "split" lentils (they're actually bright orange) cook down into a thick, porridge-like consistency, so they're perfect for thickening soups or making hummus, dips, curries, chilis, and stews.

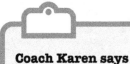

Coach Karen says

Cook without rules. Make soup!

SOUPER STUFF

Soup is made from whatever you have on hand, that is, all your nutritious leftovers and farmers market produce. Create your own signature soup that's loaded with COLORS, such as…

- **Produce** — Apples; Bell Peppers; Broccoli; Butternut Squash; Carrots; Dark Leafy Greens; Garlic; Ginger; Jalapeños; Mushrooms (shiitake, porcini, enoki); Potatoes; Pumpkin; Sweet Potatoes; Tomatoes

- **Legumes** — Beans; Edamame (shelled); Lentils; Tempeh; Tofu

- **Intact Grains** — Barley; Bulgur; Farro; Rice (black, brown, red)

Cool Your Soup Safely

Just like your sore muscles after a long day of play, you have to ice down your large batch of soup too. It's critical to cool it down *fast*. Putting the remaining hot pot of soup directly into the refrigerator won't cut it. It'll warm up your fridge (as well as whatever's in it) and leave your soup in the food danger zone (40°-140°F) for several hours. When food stays too warm for too long, bacteria can multiply rapidly.

Use the following ice cooling method for batches of chili, stews, stock, and spaghetti sauce. Here's how...

1. **Divide** large batches into chilled small containers (the flatter the better). Not only will they chill faster in a shallow pan, they'll fit more easily in the fridge.

2. **Plunge** the soup-filled containers into a sink filled with ice. Add enough cold water to cover the ice without seeping into the container.

3. **Chill** in the ice bath for about 30 minutes, and stir the soup occasionally.

4. **Refrigerate** cooled soup.

Reheat Your Leftovers Safely

Reheating your leftover soup is just as important as cooling it. To retain moisture and ensure it heats all the way through, put a lid on it when reheating. Bring it to a rolling boil. Use your food thermometer to check that your leftover soup reaches 165°F throughout.

You can usually make a double batch fairly easily and most of them freeze well too. Tuck them away in the freezer, and break them out on those days when you played too long and too hard — and can barely lift a fork, much less cook.

 TRY THESE REAL FOOD RECIPES!

Basil Tomato Corn Soup pg. 254
Black Bean Soup with Butternut Squash pg. 255

PLAY 12 — NO. 1 SEED

Eat This Food EVERY Day

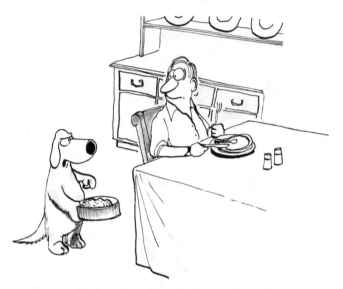

"You eat the dog food, I'll eat the steak."

Take a tip from your next best coach...your vet. Yup, you read that right. Why? Because your pooch is way ahead of the game on this. Dogs have been eating this wonder food every day, so why not you? Wouldn't you like to sport a soft, glossy coat and healthy skin? Man's best friend is slurping up flaxseed (a.k.a. linseed) — the same stuff that's been used to make linen sheets, underwear, Grandma's table-cloth, rope, and finish wood. It was even used to entomb mummies. Sound appetizing? Keep an open mind. Here's why...

Ground flaxseed is actually considered a 'functional food', which means it has physiological benefits, nutritional effects, and/or reduces the risk of chronic disease.[1]

This superseed is also known for boosting the immune system and lessening inflammation. Dietary flaxseed is a rich source of omega-3 fatty acids and lignans, which may help you to:

• **Decrease chronic inflammation.** Studies show you can reverse the plaque buildup in your arteries when you reduce inflammation.[1] Arteries harden when plaque builds up in your pipes (atherosclerosis). Some studies suggest that the omega-3s in flaxseed keep cells from sticking to the inner lining of your blood vessels. Once you unclog the plumbing, your arterial walls can heal and are better able to open and relax. This open-relax action within your blood vessels is critical if you want your heart to keep on beating.

• **Decrease total cholesterol by 7% and levels of LDL (the "bad" stuff) by 10%.** These results were indicated in a study of menopausal women who consumed four tablespoons of ground flaxseed each day for three months.[2]

Can Flax Replace Fish?

Flaxseed, fish, and walnuts are excellent sources of omega-3 fatty acids. There are three different types of omega-3 fats:

1. **ALA** = alpha-linolenic acid (from plants, e.g., flaxseeds, chia seeds, hemp seeds, and walnuts)

2. **DHA** = docosahexaenoic acid (from fatty fish)

3. **EPA** = eicosapentaenoic acid (from fatty fish)

Your body is an amazing vessel. It can convert omega-3 fats from plants to EPA and DHA through a chain of chemical reactions, mainly in your liver, although it's not able to do it very efficiently. Only a small percentage of ALA, 0%–9%, converts to DHA, and 8%–21% converts to EPA.[3] ALA cannot replace the omega-3s you get from fish, but on a positive note, studies suggest that ALA has health benefits of its own. So it's a good idea to still eat ALAs daily.

How Much ALA?

Current ALA dietary recommendations for adults by the Institute of Medicine's Food and Nutrition Board suggest a daily intake of 1.1 gm for women; and 1.6 gm for men.[4]

Coach Karen says

Try to remember the three-letter abbreviations and that ALA comes from plants; DHA and EPA come from fish.

SELECTED FOOD SOURCES OF ALA

FOOD	ALA (gm)
English walnuts, 1 oz (about 14 walnut halves)	2.6
Flaxseed, ground, 2 tablespoons	2.9
Chia seeds, 2 tablespoons	2.2
Hemp seeds, 2 tablespoons[5]	2.0
Black walnuts, 1 oz	0.8
Tofu, 4 oz	0.4
Edamame, frozen, prepared, 1/2 cup	0.3
Refried beans, canned, vegetarian, 1/2 cup	0.2
Kidney beans, canned 1/2 cup	0.1
Baked beans, canned, vegetarian, 1/2 cup	0.07
Bread, whole wheat, 1 slice	0.04

To reduce cardiovascular disease and events, the American Heart Association recommends consuming a sum total of 0.5 gm DHA/EPA per day (3.5 gm per week) *from food*. This amounts to about two servings of non-fried, fatty-type fish or about 3/4 cup of flaked fish.

SELECTED FOOD SOURCES OF EPA AND DHA

FOOD	DHA/EPA (gm)
Mackerel, Atlantic, cooked, 3 oz*	2.5
Salmon, Atlantic, wild, cooked, 3 oz	1.8
Herring, Atlantic, cooked, 3 oz*	1.7
Anchovy, 3 oz	1.4
Sardines, canned in tomato sauce, drained, 3 oz*	1.2
Salmon, pink, canned, drained, 3 oz*	0.9
Algal oil, 1 tsp**	0.5
Tofu, House Foods® with DHA from added algal oil**	0.04

Source: USDA Food Composition Databases

*Except as noted, the USDA database does not specify whether fish are farmed or wild caught.

**Algal ("AL-gl") oil is a vegetarian source of DHA/EPA derived from algae. The oil is an industrial genetically modified microalgae. Fish can't make omega-3s on their own. They get it from the algae they eat!

Load Up on Lignans

Lignans are fiber-rich COLORS *(polyphenols)* present in a wide variety of plant foods, such as nuts, seeds, whole grains, legumes, fruit, and vegetables. Studies show flaxseed lignans decreased total cholesterol and LDL cholesterol by 24%, and decreased blood glucose concentrations by 25%.[6]

These lignans (prebiotics) are a feast for your gut microbiome, and the byproducts of this gut fest (enterolignans) can potentially reduce the risk of certain cancers and cardiovascular disease.[7] Flaxseed is by far the richest dietary source of plant lignans (75-800 times more than other plant foods). Sesame seeds also contain especially high levels of lignans, but flaxseed oil does not, so feed on the seed.

Get It Ground

Buy flaxseeds ground (flaxseed meal), or get them whole, and grind them yourself. Flaxseeds have a thicker seed coat, so crushing or milling enhances their ability to be absorbed and used by your body. If you grind your own flaxseeds, just grind small batches at a time. Ground seeds are more perishable than whole.

A Tablespoon a Day Keeps the Doctor Away

Get your daily dose of omega-3s, lignans, and fiber by sprinkling a tablespoon or two of ground flaxseeds into various foods, such as yogurts, hot and cold cereals, salads, smoothies, tomato sauces, casseroles, stews, enchiladas, chilis, and intact grains. Add two to four tablespoons to a casserole that serves four. Use ground flaxseeds to replace some of the flour in your recipes. If a recipe calls for two or more cups of flour, you can replace 1/4 to 1/2 cup of the flour with ground flaxseeds.

How to Make a Flax "Egg"

Not the sort of egg to be eaten on its own, a flax egg is an inexpensive and healthy alternative to eggs in baked goods — even if you're not a vegan. It's super easy to make with just two ingredients required. Flax eggs yield a "glue-y" consistency similar to egg whites and help to bind ingredients together.

Just mix three tablespoons of water with one tablespoon of ground flaxseeds (3-to-1 ratio) in a small bowl. Stir and let the mixture stand for five minutes to thicken. Use your flax egg in waffles, pancakes, brownies, quick breads, muffins, and veggie (or even carnivore)

Coach Karen says

Prebiotics are types of dietary fiber that feed the friendly bacteria in your gut. Think of them as fertilizer for the live good bacteria and yeasts (a.k.a. probiotics) in your digestive system.

Coach Karen says

Flaxseeds make a good substitute for eggs if you have an egg allergy, you're a vegan, or simply out of eggs.

burgers. Chia seeds can also be used as an egg replacer (chia egg) using the same 3-to-1 proportions as a flax egg

Store Flax in the Fridge

Omega-3 fats are sensitive to heat, light, and air, so keep them stored in the fridge or freezer to prevent them from oxidizing and losing their nutritional potency. When mixing flax in your cooked oatmeal or other grains, cook the cereal first, *then* stir in the flax once your cereal is cooked to get the full benefits of the omega-3 fats.

The Dynamic Duo — Chia and Hemp Seeds

Along with your daily dose of flaxseeds, be sure to rotate chia and hemp seeds through your weekly training plan. These two 'super seeds' are highly nutritious and each of them has its own unique health properties. Pair them with oatmeal, yogurt, ready-to-eat cereals, smoothies, soups, salads, pancake batters, and pastas.

Chia and hemp seeds are 'complete proteins', that is, they contain all the essential amino acids that cannot be made by your body and must come from the diet. Amino acids are often referred to as the "building blocks of proteins" and promote growth (think brain, muscles, skin, hair, bones, hormones, immune cells).

Chia Seeds — Eat them ground or whole, and hydrate them for 5 minutes (e.g., in your smoothie, milk, salad dressing, pudding, fruit spread) *before* eating to better digest and absorb the nutrients.[8] *Do not eat dry chia seeds as they expand and swell after absorbing liquid.* Soaked chia seeds will take on a tapioca pudding-like texture. Chia seeds are highest in fiber and high in many bone nutrients: calcium, magnesium, phosphorus, zinc, and protein. *Ch-ch-ch-chia!*

Hemp Seeds (a.k.a. hemp hearts) — Hemp seeds are the edible fruits of the *Cannabis sativa* plant, and a great source of protein, magnesium, zinc, iron, and vitamin E. During harvesting and processing, these seeds contain less than 0.001% psychoactive compound THC and little or no CBD. According to a 2018 FDA evaluation, these amounts are low enough that they're not a concern for any group, including pregnant or breastfeeding mothers.[9]

 TRY THESE REAL FOOD RECIPES!

Fudgy Oatmeal Bars pg. 292
Vegan Hemp 'Parmesan' pg. 284

Coach Karen says
Chia and hemp seeds are rich in plant omega-3s, so store them alongside your flaxseeds in the fridge or freezer.

Coach Karen says
Protein (gm) in seeds per oz:

#1 Pepitas, **9.7**

#2 Hemp, **9.3**

#3 Flax, **6.0**

#4 Sunflower, **5.8**

#5 Sesame, **5.0**

#6 Chia, **4.0**

Coach Karen says
THC (tetrahydro-cannabinol) and CBD (cannabidiol) are found primarily in the hemp flowers, leaves, and stems, not in the hemp seeds.

PLAY 13 — WHOLE GRAIN ANALYSIS

The 5-to-1 Fiber Rule

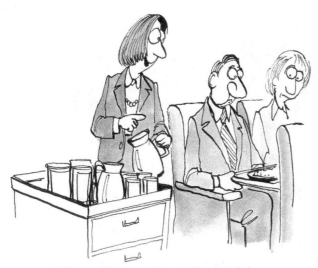

"Now that you've taken a bite
would you like to know what it is?"

Ever since your doctor told you to start eating more dietary fiber (meaning a whole lot of plants) to reduce your risk for a host of diseases, you reluctantly traded in your soft white wonder for a 21-grain brick. But your new kind of loaf may not be as healthy and whole as you might think. Shopping for whole-grain foods can be confusing with all the varying descriptors. So here's your tactical guide to help you decipher what's whole grain and healthy — and what's not.

Tactic #1: Look for "Whole"

To qualify as a whole grain, 100% of the original kernel (that is, all of the bran, germ, and endosperm) must be present. All grains start out whole, but during the refining process, the bran, germ, and up to 75% of its phytonutrients are removed (a.k.a. *refined* grains). What remains is the "flour-y" or starchy part of the grain (the endosperm), which is the largest part of the grain.

As a general rule, look for the key word "whole", such as "whole grain", "100% whole grain", or "whole wheat" when shopping for a whole grain product and see that it's listed as the *first ingredient* on the food label.

Coach Karen says

The word "whole" has to be spelled out in barley, corn, cornmeal, rye, spelt, and wheat. For example, bread made with "rye flour" is not a whole grain product.

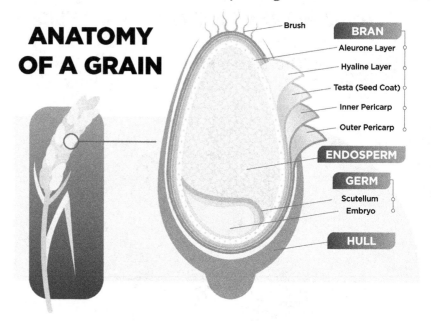

ANATOMY OF A GRAIN

- Brush
- **BRAN**
  - Aleurone Layer
  - Hyaline Layer
  - Testa (Seed Coat)
  - Inner Pericarp
  - Outer Pericarp
- **ENDOSPERM**
- **GERM**
  - Scutellum
  - Embryo
- **HULL**

Tactic #2: Apply the 5-to-1 Fiber Rule

Refined grain products give carbs a bad name. Beans, fruits, and vegetables are carbohydrates too! Many breads, bagels, breakfast cereals, crackers, tortillas, muffins, pancakes, pastries, pastas, pretzels, pizza crust, and waffles contain little or no whole grains and fiber. These starchy-type carbs break down quickly, spike blood sugar, and contribute to storing fat. So how do you spot healthful whole grain goodness? Compare the proportion of carbohydrates to fiber.

Coach Karen says

Apply the 5-to-1 Fiber Rule when shopping for starchy foods, like breads, cereals, crackers, pastas, and tortillas. The rule applies to these 'packaged' foods, not intact grains.

To figure this out, simply divide the number of carbs by the amount of fiber. If your favorite bread contains 30 grams of carbohydrate and 2 grams of fiber, the ratio of carbs to fiber is 15 to 1. Not surprising if it's made with enriched wheat flour (not whole) and sweetened with some form of sugar.

Remember, fiber slows carbs from flooding your bloodstream, which deters blood sugar spikes and fat storage, so be sure the fiber content is adequate. By checking these ratios, you'll keep a whole lot of packaged starchy foods out of your shopping cart.

But hold on...just because a carb plays by the 5-to-1 Fiber Rule, it doesn't make it healthy yet. Next, see if it meets the 1-to-1 ratio of calories to sodium. If it passes, then eyeball the ingredients. If it doesn't say "whole" and contains added sugar, starches, phosphates, and any processed ingredients (typically ones you can't pronounce), then it's not cart-worthy.

Tactic #3: Don't Get Faked Out

The following words do not guarantee that a product is whole grain, so you still have to look for the word "whole" in the list of ingredients.

Durum wheat, durum flour, or semolina — Durum wheat is a species of wheat. Also called "pasta wheat" or "macaroni wheat". Durum wheat is milled into both semolina and durum flour or durum wheat flour.

Stoneground — This term only refers to how the grains are crushed between stones during processing. It doesn't tell you if the grains are whole or stripped of any of their nutritious layers.

Organic flour — This only identifies that the flour is organic. It doesn't tell you if it's a whole grain.

Multigrain — Sounds healthy, but this mixture may be a combo of several refined grains or whole grains or a mix of both.

The following words *never* describe a whole grain:

- **All-purpose flour (a.k.a. white flour)** — This flour is made by stripping the germ and bran from the whole grains before milling.
- **Enriched wheat flour** — This is an all-purpose flour that has been fortified with additional vitamins, many of which are lost in the refining process.
- **Degerminated or degermed corn** (used in some corn meals) — Degerminated means the nutritious, oily germ and bran are removed in processing, so it's no longer an intact grain. Oils can go rancid, so this process makes the corn more shelf stable.
- **Bran**, e.g., bran flakes, bran cereal — "Bran" is often associated with healthy foods, but the bran is only a part of the whole grain.
- **Wheat germ** — Like bran, wheat germ is just part of a wheat kernel.

Tactic #4: Don't Judge a Bread By Its Color

Just because a bread is brown and contains the word "wheat" in the name, doesn't mean it's a whole grain. Brown bread could be white flour colored brown with caramel or contain other dark-colored ingredients like molasses.

Coach Karen says

If your grains look like a Cheerio, chip, or chocolate chip cookie, beware. Figure out the carb-to-fiber ratio and decide if the minute of indulgence is worth storing more fat.

Coach Karen says

Eat a diet that includes plenty of COLOR-ful intact grains, beans, nuts, and seeds.

Tactic #5: Upgrade to "Intact Grains"

Intact grains are whole grains in their original form, where you can see the actual grain. Contrast these grains with grains pulverized into a flour (that is, they're no longer intact) and used in bread, pasta, pastries, and ready-to-eat cereals.

Grains ground up into a flour are quickly converted into blood sugar (glucose) because the starchy surface area is more available to digestive enzymes. On the other hand, ground up beans, such as hummus, bean dip, chickpea flour, soybean flour, or pasta made with black bean flour, don't boost starch availability and cause blood sugar spikes like whole wheat flour and other grain flours.[1, 2]

Coach Karen says

Higher blood sugar levels increase fat storage and the risk of type 2 diabetes.

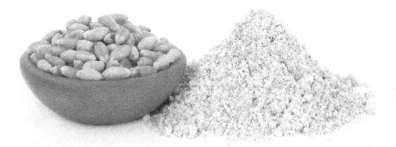

"Intact grains" are grains in their original form (left). Whole wheat flour (right) is not an intact grain.

Try these intact grains as a healthy side, breakfast porridge, or in soups, stews, salads, and stuffings:

- **Barley, hulled or hulless**
- **Cracked wheat**
- **Farro, whole**
- **Kamut® berries** — a high-protein variety of wheat
- **Millet**
- **Oat groats, steel-cut oats, and rolled oats**
- **Rice (brown, black, red)** — White rice is not an intact grain because its bran and germ layers have been removed.
- **Rye**
- **Spelt** — a cousin of wheat
- **Wheat berries**

Although quick-cooking oats are intact grains, they're the most processed with the least fiber and the most starch. During processing, these oats are steamed and rolled multiple times, which make them quick to cook and quicker at raising your blood sugar. For the biggest bang, stick with oat groats, steel-cut, or rolled oats.

The following foods are often thought of as grains. They're cooked and eaten in a similar way as grains, so they're lumped into this category, but they're actually seeds, and sometimes referred to as "pseudo-grains".

- **Amaranth**
- **Buckwheat groats** — Buckwheat is not a wheat. You may have had buckwheat in the form of "kasha" (roasted buckwheat groats) or as "soba" (Japanese noodles made with buckwheat flour).
- **Quinoa** ("KEEN-whah")
- **Wild rice** — These are the seeds of a native North American long-grain marsh grass.

Coach Karen says

Couscous may look like a grain, but it's actually a tiny flour-y pasta made from durum wheat semolina. The flour is moistened into a raw dough, tossed or spun to transform into tiny round balls, then dried.

Whole intact grains are vital to having a healthy gut microbiome — that is, the trillions of microorganisms or "microbes", such as bacteria, fungi, and viruses that live primarily in the large intestine. The fiber in whole intact grains helps produce healthy gut bacteria, which wards off chronic diseases and boost immunity.

Diets that eliminate intact whole grains (e.g., the Paleo Diet) have three potentially harmful issues: 1) lower levels of beneficial bacteria, 2) less bacteria diversity, and 3) elevated levels of TMAO.[3] If you recall in *Play 2: Free Agents*, an unhealthy gut microbiome damages your mitochondrial power plants, and reduces your ability to thrive.

Tactic #6: Know That All Intact Grains Are Not Created Equal... and That's Okay

The fiber content in whole grains varies widely.[4] But just because a grain isn't that high in fiber, it's still full of all those age-defying phyto-, macro-, and micronutrients. Also, of the following grains and pseudo-grains, amaranth, buckwheat, quinoa, and wild rice are "complete" proteins. That is, they contain all nine essential amino acids (just like animal proteins) that your body can't make on its own. So sub out some COLOR-less beef from your Power Plate, and sub in some COLOR-ful buckwheat.

GRAIN (45 gm; about 1/4 cup)	% FIBER	AMOUNT OF FIBER (gm)
Bulgur wheat	18.3%	8.2
Barley	17.3%	7.9
Rye	15.1%	6.8
Triticale	14.6%	6.5
Wheat	12.2%	5.6
Kamut® khorasan wheat	11.1%	5.1
Spelt wheat	10.7%	4.8
Oats	10.6%	4.8
Buckwheat (seed)	10.0%	4.5
Millet	8.5%	3.9
Corn	7.3%	3.4
Quinoa (seed)	7.0%	3.1
Amaranth (seed)	6.7%	3.1
Sorghum	6.3%	2.8
Wild rice (seed)	6.2%	2.8
Brown rice	3.5%	1.7

Source: USDA National Nutrient Database

Coach Karen says

Nutrients are substances that nourish plants and animals to grow and live, whereas "anti-nutrients" block the absorption of nutrients.

Coach Karen says

Unlike animals, plants are pretty defenseless against predators, but have evolved to have their own built-in defensive line. They produce anti-nutrients to repel insects, other pests, and microorganisms.[3]

Tactic #7: Eat Them Sprouted

Sprouted grains are whole intact grains (as well as legumes and seeds) that are "sprouted" in water, smushed into a dough, and baked into products like bread, English muffins, breakfast cereals, waffles, and tortillas. Sprouted grain products are not only flourless and better for your gut microbiome and immune system, the soaking and sprouting removes "anti-nutrients" like phytic ("FY-tik") acid and lectins. These compounds bind to minerals like calcium, iron, magnesium, and zinc, which can hinder your ability to absorb them — another great reason to de-flour your diet and go sprouted.[5]

However, be aware of "sprouted flour" where soaked grains are dried and pulverized into flour or bread manufacturers that toss in some sprouts with traditional flour-based bread and call it "sprouted". Currently, there is no regulation for using the term "sprouted", so you have to read the ingredient label to find out what's in the food you're buying.

True sprouted whole grain products are a good source of protein, fiber, B vitamins, and COLORS. Watch out for sprouted whole grain products that add flour, sweeteners, starch, oils, and too much sodium that negate the benefits of being sprouted. For sprouted grain product recommendations, go to pg. 211.

Sprouted rice has gained popularity and is more readily accessible. A Korean study showed eating sprouted rice is effective in increasing HDL ("good") cholesterol and other antioxidants that lower artery-clogging cardiovascular disease risk.[6]

Tactic #8: Pass on the Pearl — Go for Hulled, Dehulled, or Hulless

When buying farro and barley, be sure they're not **"pearled"**. Pearled or polished grains have been stripped of the inedible tough outer hull as well as the nutritious bran layer, leaving only a small white 'pearl' of endosperm (the starchy part of the grain).

Instead, look for **"hulled"** or **"dehulled"** farro and barley, which are minimally processed. The husky hull is carefully removed, but the bran layers, endosperm, and germ are still intact. **"Hulless"** is just a different variety of grain. It has a hull that's loosely attached to the kernel, which typically falls off naturally during harvesting, so additional processing to remove the hull is often not required. All parts of the grain in hulless grains are retained.

Read labels carefully on **"grits"**. Barley grits are created when the grain kernels are cut into several pieces. Barley **"flakes"** are like rolled oats. They're created by steaming the kernels, rolling them flat, and drying them. Be sure your grits and flakes are made from whole barley, not pearled barley.

Coach Karen says

The older Okinawans, the world's longest-lived people, eat germinated, a.k.a. sprouted, brown rice (pg. 212), which is a healthier version of brown rice with a sweet flavor and softer texture.

 TRY THESE REAL FOOD RECIPES!

Barley with Fresh Figs, Arugula, and Maple Mustard Vinaigrette pg. 275
Sprouted Grain 'Crackers' pg. 293

PLAY 14 — BREAKFAST OF CHAMPIONS

Picking a Winning Cereal

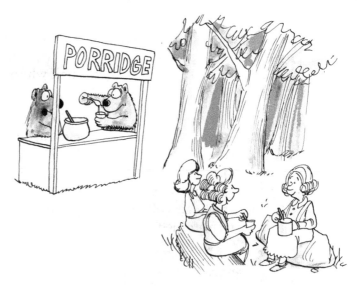

"I don't know what porridge is either, but they're all crazy for it."

Cereal is a big business with the majority of them posing as edible entertainment with their mesmeric advertising, iconic characters, and colorful packaging. The majority of them are big on refined grains, sugar, honey, syrups, sodium, and artificial colorants. So what's the attraction? Convenience — or perhaps you just can't part from your sugar-coated childhood. But if you seriously want to break loose of the aging consequences caused by a culture of convenience, trade in your Cocoa Krispies and Cap'n Crunch for something with less goo and more grit.

Why Eat Breakfast?

Several studies have associated skipping breakfast with cardiovascular disease, atherosclerosis, arterial stiffening, obesity, diabetes, unfavorable lipid profiles, and hypertension.[1] Those who miss breakfast alone or in combination with a late-night dinner have an increased risk of death from coronary events, such as heart attacks and strokes, compared to those who eat a high-energy breakfast every day. In addition to the direct association with cardiovascular risk factors, researchers found that breakfast skippers were also more likely to have an overall unhealthy lifestyle, such as a poor overall diet, frequent alcohol consumption, and smoking. They were also more likely to be overweight, obese, and hypertensive.[2]

As you sleep, your body works hard to recover from that day's marathon playdate or stress relay. By the time you wake up, your body and brain demand fuel. How well do you maintain your amazing athletic machine? People who habitually start their day without a morning meal often feel depleted, make some not-so-smart decisions as they go along, and overcompensate at night. Instead of your brain repairing, rebuilding, and restoring while you sleep, your stomach is mixing, your gut is churning, and waste is moving thanks to those late-night snacks and meals.

If you're overeating or doing some late-night snacking, it's likely you won't be hungry at the crack of dawn. But worse yet, you wake up with a **"food hangover"** — bloating, lethargy, maybe a little queasiness or indigestion, gas, and a general feeling of *blah*. You need caffeine to get the motor running, and the last thing you want is breakfast. Unfortunately, your body becomes accustomed to this erratic feeding schedule. The good news? Your appetite can change.

Coach Karen says
Refrain from overeating and late-night snacking to avoid waking up with a **"food hangover"**.

What If You're Not Hungry

Eating breakfast improves insulin sensitivity throughout the day, reduces caloric intake, increases satiety, improves dietary food choices, and helps with weight control. But just because it's 7:00 AM doesn't mean you *have* to eat breakfast...yet. If you're not ready to eat when your eyes open to the world, then wait until you're No. 3 or "Crazy Hungry" on The Hunger Scale (refer to The Hunger Scale on pg. 138). Start listening to your own hunger-satiety cues.

Be open to change. Even if you haven't eaten breakfast for the past 20, 30, or 40 years, you can still be taught new tricks. Once you start living and eating to break 100, your appetite will change too.

Breakfast of Champions — The Big Five

Not sure if your ready-to-eat breakfast cereal is championship material? To make the training table, it should meet all five anti-aging criteria:

1. **The first ingredient is a "whole" or "sprouted" grain.**
2. **Meets the 5-to-1 Fiber Rule.**
3. **Meets the 1-to-1 Sodium Rule.**
4. **Has 5 or more grams of fiber.**
5. **Has less than 5 grams of added sugar. (Better yet, *none*.)**

If you never start a play day without a mammoth bowl of "cholesterol-lowering, heart healthy" little O's, then it's time to ignore the jargon-ese and scrutinize the ingredients. Second to whole grain oats, you'll find corn starch, sugar, salt, and phosphate. Oy! All the foods to ditch! And always be aware of a brand's "multigrain" creation. Don't be surprised to find four times the added sugar and less protein in the more 'grainy' versions.

In the end, though, the best breakfast cereal is pure unadulterated whole oats and barley. That's because they contain a special kind of soluble fiber called **beta-glucan** ("GLUE-can"). This particular fiber has been shown to prevent and treat various metabolic syndrome-linked diseases, that is, abdominal fat, high blood pressure, high blood sugar, high triglycerides (blood fats), and low HDL ("good") cholesterol.[3, 4]

Clean Up Your Body with a Sponge and Broom

Coach Karen says

O-BBBOY! Remember the acronym OBBBOY for foods high in soluble fiber: **O**ats, **B**arley, **B**eans, **B**erries, **O**nions, **Y**ams.

To quickly differentiate the roles of soluble versus insoluble fiber, **soluble fiber** dissolves in water and forms a viscous (soft and sticky) gel. It's literally a **"cholesterol sponge"** that mops up potentially harmful compounds, such as unhealthy fats like LDLs in the intestine. Before they can accumulate in blood vessels and contribute to making artery-clogging plaque, the fiber gets rid of them through your back door with other waste. Your body, by the way, needs *some* LDL cholesterol to produce hormones and provide structure to cell membranes, but because excesses can accumulate in the blood vessels and promote atherosclerosis, it's been branded as the "bad" cholesterol.

In contrast, **insoluble fiber** does *not* dissolve in water, but absorbs water as it travels through your digestive tract, which eases elimination. It acts like **"Nature's broom"** and by sweeping things out swiftly, it limits the amount of time toxins lurk in your system. Your body and brain absorb toxins from the environment and from the food you eat, such as BPA, mercury, and pesticides. The faster these compounds and chemicals move through you, the time they have to do damage is reduced.

When it comes to good broom food, think wheat (wheat bran) and fibrous plants — in other words, 'roughage' — such as those with tough stalks, edible seeds, skins, or membranes. These are foods like apples (the skins), artichokes, broccoli, Brussels sprouts, raspberries, blackberries as well as nuts, corn, and popcorn.

Foods High in Beta-Glucan

Okay, back to beta-glucan. Beta-glucan is found naturally in the cell walls of cereals, certain types of mushrooms (e.g., shiitake, reishi), yeasts, seaweed, and algae. It's the main component of soluble fiber in oats and barley that gives your morning oatmeal its creamy, viscous texture. Among cereals, barley and oats contain the highest amounts of beta-glucan, which encourage the increase of beneficial gut bacteria and anti-inflammatory activity.[5]

BETA-GLUCAN CONTENT

WHOLE GRAIN	GRAMS PER 100 GM
Barley	2–20
Oats	3–8
Sorghum	1.1–6.2
Rye	1.3–2.7
Maize	0.8–1.7
Triticale	0.3–1.2
Wheat	0.5–1.0
Durum wheat	0.5–0.6
Rice	0.13

Serve up a some beta-glucans daily by including:

1. **Barley groats, hulled, hulless, or hulless flakes** — Barley groats are the whole grain form of barley (only the outermost hull has been removed). Remember to pass on pearl barley.

2. **Barley flour** — Barley flour has a mild, sweet, and slightly nutty flavor. Be sure the barley flour is ground from whole barley, not *pearl* barley.

3. **Oat groats** — Oat groats are the whole oat kernels (bran and all) that remain after the inedible husks are removed. They're chewy, nutty, and nutritious, and great for grain bowls, salads, stews, and hot cereal. They can also be ground into fresh oat flour.

Coach Karen says

If you're a sugar junkie trying to kick your candy-coated cereal habit, add a dollop of date paste (pg. 279), sprinkle of date 'sugar', or squirt of date syrup (pg. 218) to the naked oats and barley during your transition. Don't forget the berries!

4. **Steel-cut oats (a.k.a. Irish oats)** — Steel-cut oats are whole oat groats that have been cut into small pieces by steel blades. They're the most minimally processed of the family of oat cereals.

5. **Rolled oats (a.k.a. old-fashioned rolled oats)** — Oat groats are steamed, then rolled flat into flakes. Rolled oats cook faster than steel-cut oats because there's more surface area to absorb water.

6. **Oat flour** — You can make your own oat flour my grinding uncooked old-fashioned rolled oats in your food processor or blender.

7. **Oat bran** — The bran is the outer fibrous coating on the oat groat (think of the papery-thin coating on a peanut). Oat bran is lighter and finer than wheat bran and doesn't contain any other parts of the oat groat.

Break Your Fast With Beta-Glucans

Get creative with oats and barley — they're extremely versatile. Here are some ideas...

- **Add barley flakes** to homemade granola, or eat them as a hot breakfast cereal.

- **Use the flours to thicken food and drinks.** You can use these nutty-tasting oat or barley flours to thicken smoothies, yogurt drinks, soups, and stews. When you add some oat or barley flour to your morning smoothies, they'll be more satisfying and nourishing. They'll stick with you because the fiber will help slow down digestion and prevent blood sugar spikes.

- **Add cooked oats or barley to soups and stews.** Remember, soup makes a great breakfast!

- **Use them as a base for a breakfast bowl.** Makes a nice change of taste and texture from the usual rice or quinoa.

- **Make a breakfast salad** by adding cooked hulless barley or steel-cut oats.

- **Bake some banana nut breakfast muffins with barley or oat flour.**

- **Eat them 'overnight style'.** No cooking required! Instead of cooking rolled oats to hydrate and soften them, you can *soak* them overnight in the fridge. Customize this championship breakfast with your choice of toppings, add-ins, and milk or water. The flavors will fuse while you snooze and will be ready to chow down the next morning. Overnight oats are the ideal grab-and-go for those who

Coach Karen says

Overnight oats will keep for up to 2 days. If you don't add a banana, up to 4 days. Whip up several batches beforehand to always have a ready-to-eat breakfast or mid-morning snack.

feel rushed in the morning and just can't seem to carve out time to eat.

- **Rotate cooked barley with cooked oats throughout the week.** Add apples, bananas, berries, peaches, nuts, and seeds for added fiber and shower them with ground flaxseed and cinnamon.

The Bottom Line...

Most foods contain both soluble and insoluble fiber, but have predominantly more of one than the other. Fiber is linked to improved immunity and anti-inflammatory effects. So break out of bed with more fiber! Toss a handful of COLORS into your beta-glucans. Eat a sweet potato instead of sweet corn flakes. Smear avocado on your toast instead of butter. Pile berries on your plate instead of bacon. And after revving up your engine with a powerhouse breakfast, go have a great play day!

 TRY THESE REAL FOOD RECIPES!

Date Paste pg. 280
Overnight Oats pg. 237

PLAY 15 — GAME DAY ROSTER

Soy's on First

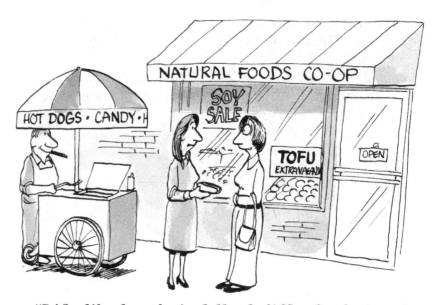

"Life, like lunch, is full of difficult choices."

Soy, the mighty bean, is a vital longevity food and has earned a top spot on The Anti-Aging Training Table. In Okinawa, the land of the centenarians, soybeans, soy bean curd (tofu), immature soybeans (edamame), and fermented soy beans (miso and natto) make up the core of their plant-centered traditional diet. Soy helps achieve a more plant-based lifestyle without falling short on protein. Eating more soy may increase your chances of crossing the century mark in relatively good health.

Why Soy Slows Aging

Soy is packed with beneficial nutrients that support the heart, brain, and muscles while reducing the risk for type 2 diabetes and some cancers. That's because soy contains:

- **Fiber**
- **Protein**

- **Omega-3 fatty acids**
- **Minerals**, such as potassium and calcium
- **WHITEs** *(isoflavones)* — Isoflavones (a.k.a.phytoestrogens), specifically, genistein, and diadzein, aren't found in any other foods. Phytoestrogens are plant-based estrogens that function similarly to estrogen in humans.

Eating tofu and other soy-based foods (not soy-based 'processed' foods) instead of animal-based proteins will lower your intake of saturated fat and cholesterol. Soy has additional health benefits that may help with the following:

- **Reduces total blood cholesterol and LDL ("bad") cholesterol** per a meta-analysis of 46 soy trials.[1]
- **Slows down bone loss**, which reduces the risk of osteoporosis.[2]
- **Eases menopausal symptoms for some women.**[3]
- **Reduces cancer risk and breast cancer recurrence.**[4]

For years, there's been confusing debate over whether breast cancer survivors should eat soy. And now that soy is more popular in the American diet, knowing whether to eat it or not is important.

How Did Soy Get a Bad Rap?

The increased risk of breast cancer and its progression is linked to estrogen, a female sex hormone. Most breast cancers are "estrogen-receptor-positive", that is, they're sensitive to estrogen, and estrogen causes cancer cells to grow. Since soybeans and soy products are the richest dietary source of plant estrogens, it was once thought that they could raise the risk of breast cancer. But, soy doesn't contain enough WHITEs *(isoflavones)* to increase this risk. Many studies, and many analyses of studies, have shown that a diet high in soy does not stimulate cancer cells.

The Soy Study

In one study, researchers examined the diets of 9,515 breast cancer patients from the U.S. and Shanghai. The study assessed the diets of these women 14.6 months after their cancer diagnosis and followed them for 7.4 years. They looked at how often they ate the soy foods, such as tofu, soy milk, cooked soybeans, miso soup, soybean sprouts, and protein shakes with added soy. The most frequently consumed soy foods were tofu and soy milk.

Coach Karen says

Try "black" soybeans. They're considered the 'Crown Prince' of beans in Japan. Low in carbs (11 gm), high in fiber (6 gm), and high in protein (11 gm), which amounts to nearly half the carbs and 2X the protein as regular black beans.

In the study, the participants' average daily intake of soy varied greatly. American women consumed an average of 3.2 mg of isoflavones, which equates to *one ounce* of soy milk. Shanghai women, on the other hand, consumed an average of 45.9 mg of isoflavones per day, or about two servings of whole soy.

The women who ate the most soy food (more than 11.83 mg of isoflavones per day), had a 27% reduced risk for breast cancer recurrence compared to those with the lowest intake of isoflavones (3.68 mg or less per day).

They also found that soy did not interfere with breast cancer drugs that lowered estrogen levels, such as tamoxifen. In fact, it revealed that soy protected against recurrence in patients who took tamoxifen.[4]

Phytoestrogens and Men

If soy contains phytoestrogens, should men and boys eat soy? No worries, soy won't feminize men. Clinical studies show isoflavones have no affect on the concentrations of estrogen and testoserone, or the quality of sperm and semen — even if more than the typical Asian dietary intakes are consumed.[6] So men, go ahead and enjoy your soy. It won't affect your masculinity or muscles.

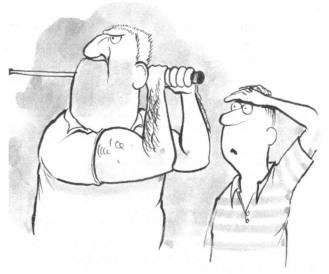

"Nice putt."

Soy Consumption (East and West)

Asians generally eat whole soy foods throughout their lifetime except for the first six to eight months of life. On the other hand, Westerners eat the most soy during the first year of life (in the form of processed soy formula), and typically eat nearly none thereafter. Studies show that women who eat less soy or start eating it later in life lack the dramatic chemoprotective effects observed in Asian women.[5]

How Much Soy Per Day

A moderate amount of soy is one to two servings per day of minimally processed forms of soy. Good sources include: tofu, tempeh, edamame, miso, and unsweetened soy milk.[7] Avoid soy 'Frankenfoods', e.g., soy hot dogs, bologna, and bars, because like other highly processed foods, they're lower in nutrient density than nutrition from the whole soybean. Processing affects the nutritional quality of soy by removing the protein from the other enzymes and bacteria needed for digestion.

In 1999, the U.S. Food and Drug Administration (FDA) determined 25 grams of soy protein a day, as part of a diet low in saturated fat and cholesterol, may reduce the risk of cardiovascular disease. Since then, numerous additional studies have been published to further support soy as a heart healthy food. Here's how soy sizes up.[7]

PROTEIN AND ISOFLAVONE CONTENT IN SOY

SOY FOOD	PROTEIN (grams)	ISOFLAVONES (mg)
Tempeh, 3 oz	13	51.5
Tempeh, cooked, 3 oz	13	30.3
Soy nuts, 1 oz (about 1/4 cup)	12	41.6
Edamame, cooked, 1/2 cup	11	16.1
Tofu, 3 oz (1/3 cup)	8	19.2
Soy milk, 1 cup, unsweetened	7	6.2

NOTE: Isoflavone content can vary considerably between brands. Consider the above list as a guide.

Studies have shown that consuming up to three servings per day of soy (equivalent to 75 mg of isoflavones) does not increase the risk of breast cancer. Consuming even four servings of whole soy, or 100 mg of isoflavones, a day is "recognized as safe".

Tofu Tidbits

Tofu is made by soaking, cooking, blending, and straining mature soybeans, which are yellow. On the other hand, edamame ("eh-da-MAH-meh"), which literally means "stem bean" in Japanese, are whole young soybeans in the pod, which are green. Since tofu is made with the mature soybeans, tofu is naturally creamy white in color.

No colorants are ever used to make tofu. The liquid that comes out of the strained beans is soy milk. The soy milk is then solidified with a coagulant. Wait 15 minutes, and voilà!...You have tofu!

Soy Supplementing

The researchers warned that soy isoflavone extracts and supplements are not recommended for reducing the risks of breast cancer because the amount and type of isoflavones in them may differ from actual soy foods. Your body may process the highly processed supplemental form of soy differently from soy in its natural form.[4]

Concentrated forms of soy (soy protein isolate) contain higher levels of isoflavones, but lack the healthy constituents. That's because foods high in these WHITEs are often rich in nutrients and fiber. Soy protein isolates are used in supplements, protein powders, meat substitutes, and infant/toddler formula. Remember, supplements are not regulated by the FDA. Some studies suggest an increased risk of breast cancer with isoflavone supplements in women who have a family history of breast cancer.[8] Be sure to check with your oncologist with any concerns.

Oh Boy, More Soy!

Think outside the carton. Here are some fun and offbeat ways to slip in more soy.

Breakfast

- Hot cereal cooked with smashed tofu
- Smoothies and shakes made with soy milk or silken tofu
- Tofu scramble
- Waffles or pancakes made with soy milk or dry soy milk powder

Main Dishes

- Bowls
- Burritos, tacos, and bean burgers
- Chili, curries, soups, stews, and stir-frys
- Edamame or soybean pasta
- Grilled kebabs
- Lasagna or stuffed pasta shells
- Meat-less loaf
- Miso soup

Coach Karen says

Stick to eating whole soy foods like soy milk, soy nuts, tempeh, and tofu, and avoid highly processed soy foods and supplements.

Salads

- Homemade mayonnaise
- Deviled egg-less salad
- Dressings, sauces

Salad Toppings

- Edamame, shelled
- Marinated tofu cubed or crumbled
- Roasted soy nuts

Sandwiches

- Barbecue-seasoned tofu slabs
- Grilled tofu
- Peanut butter-tofu spread

Side Dishes

- Mashed potatoes
- Stuffed peppers

Desserts

- Brownies, cookies, muffins

Coach Karen says

By making your own soy nuts, you control the salt and oil. They make a great snack when you crave something crunchy. Also, toss them into cookies, brownies, and on salads.

 TRY THESE REAL FOOD RECIPES!

BLT pg. 265
Cajun Soy Nuts pg. 287
Chipotle Mayo pg. 277
Eggless 'Egg' Salad pg. 266
Korean-Style Tofu Bowl pg. 259
PB&T pg. 267
Plant-Powered Pizza pg. 269
Steely Protein Oats pg. 239
Tofu Dill Dip pg. 281
Tofu Lettuce Wraps pg. 273
Tofu Mayonnaise (No Oil) pg. 281
Tofu 'Ricotta' pg. 283
Tofu Tacos with Citrus Salsa pg. 274

PLAY 16 - SPORTS NUTS

What's Your Nut Knowledge?

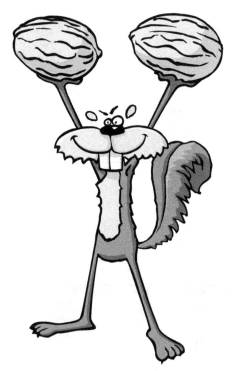

❝Peanuts, here!" Can't bear to watch baseball without your favorite ballpark staple? If you thought nuts were off limits in your quest to lose weight, here's some good news. The fiber will help fill you up, and the healthy fat will help keep you satisfied longer. Just don't go overboard, and mind your handfuls.

Nuts are rich in unsaturated fats, fiber, vitamins, and minerals as well as anti-aging WHITEs *(polyphenols)*. Here's how you can benefit and enjoy them.

- **Go nuts! Eat one ounce of nuts per day** — This amounts to approximately 1/4 cup or one "handful". But if your hand is the size of a baseball mitt, it's better to weigh or measure out a serving.

Stick with this amount to limit total fat and calories. There's one exception: Brazil nuts.

- **Limit Brazil nuts to no more than one to two per day** due to the unusually high levels of selenium (an essential mineral). One Brazil nut contains 70-90 mcg of this mineral and the Recommended Dietary Allowance (RDA) for adults is 55 mcg with a tolerable upper limit of 400 mcg for adults. Too much selenium can cause gastrointestinal distress, hair loss, white spots on nails, fatigue, and irritability.

- **Avoid roasted, canned, and packaged nuts or trail mixes that have been processed with oil and salt.** Buy your nuts raw and roast them at home without the additives. Make your own mix for hittin' the trail.

MUSCLE-BUILDING PROTEIN AND FIBER IN NUTS

NUT (1 oz)	PROTEIN (gm)	FIBER (gm)
Pepitas, 1/4 cup	9.0	2.0
Peanuts, 28	7.0	2.4
Almonds, 24	6.1	3.6
Pistachios, 49	6.0	3.0
Sunflower seeds, 1/4 cup	5.5	3.2
Cashews, 18	5.2	0.9
Hazelnuts, 21	4.3	2.8
Walnuts, 14 halves	4.3	1.9
Brazil nuts, 6	4.1	2.1
Pine nuts, 167	3.9	1.1
Pecans, 19 halves	2.7	2.7
Macadamia nuts, 10-12	2.2	2.4
Brazil nut, 1 kernel	0.7	0.4

Source: USDA National Nutrient Database

Raw vs. Roasted

Roasting can bring out the flavor and crunchiness in nuts as the heating removes some of the water. Just keep in mind that the healthy fats are sensitive to heat. It's best to eat your nuts raw as roasting can damage or oxidize their healthy fats. Store them in the fridge because nuts are also vulnerable to light and oxygen.

On those occasions when you want some toasty tree treats, here's how it's done. To control your portions, roast one serving of nuts at a time.

Coach Karen says

Serve up this "retro" snack, and slow yourself and your guests down with unshelled nuts. Present them in a big wooden bowl with a vintage nut cracker and pick set. Pair nuts with some sliced fresh fruit, like apples, apricots, peaches, or pears.

Coach Karen says

Don't buy nuts or seeds that have been displayed in the sun or stored in open bins. Exposure to heat, oxygen, and light can degrade their healthy fats.

Toss some shelled nuts (no shell) in a dry skillet over low to medium heat until lightly toasted. No oil is necessary. Keep the nuts moving to prevent burning and to toast evenly (about several minutes). Nuts should turn a light brown. Dark roasted nuts may contain very high levels of potentially cancer-causing acrylamides, so to minimize their formation, keep the roasting temperature low, and don't roast too long.

Mix Nuts with Other Water-Rich COLORS

Nuts are nutrient- and calorie-dense foods. That is, they're packed with healthy goods and a lot of calories per bite. By combining nuts with water-rich foods like fruits and vegetables, cooked intact grains, or yogurt, they take longer to eat and are more filling and satisfying.

- Add walnuts to oatmeal, smoothies, salads, and veggie wraps.
- Snack on fresh apple slices and nuts instead of chips or crackers.
- Sprinkle toasted, slivered almonds, or hazelnuts over Brussels sprouts, green beans, or asparagus.
- Stir roasted pine nuts into pasta dishes.

Nut-rition — When eaten in moderation, studies show eating foods rich in monounsaturated fatty acids (MUFA) instead of saturated fats is associated with improved cholesterol levels in your blood, which have a beneficial effect on heart disease and type 2 diabetes risk factors.[1] Listed in order of highest in monounsaturated fats to lowest.

Coach Karen says

Combine dry, dense nuts with water-rich foods, like strawberries, pears, rice, apples, oatmeal, salad greens, and yogurt.

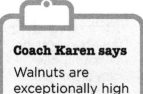

Coach Karen says

Walnuts are exceptionally high in omega-3 fats.

NUT (1 oz)	% MUFA	KERNELS PER OZ	CALORIES	CARBS (gm)
Macadamia nuts	78%	10-12	204	4
Hazelnuts	75%	21	178	4.5
Almonds	63%	24	164	5.5
Pecans	57%	19 halves	196	4
Cashews	54%	18	157	8.5
Pistachios	53%	49	158	8
Peanuts	49%	28	161	6
Brazil nuts	36%	6	186	3.5
Pine nuts	27%	167	191	3.5
Walnuts	14%	14 halves	185	4

Source: USDA National Nutrient Database

Nuts in Flour Form

Unlike grain flours made from whole wheat and rice, nut flours (e.g., almond and hazelnut flours), are low in carbohydrates plus high in fiber and healthy fat. Because of that, by subbing out grain flour with nut flour, you can avoid blood sugar spikes and rapid dives. These rises and falls increase the inflammatory response and leave you tired, hungry, and craving more sugar and calories.

Nutty Tactics

Buy nuts that are in air-tight, sealed packaging to prevent oxygen from slipping through. The healthy fats are sensitive to heat, air, and light and are highly prone to becoming rancid. Once you bring them home, store them in the fridge or freezer — not your pantry. As nuts age, the rancidity will give them a "paint" smell. Take a whiff before eating to be sure there's no off-putting or bitter aroma.

Storing Nuts

Store nuts in the refrigerator for up to a year in odor-tight, moisture-free containers, such as glass jars or vacuum-sealed bags. For longer term storage, freeze them for up to two years. Due to their high-fat content, nuts can become rancid quickly, and rancid oils not only taste and smell bad, they're pro-inflammatory. Light, heat, and air speed up the time it takes for nuts to spoil.

Nut Life

Nuts keep longer if they're:

- **Whole** — Chopped or ground nuts have a shorter shelf life.

- **In their shells**

- **Raw** — Rancidity occurs when oils are exposed to prolonged light and heat, so roasted nuts will go rancid more quickly since they've been treated with heat.

- **Almonds** — Pecans, walnuts, and peanuts are more prone to spoilage.

Coach Karen says

Nuts are like magnets for any kind of odor due to their fat content. Store all nuts in sealed containers and away from strong odors.

 TRY THESE REAL FOOD RECIPES!

Cocoa Nuts pg. 291
Five-Minute Almond Milk pg. 244
Walnut Cilantro Pesto (No Oil) pg. 285

PLAY 17 — HOW TO LOSE WEIGHT WITHOUT LOSING YOUR MIND

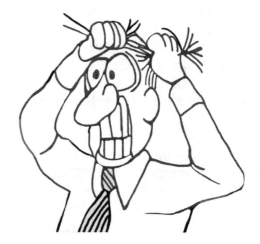

Losing weight should be simple, but it's become so darn complicated. You're constantly *COUNTING*. You're counting your 'points', carbs, calories, and even how many strawberries you're allowed to eat. After a long day of golf on a torturous course and adding up all your strokes, penalties, and lost balls, you've had it with counting.

From the time you wake up to the time you go to sleep, on a typical diet, you are on a rigid dietary budget. What could be more exasperating? If you're like most people, restriction and restraint bring about stress — a precursor to emotional eating. No wonder dieting is a great way to *gain weight*. What ever happened to the simple pleasure of eating?

Math Made Easier

If you used to break out into a cold sweat when you walked into math class, brace yourself...because losing weight now is ALL about the math. But thanks to the hundreds of apps, calculators, and products on the market, you no longer have to tally every calorie you buy, burn, chew, and crave...it's all done for you. Does that make it better? NO. It's made weight management a technological obsession. It's now easier than ever to get an up-to-the-minute score on your "perceived" success — or failure.

The Three D's

Dieting. Ugh. Diets are things you feel you have to go on, but can't wait to get off. Your eating plan should be something you can sustain for life. It doesn't start on a Monday morning and end by Friday afternoon. Dieters usually strive for perfection and feel failure if they falter. That's why diets often lead to the three destructive D's: Deprivation, Defeat, and Depression — all of which lead to harmful emotional and binge eating.

Exercise Needs Energy

Consciously restricting calories and fighting the drive to eat when hungry is counterproductive to healthy exercise. Your body is not meant to be more active when it's in a state of chronic hunger. Will power can only go so far before your physiological demands and psychological needs take over.

How to Be a Good Loser

The Athletes in Aprons approach to eating is *simple*. It includes lots of whole plant foods and rejects the culture of convenience, that is, refined packaged food. It opposes the small-portion, live-with-hunger handcuffs, and focuses on de-aging your body and brain. You do not starve, calorie count, or consciously limit your calories — nor must you exercise on limited energy.

You can cut your calories simply and sensibly without triggering your appetite and without endless calculations. The key is to apply the following six winning strategies:

1. **Slow down.** The yellow flag is waving! Pay attention and eat mindfully. Trade in your shovel for a smaller fork, and put it down between mouthfuls. Savor every bite. Eating is a full sensory experience. Enjoyment comes from the appearance, aroma, feel, and taste of your food. It takes 20 minutes for your brain to get the message that you just ate. If you're a speed eater, you may be on your third helping before your brain gets the message that it's feeding time.

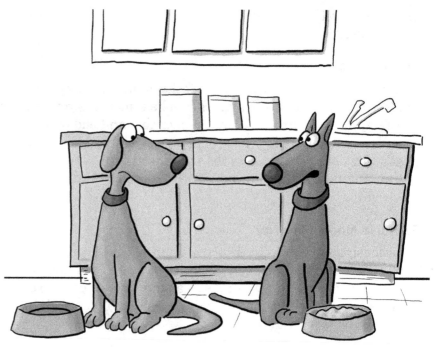

"You see, I don't believe in eating fast.
I believe in savoring. I ... hey, stop looking at my food!"

2. **Ditch the now-or-never mentality.** Lack of availability drives uncontrolled overeating (a.k.a. binge eating). Besides, "never" eating your favorite foods again is a little unrealistic. Really, will you *never* eat ice cream again after Monday — when you start your diet…again? Or will you *never* see another turkey and pumpkin pie until next Thanksgiving? The now-or-never mentality is the #1 dieting mindset that causes you to lose your mind, binge eat, and *gain* weight.

3. **Bury the all-or-nothing approach.** This perfectionistic attitude usually results in achieving nothing. Perhaps at the beginning, you're on a roll with a perfect winning streak, but after one little slip, you feel like a failure (that is, *im*perfect), so you throw in the towel, and before you know it, you're backsliding all the way to where you started — or worse. Remember, the goal is progress, not perfection.

4. **Choose First-String Foods.** These top picks consist of "high-volume" whole foods — that is, plants that contain a lot of friendly fiber or a lot of water (so they're naturally low in calories). Water and fiber fill you up, and keep you satisfied longer.

5. **Always start your lunch and dinner with a bountiful green salad or bowl of COLOR-ful soup.** Just steer clear of dressings and soups brimming with cream, fat, salt, and sugar.

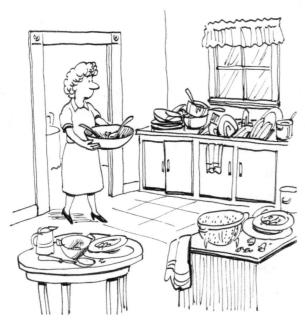

It was a great salad, but it should not have taken every bowl in the house.

6. **Swap out dense for water-rich.** Choose soups over casseroles, fresh fruit over dried, tofu over cheese, and salads over subs. Here's how it's done...

   • Eat oatmeal made with lots of water or milk. Add fresh water-rich fruit, like berries, mangos, and bananas.

   • Make a 'tall' sandwich piled high with vegetables (e.g., tomatoes, lettuce, onions, sprouts, and cucumbers).

   • Dunk your vegetables in fresh salsa. Sideline the ranch and bleu cheese that coat your veggies in fat.

   • Top your basics, like barley, brown rice, quinoa, or baked sweet potato, with lots of herbs and seasonal veggies.

   • Build your stews and soups with water-rich beans instead of dense meat. Toss in loads of veggies. Add more vegetable broth and/or water. For a "creamier" texture, add puréed vegetables like butternut squash or red lentils instead of butterfat.

Coach Karen says

Dry beans absorb a lot of liquid, so cooked beans are a satisfying water-rich food. They expand to about 3.5 times their original volume when soaked and cooked.

- When eating out, request a double or triple order of vegetables with your entrée instead of a side of buttery mashed potatoes, cheese-y au gratins, or greasy fries.

- Bench the fettuccine with artery-bustin' Alfredo. Top spiralized vegetables, spaghetti squash, or a protein (legume) pasta with a zesty RED sauce and veggies.

Grand Slam Doubles

If you eat a dry food like dried fruit, bread, or popcorn, pair it with some fresh COLOR-ful, water-rich fruit or veggies. The result? A higher volume meal or snack that's more satisfying and phyto-rich. Here are some winning combinations:

- Popcorn + pear
- Fig + cooked kale
- Baked tortilla chips + bean dip and salsa
- Ready-to-eat breakfast cereal + berries
- Whole grain toast + puréed fresh fruit
- Almonds + banana

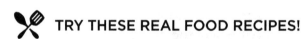 **TRY THESE REAL FOOD RECIPES!**

Chocolate Hummus pg. 232
Spiced Apples with Cinnamon Crunch pg. 297

PLAY 18 — THE FIVE-POUND PAYOFF

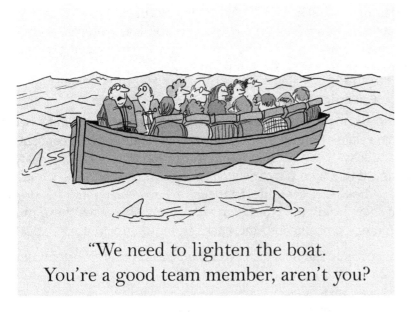

"We need to lighten the boat.
You're a good team member, aren't you?

I f you resolved to lose weight as a part of your get-healthy game plan, but have yet to reach your goal, here's some good news. You really don't have to lose that much to reap huge health benefits.

How Losing Five Pounds Boosts Your Health

If you've ever bemoaned, "I *only* lost five pounds!", then you'll be happy to know you hit a home run — with the bases loaded. Keep in mind that what you see on the scale reveals ONE thing about you (and only one thing)...and that's the amount of mass you're hauling around town.

Listen, losing five pounds does a whole lot of good — but involves things you don't see on a scale. The scale doesn't tell you that your arteries are getting less stiff, inflamed, or clogged. It doesn't tell you that you're getting more oxygen-rich blood and glial cells (your brain's clean-up crew) to that cluttered locker room upstairs. It doesn't tell you that you're pulling ahead in the free radical race. Shedding five pounds can lower blood pressure, reduce chronic inflammation, improve urinary incontinence, and improve or prevent painful arthritis. So the next time you pass a mirror, do a victory dance, and give yourself a high five for losing five pounds.

Lower Blood Pressure

The American Heart Association says if you're overweight, losing five pounds can help lower blood pressure.[1] By lowering your blood pressure alone, you reduce your risk of stroke, heart disease, heart failure, and kidney failure. That's HUGE. According to the National Heart, Lung and Blood Institute, for every 20 pounds you lose, you can drop systolic blood pressure 5-20 points (the top number in your blood pressure reading). Drop a pound, drop a point.

Reduce Chronic Inflammation

Carrying extra pounds fires up chronic inflammation.[2] That's because fat tissue releases many inflammatory compounds. High concentrations of this systemic accelerant floating around in your bloodstream are believed to play a part in causing insulin resistance — creating a cascade of health effects intertwined with overeating and fat storage. Studies show losing an average of six pounds decreases these pro-inflammatory proteins and increases immune function.

In another study published in Nutrition Research, the researchers found that inflammation increases after eating high-fat and high-carb meals as well as foods that contain AGEs. Healthy eating patterns, such as consuming whole grains, vegetables, fruits, fish, vitamin C, vitamin E, and REDs *(carotenoids)*, lowered it.[3] Lose weight, and your cells will chill out.

Improve or Prevent "Wear-and-Tear" Arthritis

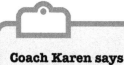

Coach Karen says

Osteoarthritis is the leading cause of disability in the U.S.

When you carry extra pounds, it puts grimace-worthy pain and pressure on your joints and puts you at risk of osteoarthritis (often referred to as a "wear-and-tear" disease). In knee osteoarthritis, the cartilage in the knee joint gradually wears away. As the cartilage disintegrates, the protective space between the bones decreases. Whether you're jumping up to catch a frisbee or just standing on one leg, deterioration of this shock absorber can result in bone rubbing on bone, and thus, pain, stiffness, loss of movement in the affected joint, and bony spurs that press on nerves.

Wake Forest University conducted an 18-month diet and exercise study on sedentary, overweight, older adults with symptomatic knee osteoarthritis. They concluded that for each pound of weight lost, each knee bears four pounds less pressure per step.[6]

Improve Urinary Incontinence (UI)

Added to the long list of health benefits of losing five pounds is reduced urinary incontinence (involuntary urination). Studies estimate about 25% of American men and 50% of women age 65 years old and older (not living in care facilities) have a problem with leakage.[4] These rates increase with age although UI is not considered a part of natural aging. Keep this in mind while keeping your eye on the 100th year prize. Act now. Get surgery or physical therapy (if recommended), shed extra pounds, keep your muscles strong, and feed your body well.

CAUSES AND CURES FOR URINARY INCONTINENCE

Gravity, aging tissue, and hormonal changes all contribute to urinary incontinence. Pregnancy is problematic. Think about the pressure a 6-pound bowling ball in your abdomen would have on your bladder. Oh, and then there's childbirth. This laborious (no pun intended) activity weakens or stretches the entire pelvic floor which can cause a future of leaks when sneezing, coughing, laughing, and jogging. But before swearing off laughing and making babies, losing five pounds can reduce the stress on the pelvic floor and reduce incontinence significantly.

A UCSF study of over 338 women (average age of 53) strongly suggests weight loss decreases incontinence episodes. They found that those who lost an average of three pounds reported 28% fewer urinary incontinence episodes. Those that lost 17 pounds had 47% fewer episodes. These outcomes improved quality of life significantly — more proof that shedding five pounds of visceral fat (fat that wraps around your internal organs) can relieve intra-abdominal pressure on the bladder and pelvic floor.[5]

Weight loss is an effective, nonsurgical, and noninvasive treatment and should be considered a first-line therapy for incontinence. Incontinence drugs have uncomfortable side effects. Those that take them complain of dry mouth, dry skin, dry eyes, constipation, and upset stomach. They say the parched, dry mouth is especially unpleasant when working out (breathing more through your mouth dries it out even more).

Coach Karen says

It has been reported that 50% of women discontinue drug treatment within one year because of the side effects.

Joint Care is Essential to Longevity

Your joints are in charge of *so* many of the daily movements that enable you to be functionally independent — from walking, sitting, standing, kneeling, lunging, lifting, and carrying heavy things. Aim for losing a little weight versus a lot. It's less daunting and the scientific evidence is clear. You'll receive the health payoffs long before you drop large amounts of weight. Losing five pounds would:

- Reduce 20 pounds of pressure bearing down on each knee per step taken, which can lessen pain.
- Reduce 40,000 pounds of accumulated pressure on each knee per mile walked, assuming 2,000 steps a mile. (20 pounds of reduced pressure multiplied by 2,000 steps)
- Reduce 30 pounds of pressure off the hips.

Things that Weigh Five Pounds

Compare five pounds to some of these tangible items, and your five-pound weight loss will feel that much more substantial:

- 7 golf clubs
- 8 tennis racquets
- 5 footballs
- 2-1/2 Major League Baseball bats
- 5 pints of water
- 15 medium Russet potatoes
- 500 sheets of paper (1 ream)
- 20 medium bananas
- 5 cans of beans
- A Chihuahua
- A pair of men's size 10 hiking boots
- A brick

 TRY THESE REAL FOOD RECIPES!

Eggless 'Egg' Salad pg. 266
Tofu Mayonnaise (No Oil) pg. 281

Coach Karen says

Walking on an incline, going up/down stairs, getting in/out of a chair or car can put 3-5X your body weight, or more, on weight-bearing joints (knees, hips, ankles).

Coach Karen says

Your joints are like the tires of your car that carry the full weight of your vehicle. Over time, the tires wear down. A bigger, heavier car needs bigger, sturdier tires, but unlike a car, you can't buy bigger joints.

A competitive world offers two possibilities. You can lose. Or, if you want to win, you can change.

LESTER THUROW

PLAY 19 — FUMBLES AND FIXES

Why You're Not Losing Weight

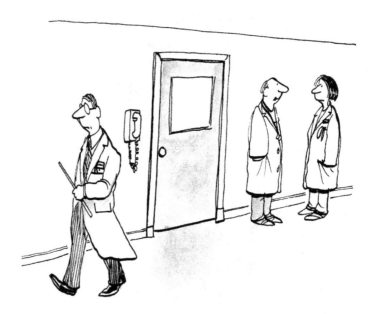

"Some patients like the magic wand prop."

If you're a veteran dieter and exerciser, you've likely concluded the scale is one of the toughest opponents you've ever had to face. Maybe you've triumphed, but maintaining the loss is not an easy feat. Losing weight is complicated, and here are the top 15 reasons why you may not be succeeding.

1. You're an active couch potato.
2. You eat too much, and eat too fast.
3. You're too stressed out.
4. You don't sleep enough.
5. You undereat and overexercise.

6. You eat mindlessly.

7. You're not drinking (or eating) enough water.

8. You're missing your workouts.

9. You're too impatient.

10. You're not cooking enough.

11. You blow it with your buddies on the weekends.

12. You've hit a wall.

13. You reward yourself with food.

14. You have a medical condition.

15. You don't plan.

1. You're an active couch potato.

Fitness is no longer measured by how much time you spend working out, running around a tennis court on weekends, or swinging a golf club a couple times a week. It's quantified by how much time you spend sitting as well.[1] Are you sitting six or more hours a day? Think about how much time your spend on your toosh — sitting in your car, sitting at your desk, sitting in meetings, sitting to eat, sitting with your laptop, and sitting on the sofa. If you exercise, but still sit more than six hours per day, consider yourself an active couch potato.

Chronic sitters tend to have other unhealthy behaviors, such as watching more TV and snacking more too. Sitting in itself has serious metabolic consequences, such as increased insulin resistance, elevated C-reactive protein (an inflammatory marker), excess abdominal fat, and abnormal cholesterol, triglycerides, blood sugar, and resting blood pressure — all pointing to an increased risk for chronic age-related diseases. Conversely, men and women who spend the least time sitting are leaner, less likely to have smoked, and eat fewer calories.

Spending too much time sitting has the following distinct physiological effects:

- The circulatory system (blood, oxygen, and vital nutrients) slows down.
- Energy expenditure decreases (fewer calories burned).
- Enzymes that break down fat drop by 90%.
- HDL ("good") cholesterol) production drops by 20%.
- Risk of diabetes increases 24%.[2]

Coach Karen says

Take frequent breaks from sitting. Whether you're sitting to work, study, craft, play video games, or just watch TV, follow the "20-8-2" movement pattern.

If your work requires a lot of sitting, your health is affected by how long you sit at your desk as well as how many breaks you take.[3] To survive a sedentary job, **sit for 20 minutes, stand for 8, then move for 2**. Moving is critical for blood to circulate throughout your muscles and back to your heart. By following the 20-8-2 movement pattern every 30 minutes, a 7.5 hour workday would equate to 5 hours of sitting, 2 hours of standing, 30 minutes of moving, and 16 sit-to-stand changes.

2. You eat too much and eat too fast.

These two habits go hand-in-hand. You eat too much because you devour more calories per minute. A study showed that fast eaters were heavier than those with a lower body mass index (BMI). Men also tend to eat faster than women. On the average, men wolf down 80 calories per minute versus women who eat 52 calories per minute.[4] Think of eating as a slow distance race, not a sprint!

Here are some tips to reduce your speed:

- Relax before eating. When stressed, you tend to eat fast.
- Use smaller utensils or chopsticks, and savor each bite.
- Sip water between bites to help fill you up and slow down your eating pace.
- Toss on some heat, like hot sauce or habaneros. They're bound to make you stop and take notice.

3. You're too stressed out.

Cortisol is your body's main stress hormone. Think of it as your built-in alarm system that goes off when you're under pressure or danger. If you're under constant stress, that alarm button stays on, which can derail many of your bodily functions and lead to health issues, including weight gain, heart disease, and memory problems.

Excessive stress not only leads to eating too fast, it contributes to storing more abdominal fat — that infamous 'paunch' that appears with age. Studies show greater exposure to cortisol contributes to greater depots of central fat and greater risk of disease.[5, 6] Identify your sources of stress and come up with ways to cope with and/or eliminate the stressors in your control, and let go of the ones you can't control.

Do you have cravings for foods like chocolate, ice cream, cookies, chips, pizza, and fast food — even if you're not physically hungry? Studies show chronic stress has a direct effect on food cravings (foods high in fat, sugar, and carbohydrates), and these food cravings have a direct effect on body weight.[7] People often regard giving into their food cravings as a personal weakness and lack of willpower, but it's very possible this food craving phenomenon is triggered by chronic stress.

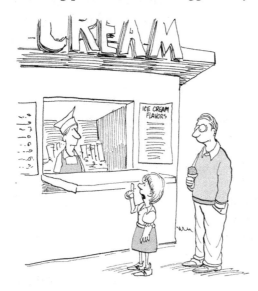

"Better make mine a double.
It's been a tough day."

In order to stop eating emotionally, you must first recognize that stress is feeding your need for comfort food. Pay attention to your eating behaviors — that is, when, why, and what you eat. Are you craving high-fat, high carbohydrate foods when you're stressed out? Notice specific food cravings, emotions, and triggers. When you start seeing a cyclical pattern of stress eating, then, and only then, can you address and manage your food cravings.

In the meantime, incorporate ways to relax rather than reflexively grab your comfort foods. Get to the root of your stress, and find ways to resolve the problem. Practice deep breathing exercises and take time to clear your head. Even in your most wound-up moments, you can teach your body to voluntarily (and eventually automatically) relax.

4. You don't sleep enough.

Do you find yourself sleeping less and eating more? If so, there are two things that are working against you. First, if you're a night owl, then you're probably more likely to do some late-night snacking, which means more calories. Second, a lack of sleep affects your circulating appetite hormones. Sleep deprivation triggers increased levels of

Coach Karen says

Men and women who sleep 7 hours per night have lower mortality rates from heart disease, cancer, and stroke compared to those who sleep 8 or more or 6 or less hours per day.[10]

ghrelin and decreased levels of leptin, resulting in feeling hungry and not feeling full — a physiological fiasco when it comes to weight control.[8]

Men who don't sleep enough have been shown to eat as much as 550 more calories a day.[9] Keep that up everyday, and you'll gain just over 57 pounds in a year. That's like carrying two full sets of golf clubs. How would your knees and back feel carrying around that kind of load 24/7?

Coach Karen says

Ghrelin (the "hunger hormone") is produced in your gut and tells your brain to seek out food. Leptin (the "satiety hormone") is produced by fat cells and signals that you have enough energy stored in your fat tissue, and you feel satisfied.

Coach Karen says

Melatonin production declines with age, which could explain why the older you get, the more difficulty you have falling asleep, staying asleep, and/or falling back to sleep.

WHEN COUNTING SHEEP DOESN'T WORK

If you have trouble falling asleep, be sure your room is void of all light. Wear a sleep mask. When the brain senses pure darkness, it produces and releases melatonin — your body's homegrown sleeping supplement. Even bits of light from your alarm, phone, and TV can throw off melatonin release. Same thing applies when you get up to go to the bathroom, and your brain senses light again.

Melatonin is a hormone produced in a part of the brain called the pineal gland. This gland regulates sleep and wakefulness (the sleep-wake cycle). Melatonin production and release increase when it's dark and decrease when it's light. Over-the-counter melatonin supplements are available, but if you take medications, talk with your doctor before taking a melatonin supplement. Try the sleep mask first to increase melatonin naturally.

5. You undereat and overexercise.

Stop being a human yo-yo. Lose weight by eating — not starving. Your body isn't meant to be more active when it's chronically hungry. Also, when you go overboard with exercise, you may burn more calories, but you negate the effort by eating more. Moderate levels of exercise won't affect your appetite, but if you ramp it up and burn more than 500-600 calories exercising, you'll likely increase your need to eat.

6. You eat mindlessly.

You're stuck on autopilot. You'll eat willingly even if you're not hungry. Some common scenarios that trigger this spontaneous reflex include:

• Walking past the concession stands at the stadium

- Driving by your favorite drive-through
- Passing a bowl of M&M's or chips
- Strolling through Costco when they dish out free samples
- Watching ESPN from your cushy recliner
- Sitting next to humongous platter of nachos

Take notice of your satiety level. To shed your surplusage, thinking about how you eat is just as critical as *what* you eat. Remember your brain is about 20 minutes behind your stomach. If you eat until you're 100% full, in 20 minutes, you'll cross over into being really stuffed. So eat until you're pleasantly full, but not stuffed — that is, you're a No. 6 on The Hunger Scale.

The Hunger Scale Habit

Tune out external cues, like 'food pushers' and when it's "time" to eat. Cue in to when your stomach says it's time. Practice 'The Hunger Scale' habit by listening and rating your own hunger and satiety signals.

During the day, stay between a No. 3 (Crazy Hungry) and No. 6 (Satisfied and Light). When you do, you'll get reacquainted with your own hunger and satiety signals and become an "intuitive eater" versus a "dieter". The Okinawans, some of the healthiest, longest living people in the world, do it too. They call this practice "hara hachi bu", which is Japanese for "eat until you're 80% full".

So what does 80% full feel like? Stop eating when you feel you can still eat a few more bites, but don't. If you keep eating, you'll cross over into No. 7 and feel full. You'll know you hit No. 8 if you have to unbutton your pants to just breathe.

Coach Karen says

Eat until you feel satisfied and light, that is, 80% full or No. 6 on The Hunger Scale.

THE HUNGER SCALE

DESPERATE

1 You're ravenous, dizzy, weak, shaky. You're so hungry you'll eat year-old Slim Jims you found in your golf bag or lint-covered mints buried at the bottom of your purse or pocket.

Your stomach is growling a lot, your brain demands energy, and your head aches. You're irritable, beyond hungry, and eyeing Benji's peanut butter biscuits.

2 **UNCOMFORTABLY HUNGRY**

CRAZY HUNGRY

3 Your stomach is beginning to growl. You have hunger pangs. The urge to eat is strong. You can't concentrate on simple tasks, such as complaining about your botched two-inch putt.

You're beginning to feel hungry. It's time to think about what to eat. You can wait, but when asked if you want a 6" or footlong sub, you reply, "Both."

4 **A LITTLE HUNGRY**

NEUTRAL
(Neither Full Nor Hungry)

5 You're not preoccupied with eating. "My mind is on my game, not food."

You are pleasantly full, and think, "I could still eat a few more bites…"

6 **SATISFIED & LIGHT**

FULL

7 You feel slightly uncomfortable. You won't be hungry for 3 to 4 hours. You're able to make it most of the way home from a restaurant without digging into your doggie bag.

You feel stuffed, and you're busting out of your pants. You don't want anything else, and declare, "I can't eat another bite… Oh look, pie!"

8 **VERY FULL**

VERY UNCOMFORTABLY FULL
(Thanksgiving Full)

9 You feel heavy. Your stomach aches. This time, you really can't eat another bite!

You are physically miserable. You can't move. You feel so full you may lose your cookies. **10** **PAINFULLY FULL**

7. You're not drinking (or eating) enough water.

Your pee color is a good barometer for your level of hydration. It should be a pale straw color. If it's looking more like apple juice or honey, start drinking! A good rule of thumb is to drink half your weight in ounces. For example, if you weigh 160 pounds, try to drink 80 ounces of water per day, which is 10 cups. If you add in some sweaty exercise, you'll need to drink even more.

Oftentimes, the body confuses thirst with hunger. If you catch yourself yearning for 'something', yet nothing in particular, your body may be craving fluids. Drinking the amount of fluids you need per day may be difficult, but you can also *eat* them. Fruits and vegetables are water-rich, so they're low in calories and fill you up — another great reason to eat your COLORS every day.

WATER CONTENT IN PRODUCE

%	VEGETABLES	%	FRUIT
97%	Cucumber	92%	Watermelon
96%	Iceberg lettuce	91%	Star fruit
96%	Celery	91%	Strawberries
95%	Romaine lettuce	91%	Grapefruit
95%	Radishes	90%	Cantaloupe
95%	Tomatoes	89%	Peach, nectarine
95%	Zucchini	88%	Orange
94%	Bell peppers	87%	Plum
94%	Tomatoes	86%	Raspberries
92%	Cauliflower, mushrooms	86%	Apple, pear, apricot
91%	Spinach	84%	Blueberries
91%	Broccoli	81%	Cherries, grapes
89%	Baby carrots	75%	Banana

Source: USDA

Water is a natural appetite suppressant, but even more importantly, studies have shown that you store more fat when you drink less water and deposit less fat when you drink more. That's because your kidneys can't function without enough water. When that happens, your liver has to pinch hit, which takes it away from doing its real job of breaking down fats and producing energy. Drink less water and your liver metabolizes less fat.

Coach Karen says

If you sweat buckets, then weigh yourself before and after your workouts. For every pound lost, drink 16-24 oz (2-3 cups) of water.

8. You're missing your workouts.

Are being too busy, too tired, or too lazy causing your workout lapses? Remember, exercise is a part of your anti-aging strategy. When you feel like quitting, think about why you started training in the first place, and refresh your personal goals. Establish a game plan that drills down on your goals, obstacles, and specific courses of action. Make your playbook visible. Pin your goals to your TV, couch, mirrors, pantry, fridge, and phone.

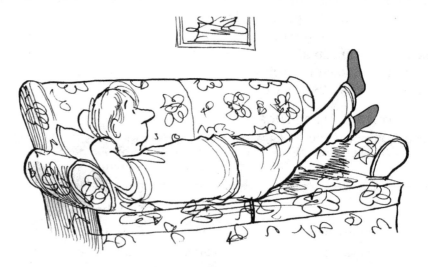

**The Procrastination World Championships
were only a month away.
He never trained so hard.**

9. You're too impatient.

Get out of the "Amazon Prime mindset". Instant gratification doesn't belong in the weight game. You can't get what you want overnight. Give yourself enough time to see results. Weight loss is a slow process, but many positive changes are taking place under your uniform that you don't see on a daily basis.

10. You're not cooking enough.

Eating out can sabotage routine food decisions. According to the National Weight Control Registry that studies successful 'losers', people who follow a consistent daily meal pattern were leaner than those with an inconsistent, random, or chaotic meal pattern. Learn to cook. Keep it simple. With the right tools, staples, and recipes, you can assemble some healthy fuel fast. Flip to **Play 29** on pg. 228: **Real Food Recipes for Longevity Jocks**, and start stirring up some good eats.

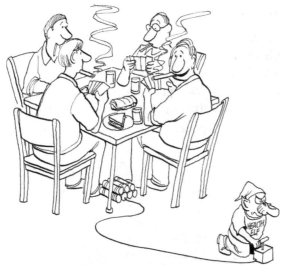

"Hey, the little guy's kind of cute."

11. You blow it with your buddies on the weekends.

Think of weight loss like any sport. Participation requires a good deal of discipline in addition to commitment, vigilance, and perseverance. You may be lured to break from training, but stay focused on your goals. Don't throw in the towel if you're not beating the weight battle. Focus on being consistent. Ball players strike out once in a while, but when they're consistently getting hits on other days, they maintain a solid batting average.

12. You've hit a wall.

Weight loss plateaus are inevitable. It's just a part of the game — like landing in a sand trap once in a while. It's frustrating, but with some skill and will, you'll get yourself out and back on course again. The human body is very adaptable and becomes very efficient at performing what it is required to do. That's basically a good thing, but if you want your body to change, you have to keep challenging it. This is a good time to switch up your exercise routine. Your body has adapted to what you've been doing. Add some higher intensity interval training, resistance, and functional fitness training. Remember, if you challenge your body, you'll change your body.

Keep in mind that about 25% of your weight loss is muscle loss. Also, as your body shrinks in size, some organs like your liver, spleen, kidney get smaller too, so your muscles support a lighter load. These physiological events (more muscle lost and fewer muscles at work) can

Coach Karen says

Exercise and nutrition are intimately related. It's not possible to work off a poor diet.

lower your basal metabolic rate and reduce the number calories you need to maintain your new weight.

As you go through the shrinking phase, but you've hit a weight loss wall, you may have to reevaluate how much food you're taking in and how much you're doing to build more mass — yeah, *muscle*! Excessive muscle loss can degrade your physical function, particularly as you age, and can mean the difference between being functionally independent and needing a caregiver.

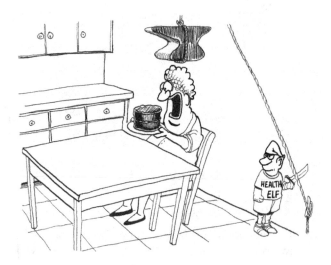

13. You reward yourself with food.

Does this sound familiar? "I've been *really* good. I stuck to my diet, so *I deserve* to eat this _____," (fill in the blank). If that's you, TIME OUT! Once you start justifying food as a reward for "good" behavior — whether it's related to diet, exercise, family, work, whatever — you must readjust your mental game IMMEDIATELY, or you'll unravel everything you've accomplished so far. Think about it...when you're "good" just some of the time, you must be "bad" the rest of the time. Negative self-talk leads to emotional (stress) eating. Reward accomplishments with tangible things that don't go into your mouth. Instead, think massage, a bike ride, new sports paraphernalia, or just some stress-free time studying the weekend stats and standings.

14. You have a medical condition.

Check with your physician to see if you have a thyroid disorder, heart condition, or if your medication could be boosting your appetite or slowing your metabolism.

15. You don't plan.

Would any competent coach enter the competitive field without a game plan? Do YOU ever play your sport without a plan? No way! You figure out how, when, where, and who you're going to play against. You get the right equipment, don the right clothes, check the weather, and even come up with a Plan B if things change. But when it comes to what you're going to eat for lunch or dinner, do you have a plan, or do you succumb to driving through the local burger joint?

Not having a plan is a sure way to sabotage your healthy habits. You've proven that you're capable of planning. It's just a matter of applying those skills and figuring out how you're going to feed yourself.

 TRY THESE REAL FOOD RECIPES!

Raspberry Champagne Vinaigrette pg. 252
Roasted Kabocha and Apple Soup pg. 262

PLAY 20 — BUILDING YOUR BODY AFTER 50

How to Reverse Muscle Loss

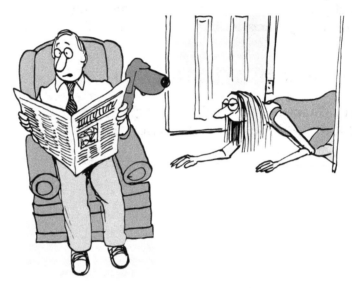

"How was Pilates?"

In the 1990's, approximately 4% of the U.S. population was over age 65; today, that number has climbed to 17% and is expected to reach 23% by 2060.[1] Between ages 30 to 70, men lose an average of 23% of their lean body mass (muscle) and women lose about 22%. That means, if you thought you were 180 pounds of USDA Prime in your 20's — 153 pounds of meat and 27 pounds of marbling, then at age 50, you could very well be a reconstituted version of your old self. You may still be holding at 180 pounds, but with age, no exercise, and insufficient protein, you may be a wee 118 pounds of beef and 62 pounds of fat!

Help! I'm Shrinking!

If you're not filling out your muscle shirts like you used to, this is the beginning of your transition from fit to frail. As you age, you're at risk for muscle atrophy (wasting away) due to inadequate nutrition and inactivity. Maybe your drive to eat has waned, or arthritic knees and hips are slowing you down. Inevitably, your muscles start to shrink from both the lack of use and lack of nourishment. Add to that, older muscles are less responsive to exercise when it comes to growth (hypertrophy), but no worries, aging muscles can still adapt positively to resistance training — it just takes more diligence.

The diets of about one-third of older Americans are nutritionally deficient, resulting in sarcopenia, a condition that affects their ability to perform activities of daily living.[2] Changes in the size and number of muscle fibers contribute to sarcopenia.

At around age 50, muscle atrophy becomes most noticeable. Gait slows down, going up and down stairs is hard, swiftly getting down and up from the floor is history, bending down to tie shoelaces is an aerobic feat, and the hardship list goes on. By age 85+, half of this group needs some assistance with everyday activities (from dressing to toileting), and falls are more likely.

Components of Frailty Syndrome

- Sarcopenia (a 3% to 8% reduction in muscle mass per decade)[3]
- Osteoporosis (loss of bone mineral density)
- Muscle weakness, a.k.a. muscle fatigue or "lack of strength"
- Diminished healing power (slower recovery overall and less likely to recover completely from physical injuries or accidents)

Causes of Malnourishment in Older Adults

Strength improves significantly when muscle fibers grow in size, but in order for muscle growth and maintenance to occur, older adults need to consume adequate amounts of protein. Older adults tend to experience the following, which affects their intake of adequate protein:

- Reduced appetite (which could be due in part to a slower metabolism and inactivity)
- Dental issues
- Impaired smell and taste
- Swallowing and digestive problems
- Limited financial resources
- Physical disabilities and mental disorders that limit shopping and food preparation
- Chronic dieting

Coach Karen says

Sarcopenia (sar-ko-PEEN-ya) is the loss of skeletal muscle mass, strength, and function — a consequence of normal aging.

Coach Karen says

Research studies link gut microbiome with physical frailty. Changes in your gut-friendly bacteria are associated with chronic inflammation and the progressive loss of muscle/bone mass, resulting in decreases in functional mobility and strength.[10, 11]

Improve Quality of Life With Food

The longer you live, it's essential to place diet, exercise, and physical activity high on your list of priorities. These elements can improve not only your overall health, but your quality of life. Resistance training and the quantity, quality, and timing of protein consumption are all important factors in reversing muscle loss, recharging resting metabolic rate, and increasing fat loss.

Functionality Improves With Adequate Protein Intake

You need key nutrients to sustain overall body function and enough energy (calories) to fuel your tank. A 2018 study followed over 2,900 men and women (aged 26 to 81 at baseline) for 23 years. The subjects in the study were tested for quadriceps (thigh) strength, grip strength, and walking speed to assess their physical function, frailty, disability, and mobility. They found that those who ate the most protein — at least 1.2 grams of dietary protein per kilogram (0.55 per pound) of body weight per day — reduced their risk of becoming functionally impaired by 30% compared to those who ate the least amount (less than the RDA).[4]

Animal or Vegetable — Which Protein Is Best for Muscle Building?

Chronic inflammation disrupts normal muscle breakdown and body building, and results in muscle loss. Inflammation is linked to chronic diseases, such as heart disease, diabetes, arthritis, inflammatory bowel diseases, osteoporosis, and Alzheimer's. Researchers found that C-reactive protein, an inflammatory blood biomarker, predicted sarcopenia in over 11,000 older adults.[5] Saturated fats (found in animal fats and tropical oils), sodium, and sugar promote tissue inflammation. Plant-based, antioxidant-rich proteins possess anti-inflammatory properties. So in contrast to animal proteins that boost inflammation, plant proteins fan the flames.

From Beef to Belief

Keep your chin up! You can add years to your life, but even more importantly, you can still add life to those years. Being able to swing a club, racquet, and bat, or hike, bike, and take care of your own needs are all possible. Exercise is an amazing fix, but you cannot make physiological gains (and reduce those aches and pains) without properly nourishing your body. Similarly, it's not possible to build on your resilience by eating well and not working out. **Like good food, movement is medicine too.**

It all comes down to belief. Believing that you can do certain things is vital to achieving your goals and to attaining (and sustaining) functional longevity. With regard to exercise, target mobility, stability, and strength; then cultivate the belief that you can train and gain muscle through gradual progressions. Dive in slow. Raise the bar slowly. Think like a child. A child doesn't know doubt.

> *When a child learns to walk and falls down 50 times, he never thinks to himself: "Maybe this isn't for me?"*

Weight Loss = Muscle Loss

Older adults (50+ years old) especially need to watch their protein intake when restricting calories to lose extra pounds. That's because a whopping 25% of weight loss comes from muscle loss, which contributes to age-related decline, a slower metabolism, and a greater accumulation of body fat. It's possible to simultaneously lose fat mass and lose less muscle mass, but to do this, you'll have to strength train AND consume optimal protein.

Protein + Strength Training After 50

Resistance exercise paired with optimal dietary protein intake can maintain muscle function.[3] Keep in mind that "adequate" intake is not optimal intake. Older aging bodies aren't as efficient at processing protein and need more of it for optimal muscle maintenance, bone health, and other essential physiological functions. But one-third of adults over age 50 don't even meet the RDA for protein.[3]

Feed Your Muscles, Not Your Fat

If you want to know if your protein intake is in the ballpark, you'll have to factor in your body weight. However, if you're overweight, use your "ideal" body weight instead of your current body weight. The objective is to grow more muscle, not store more fat.

Coach Karen says

Muscle is 22% protein and 78% water. It needs adequate protein and water to grow.

Coach Karen says

Simply speaking, optimal protein intake for muscle maintenance calculates to about 15% to 25% of your total daily calories per day.

PROTEIN RECOMMENDATIONS (BREAK OUT YOUR CALCULATOR)

Keep in mind that the following protein recommendations can be met with *real* food — not protein or amino acid supplements.

Healthy adults under 50 years old need 0.8 grams of dietary protein per kilogram of body weight per day. If calculating your daily protein needs per pound of body weight, multiply your body weight in pounds by 0.36 grams. This is the Recommended Daily Allowance or RDA. That means, for someone who's **ideal body weight** is 150 pounds (or 68 kg), calculating the daily dietary protein requirement would look like this:

- 68 kg x **0.80 gm** = 54.4 gm protein/day OR
- 150 lb x **0.36 gm** = 54.0 gm protein/day

Athletes and older adults need more protein. Here's how much more...

Endurance and strength-trained athletes need 1.2 to 1.7 grams of dietary protein per kilogram (or 0.55 to 0.77 grams per pound) of body weight per day.[6] Depending on the athlete's "trained" status, training, carbohydrate availability, and energy availability, daily protein intake may need to be as high as 2.0 grams of dietary protein per kilogram (0.9 grams per pound) of body weight at times.

Healthy older adults (50+ years old) need 1.0 to 1.5 grams of dietary protein per kilogram (0.45 to 0.68 grams per pound) of body weight per day.

Older adults (50+ years old) with an acute or chronic illness* need 1.2 to 1.5 grams of dietary protein per kilogram (0.55 to 0.68 grams per pound) of body weight per day.

An increase in daily protein intake may be indicated to offset the elevated metabolism of inflammatory conditions.[7] For those with a severe illness or injury, an even higher intake of protein may be indicated.

Caution! Always check with your physician before increasing your protein intake to identify any silent underlying disease. These recommendations do NOT apply to patients with kidney disease, and particularly if not on dialysis.

A Sample Plant-Based Protein Menu

Now let's put this into context using a healthy 150-pound older adult as an example. Optimal protein works out to 68 to 102 grams per day, so a typical day's menu of three meals and two snacks might break down to 15-25 grams protein per meal + 10-13 grams protein per snack. Here's a sample menu for inspiration:

Coach Karen says
Keep protein at the forefront of your mind. Each meal should be based on protein. Eat some protein every 3 hours or so.

Breakfast

- Steel-cut oats with walnuts and flaxseed + soy milk
- Blackberries

Morning (or Pre-Exercise) Snack

- Almond milk Greek yogurt, unsweetened, plain + muesli
- Fresh berries

OR

- Tofu smoothie with berries + chia seeds + spinach
- Roasted soy nuts

Lunch

- Split pea soup
- Sprouted whole grain bread
- Orange

Afternoon (or Pre-Exercise) Snack

- Hummus with fresh veggies
- Sprouted whole grain pita

OR

- One slice sprouted grain bread with peanut, almond or sunflower seed butter
- Sliced banana + cinnamon

Dinner

- Soybean pasta with broccoli marinara
- Arugula salad with peaches, sliced almonds, and Pomegranate Balsamic Vinaigrette (recipe on pg. 250)
- Mango Berry Freeze (recipe on pg. 246)

Post-Exercise Drink

Drink during the first 30 minutes after strength training.

• Chocolate Recovery Milk (recipe on pg. 241)

Is More Protein Better?

Multiple studies show that protein overfeeding from protein supplements does NOT lead to better results. Subjects in one study were fed nearly four times the recommended daily allowance of protein. Another study had resistance-trained subjects consume five and a half times the RDA. The results? The extra protein had absolutely no effect on building more muscle.[8] So eating more beef won't make you more beefy. It won't enhance your performance. It won't overhaul your body composition either, that is, it won't improve your percentages of muscle and fat.

Muscle Recovery

Coach Karen says

Refuel, Recover, and Rebuild.

If your idea of recovering from a round of exercise is a beer in the clubhouse or a Reuben in your recliner, then read on. To prevent injury caused by the stress of exercise, you have to let the ol' bod repair and rebuild itself. Otherwise, your muscles, tendons, and ligaments are unable to perform optimally during the next bout of exercise.

Coach Karen says

Plan your post-exercise meals and snacks — especially if you're trying to lose weight. If you deplete your energy stores after exercising, you'll be inclined to grab the first food available, which may not be in your fitness plan.

Muscles may get a little sore within 24 to 48 hours after an intense (or a new) workout. That's because cellular waste products build up in muscle cells and cause inflammation, or because all that lifting and lunging you did caused micro-tears to occur within your muscle fibers. To minimize muscle soreness the next time you flex your muscles and to maximize recovery, feed yourself well, get sufficient sleep (7 hours)[9], rest at least 48 hours between higher intensity exercise of the same muscle groups, and hydrate, hydrate, hydrate!

Easily Add More Protein

Fitting in more protein need not to be complicated or overwhelming. Here's how to seamlessly bump up those grams per day without disrupting your normal routine...

• **Add Greek yogurt:** Toss in some nuts, chia seeds, and berries. Add it as a topping for baked potatoes, and use it as a base in dressings/sauces.

• **Prep tempeh strips:** Grill, bake, or sauté in advance, and store in the fridge for some ready-to-eat protein.

- **Keep naked (raw, unsalted, unflavored) nuts and seeds handy:** Add crunch to salads, cereals, yogurt, stews, stir-fries, and entrées. Add tahini (sesame seed paste) to salad dressings instead of oil. Swirl nut butter into oatmeal.

- **Add cooked beans and peas to anything:** Pile them on salads, pastas, in soups, and homemade veggie burgers. Keep some conveniently stored in an airtight container in your fridge.

- **Add lentils to soup:** Toss in a handful of lentils during prep. Use creamy cooked red split lentils to thicken soup.

- **Be creative with tofu:** Use it in scrambles, stir-fries, pizzas, chilis, cookies, smoothies — just about anything!

- **Choose quinoa or black rice over brown rice:** Enjoy them on the side, in your salads, soups, muffins, pancakes, and homemade veggie burgers.

- **Pick legume pasta over quinoa:** Power up meals with these pastas that pack in lots of protein.

- **Try more intact grains:** Expand your horizons with other intact grains, such as amaranth, Kamut®, and teff.

- **Spread hummus around:** Add a layer to sandwiches, celery sticks, and crackers.

- **Use nutritional yeast:** At five grams of 'cheesy' protein per two tablespoons, sprinkle it generously on popcorn, potatoes, pasta, and roasted veggies.

- **Be generous with chia seeds:** Sprinkle in smoothies, cereals, salad dressings, and baked goods.

Upgrade to a plant-centered eating plan with fiber-rich plant-based proteins. Here's how they size up to an ounce of fiber-free meat that contains 7 grams of protein.

HIGH QUALITY PROTEIN SOURCES

SOYBEANS	PROTEIN (gm)
Soybeans, 1 cup cooked	30
Tempeh, 4 oz	22
Edamame, 1 cup	18
Soybeans, 1/2 cup cooked	15
Tofu, extra firm, 4 oz	11
Soy nuts, 1/4 cup	10

SOYBEANS	PROTEIN (gm)
Tofu, firm, 4 oz	9
Tofu, medium firm, 4 oz	8
Tofu, soft, 4 oz	7
Soy milk, unsweetened, 1 cup	7
Soy yogurt, plain, 5.3 oz	6

OTHER LEGUMES 1 cup cooked	PROTEIN (gm)
Hummus	19
Lentils	18
Split peas	16
Cannellini beans	16
Chickpeas (garbanzos)	15
Kidney beans	15
Lima beans	15
Pinto beans	15
Black beans	14
Great Northern	14
Vegetarian baked beans	14
Black-eyed peas	13
Fava beans (broad bean)	12
Peas, green	8

WHOLE GRAINS, PSEUDO-GRAINS 1 cup cooked	PROTEIN (gm)
Spelt berries	11
Kamut (Khorasan Wheat)	10
Teff	10
Amaranth	9
Quinoa	8
Farro	8
Muesli, 1/2 cup, uncooked	8
Barley, hulled	7
Oat bran	7
Wheat berries	7
Millet	6
Oatmeal	6

WHOLE GRAINS, PSEUDO-GRAINS 1 cup cooked	PROTEIN (gm)
Buckwheat grout, whole (Kasha)	6
Bulgur	6

RICE 1 cup cooked	PROTEIN (gm)
Black rice	9
Wild rice	7
Red rice	6
Brown rice	6

PLANT-BASED (NON-SOY) YOGURT	PROTEIN (gm)
Almond milk Greek yogurt, unsweetened plain, 5.3 oz	11
Oat milk yogurt, unsweetened plain, 6 oz	6
Almond milk yogurt, unsweetened plain, 5.3 oz	4
Cashew yogurt, unsweetened plain, 5.3 oz	3

PASTA/BREAD	PROTEIN (gm)
Liviva™ organic soybean or edamame pasta, 2 oz uncooked	23
Buckwheat soba, 2 oz uncooked	7
Ezekiel 4:9® sprouted whole grain tortilla, 1 large	6
The Organic Pantry® Turmeric Flaxseed Crackers, 4 crackers	6
Ezekiel 4:9® sprouted whole grain bread, 1 slice	5

NUTS AND SEEDS	PROTEIN (gm)
Pepitas, 1 oz, 1/4 cup	9
Peanut butter, 2 tablespoons	8
Hemp seeds, 2 tablespoons	6.6
Chia seeds, 2 tablespoons	6
Almonds, 1 oz, 24 nuts	6
Sunflower seeds, 1 oz, 1/4 cup	6
Almond butter, 2 tablespoons	6
Pistachios, 1 oz, 49 nuts	6
Cashews, 1 oz, 18 nuts	5
Walnuts, 1 oz, 14 halves	4

NUTS AND SEEDS	PROTEIN (gm)
Flaxseed, ground, 2 tablespoons	3
Pumpkin seeds, 1/4 cup	3
Pecans, 1 oz, 19 halves	3
Macadamias, 1 oz, 10-12 nuts	2

FRUITS AND VEGETABLES 1 cup	PROTEIN (gm)
Guava	4
Potato, baked, cubed	3
Brussels sprouts, cooked	3
Asparagus	3
Broccoli, raw, chopped	2.5
Sweet potato, baked, cubed	2
Apricots	2
Kiwi	2
Blackberries	2
Cauliflower	2
Banana	1.5
Cantaloupe	1.5
Raspberries	1.5
Peaches	1.5
Mustard greens, chopped	1.5
Alfalfa sprouts	1.5
Orange	1.5
Dark leafy greens, raw (e.g., arugula, spinach)	1
Blueberries	1
Bok choy (Chinese cabbage), shredded	1
Collard greens, chopped	1
Watercress, chopped	1

Coach Karen says

While vegetables don't contain significant amounts of protein, every bit counts. Besides, they add to your COLOR scheme with few calories.

Source: USDA National Nutrient Database

 TRY THESE REAL FOOD RECIPES!

Cilantro Lime Farro pg. 279
Steely Protein Oats pg. 239

PLAY 21 — EXTRA INNINGS

Pre- and Post-Game Snacks

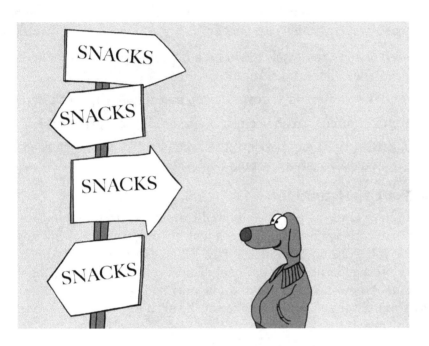

If you're first out of the gate to hit the slopes, court, field, or course, remember, your performance is the aftereffect of what you feed yourself. Don't skimp here. Cash in on some COLORS instead of a dense, sticky hockey puck (a.k.a. energy bar). Quality carbs, protein, and healthy fats provide the gas you need to get you going, and even more importantly, keep you going.[1] Include these macronutrients plus fluids in your pre- and post-game snacks. The amounts you require will vary depending on the activity and your body's own requirements. Here's why you need them:

1. **Carbohydrate** — Needed to replenish the energy stored in your muscles and liver. Carbs are your body's preferred source of fuel for almost every sport or type of exercise.

2. **Protein** — Needed for muscle repair and building new muscle.

3. **Fat** — Needed to provide energy, maintain healthy cell membranes, and absorb essential fat-soluble vitamins (vitamins A, D, E, and K).

4. **Fluid** — Needed to achieve optimal rehydration.

Pre- and Post-Game Snacks

A combination of carbohydrates, protein, and a little healthy fat about 30-60 minutes pre-game time will provide you with what you need to sustain your energy and provide what you need for optimal recovery as well. Eat post-game snacks or your Power Plate meal within two hours after exercise. Some ideas for snacks:

- 1 slice of sprouted whole grain bread, 2 tablespoons nut or seed butter, sliced banana, cinnamon
- 5.3-oz Greek almond yogurt, 1/4 cup muesli, 1/4 cup fresh berries
- 1/2 cup hummus, fresh veggies, 1 sprouted whole grain pita
- Smoothie (e.g., 1 cup berries, 2 oz. tofu, 1 tablespoon chia seeds, 1 cup spinach), roasted soy nuts

Pre-Exercise Hydration

When you're working out, sweaty and thirsty, you're likely to think about drinking some water. But it's just as important to think about it *before* you work out and here's why. When exercising, your muscles contract and generate internal heat. To prevent overheating, the heat must be promptly dissipated via your body's cooling mechanism (sweating). Sweat cools the surface of the skin and decreases your body temperature.

Maintaining good hydration levels during exercise is critical to regulating body temperature (thermoregulation) and regulating blood pressure. When you're dehydrated, your body's mechanism to get rid of heat shuts down, which can result in heat exhaustion or worse yet, heat stroke.

By keeping your body adequately hydrated, you can perform at your optimal level. Without adequate water, neuromuscular activity slows down, which affects how fast and how hard your muscles can contract. As a result, you can experience a loss of strength, reduced endurance, and/or slower reaction and response times.

But I'm Not Thirsty...

As adults age, the body is less able to recognize dehydration due to diminished thirst perception. That means, the initial thirst signals

Coach Karen says

Exercise and nutrition are like two wheels on a bicycle. If one is faulty or inadequate, you end up with a dysfunctional bicycle.

aren't triggered and sent to the brain. So, oftentimes older adults can become easily dehydrated. It's important to be constantly aware of how much water you drink each day and especially critical when you're exposed to heat, humidity, and exercise, or lose fluids from diarrhea and/or vomiting.

If you just can't swallow another ounce of water, *eat your fluids*. Fruits and vegetables make excellent snacks with their high water content. Chow down on some hearty stalks of broccoli or carrot sticks — they're 90% water! These foods help replace lost fluids while being a valuable carbohydrate and nutrient source.

Why and How to Pre-Hydrate

Never begin exercising if you're thirsty (a sign of dehydration). As a general rule, start drinking five to seven milliliters (ml) of fluid per kilogram (kg) of body weight two to four hours before game time. That means, if you weigh 150 pounds (68 kg), you should drink 341 to 476 ml — or about 11-1/2 to 16 oz. Simply put, the average-sized person should drink about **1-1/2 to 2 cups pre-exercise**. By doing so, you'll allow time for your kidneys to process the fluid and get rid of any excess. Then drink a little more five to fifteen minutes before your start time.

Hyperhydration

Drinking too much fluid can cause the spaces in and around your cells to expand. Studies show being over-hydrated has no clear physiological or performance advantage over being in a normal state of hydration. Excessive fluid intake can result in hyponatremia (a.k.a. "water intoxication") and is more common in marathons or other prolonged activities. In this condition, sodium levels in the blood become dangerously diluted and can be fatal. Signs and symptoms may include nausea, vomiting, headache, confusion, muscle spasms or cramps, fatigue, seizures, unconsciousness, and coma.

Replenish Fluids

The time to keep up with replenishing the fluids you lose through sweating is during *and* after your workouts. Sip on small amounts of water throughout your training and physical activity. The amount (anywhere from 1-1/4 cups to 10 cups of water) will depend on the intensity and duration of the exercise, your fitness level, and environmental factors, such as heat, cold, humidity, and altitude.

By staying hydrated during your workout, you'll support your recovery and will naturally perform longer, harder, and faster. If you tend to sweat bullets or buckets, it's best to weigh yourself before you exercise and then right after you exercise. For every pound of weight you lose (which is water, by the way), you need to drink 2 to 3 cups of water. Monitor your hydration status by checking the color of your pee. It should be light yellow (like lemonade). If it's dark yellow (like apple juice), drink an additional 1 to 1-1/2 cups of water.

If you quench your thirst with alcohol while attempting to set a new personal record, forget about it. Not only does alcohol slow your reflexes, impair decision-making, and dull fine muscle control, the alcohol dries you out! If you're not supplementing with lots of water, don't cry when you swing and miss or throw a gutter ball.

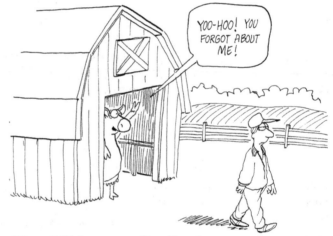

The milking was finally done ... or was it?

Chocolate milk, low-fat, organic 1 cup*

Calories. **170**
Carbs. . . . . .26 gm
Protein. . . . . .9 gm
Fat . . . . .3 gm
 (2 gm saturated)
Sodium . . . . 200 mg

Contains cocoa processed with alkali.

Chocolate Recovery Milk, organic, 1 cup*

Calories. 177
Carbs: . . . . 25.5 gm
Protein. . . . . .9 gm
Fat . . . . .4 gm
 (0.5 gm saturated fat)
Sodium . . . . .75 mg

Contains non-alkalized cocoa.

Milk... Does It Do Your Body Good?

Milk is an excellent post-game source of fluid, carbohydrate, protein, and essential vitamins and minerals. In fact, low-fat chocolate milk makes an effective recovery drink with its ideal balance of macronutrients. Studies revealed a greater increase in lean body mass and muscle growth in resistance exercisers who drank milk during recovery compared to those who drank commercial sports drinks.

But cow's milk has been shown to raise serum concentration of **insulin- like growth factor-1 (IGF-1)**. IGF-1 is a hormone associated with rapid growth, rapid weight gain, and cancer cell growth. In particular, it's associated with an increased risk for several common cancers, including cancers of the prostate, breast, colorectum, and lung.[2]

So, instead of chugging a carton of chocolate moo, mix up a glass of Chocolate Recovery Milk to drink during the first 30 minutes after exercise. It contains the perfect balance of macros without added refined sugars, oils, salt, phosphates, and growth hormones. Natural (non-alkalized) cocoa powder contains higher levels of COLORS *(flavanols)* than cocoa treated with alkali (Dutch-process). The COLORS reduce inflammation and dilate (widen) blood vessels. Treating cacao with alkali reduces their COLOR content.

The Window of Metabolic Opportunity

After playing hard or working out, your body is starved for nutrients and quickest at absorbing them during the first 30 minutes post-exercise and at two-hour intervals for four to six hours. This is especially true following heavy resistance exercise (strength training) aimed to increase body mass and muscle growth.

Packing in some protein within this window boosts muscle building and may delay the onset of sarcopenia and slow its progression.[3] Studies show that eating some protein 30 minutes to two hours after a weight training session enhances muscle-building effects. Waiting too long to eat can impair your performance and function. Also, the earlier you eat carbohydrates within this window, the faster you'll replenish your energy stores. Once depleted, it generally takes 24 hours to fully replenish these reserves.

Coach Karen says

In general, it's good practice to consume a high-quality carbohydrate snack or meal with some protein during the hours following exercise.

 TRY THESE REAL FOOD RECIPES!

Chocolate Recovery Milk pg. 241
Tropical Berry Quinoa Salad with Zesty Citrus Dressing pg. 252

PLAY 22 — BASIC TRAINING

Bowl Like a Pro

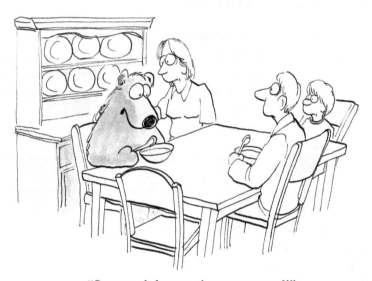

"Someone's been eating my oatmeal!"

Hungry but not ready to trade in your baseball cap for a chef's hat? No worries. Here's your chance to do some no-sweat cooking. All you have to do is grab a bowl, and build on one of the four "basics" (intact grains, potatoes, legumes, or soba). With this approach, you can create your own meal in minutes. When you follow the fundamentals, and keep your locker stocked with an ample supply of staples, you can stick to your anti-aging game plan. You probably won't even get your apron dirty!

Why Food Tastes Better In a Bowl

When you eat from a bowl, you hold the bowl in your hands. It creates a feeling of coziness. Holding your food close to you while eating it can make the experience more intimate. That is, you connect your body to your food using all your senses in the present moment (mindful

> **Coach Karen says**
>
> Think Power Plate. A healthy bowl is basically a Power Plate in a bowl!

eating). Bowl-inspired meals are more informal, organic, and less rigid than eating off a plate with a fork and knife. Also, the bowl's high sides keep the ingredients inside, and you can easily mix all of its contents and entangle all the flavors and textures. Bowls allow you to grab bites of food more efficiently with its curved edges. You're not chasing food around on a plate and having to bring food neatly from the plate to your mouth, which makes bowl-ing a more relaxing way to eat. So build your bowl, get comfortable, and dig in!

THE METHOD (HOW TO BOWL)

1. **Start with a good size serving bowl.** Use one that is deep enough to contain your basic and toppings. Japanese donburi ("DOHN-boo-ree") bowls are the perfect size and height. They're about 6.25" in diameter and 3.25" high and hold 32-ounces (pg 205).

2. **Toss in one of the four basics.** This is the foundation of your bowl. Leftovers as well as cooked frozen grains are an easy way to bowl.

3. **Use a variety of toppings** (leaves, protein, leftover veggies, fruit, locker room staples, crunchies, fresh or dried herbs, and sauce).

4. **Make it COLOR-ful.**

5. **Include local, seasonal produce.** When you eat with the seasons, your food will be COLOR-ful, interesting, and have maximum nutritional value. Research shows that dark leafy greens are linked to a reduced risk of heart disease, certain cancers, macular degeneration, type 2 diabetes, osteoporosis, and memory loss.

6. **Eat your leaves chopped.** Salad greens can be more flavorful and are easier to eat when chopped. That's because each forkful delivers a snippet of all the ingredients, such as the leaves, protein, veggies, crunchies, and sauce, versus whatever lands on the large leaves. Chop them up with a pair of sharp kitchen shears...and do it right in the bowl. Just dig in and start snipping. No need to pull out the chopping board for this.

Coach Karen says

Donburi is a Japanese "rice bowl meal" where a bowl of rice is topped with a seasoned protein (meat, tofu, or seafood), vegetables, and a flavorful sauce. It's Japan's classic comfort food.

Coach Karen says

Farro (not pearl) is hearty and chewy with a rich, nutty flavor. It's one of those grains that tastes good with just about anything.

Coach Karen says

Soba from Eden Foods® is made in Japan with 100% organic buckwheat flour. Contains no gluten, so it's more fragile if overcooked. Many companies make soba from a combo of wheat and buckwheat flours, 70% and 30% respectively.

THE BASICS

Basic #1: Intact Grains — barley, rice (black, red, brown, or wild), bulgur, corn (polenta), farro, steel-cut oats, quinoa. Cook a pot of intact grains, and you'll be set for several days. If you freeze extra cooked grains in individual serving packs, you'll always have a basic for later. Think outside of the rice bowl. Farro, quinoa, barley, and even steel-cut oats make great basics.

Basic #2: Steamed and Baked Potatoes — white, gold, sweet, and purple spuds. Steam and bake several potatoes at once, and keep leftovers in the fridge to use as a basic for meals or snacks.

Basic #3: Legumes — tofu, tempeh, beans, lentils, split peas, edamame, edamame pasta, soybean pasta, lentils, lentil pasta. Beans, lentils, split peas, tofu, and tempeh pack in lots of protein, fiber, and antioxidants.

Basic #4: Soba (Japanese buckwheat noodles) — Authentic soba is made from just buckwheat flour and water. Buckwheat is a relative of rhubarb and rich in a variety of plant compounds. It contains more antioxidants than many common cereal grains, such as barley, oats, wheat, and rye.[1, 2] The noodles are thin, like spaghetti, and brown in color. Buckwheat flour is more delicate to work with, so many packaged brands add wheat flour for stability.

Cook up some extra noodles for assembling a quick, healthy bowl the next day. In Japan, soba is served in a hot savory broth, and during hot summers, it's served chilled, called "zaru soba", with a soy sauce-based dipping sauce.

Basic Serving Sizes

- Intact grains: 1/2 cup cooked
- Potato: 1 medium baked; 1 cup diced or mashed
- Legumes: 1/2 cup cooked beans or lentils; 4 oz tofu; 1 cup cooked legume pasta (2 oz dry)
- Soba: 1 cup cooked (2 oz dry)

THE TOPPINGS

For inspiration, toss in some of these components to build your bowl layer by layer:

Leaves

Leafy greens (greenhouse-grown or "live" and hydroponic are best):

- **Lettuce** — Romaine, butter, and red or green leaf lettuces (the darker or redder, the better)
- **Greens** — Spring mixes, arugula, baby spinach and kale mixes, baby spinach and arugula mixes, beet greens, bok choy, cabbage, collards, kale, Swiss chard, turnip greens, watercress, and other "Power Green" mixes, such as baby spinach, baby read and green chards, and baby kale

Protein

- Edamame, tofu, tempeh
- Black beans, cannellini beans, garbanzo beans, red beans, peas, lentils
- SMASH (fresh or canned, wild)
- Hemp seeds, chia seeds
- Croutons made from sprouted whole grain bread
- Hummus

Leftover Veggies (steamed, raw, roasted, or grilled)

Fruit (fresh or frozen)

- Apples, pears, Asian pears, grapes, cherries, berries
- Citrus fruits, e.g., blood orange, grapefruit, mandarin orange
- Tropical fruits, e.g., kiwi, mango, papaya, pineapple
- Persimmon (Fuyu), pomegranate arils, watermelon
- Dried fruits, e.g., apples, apricots, figs, mulberries, raisins

Locker Room Staples

- Artichoke hearts, hot green chiles, low-sodium olives, water chestnuts

Crunchies

- Freeze-dried fruits and vegetables
- Nuts and seeds, soy nuts

Coach Karen says

Leafy greens have a healthy nutritional profile, but each kind has its own unique superpowers, so be sure to include a variety in your rotation.

Coach Karen says

Rinsing canned beans will reduce the sodium content by about 40%.

Coach Karen says

Trade in your cereal bowl for a salad bowl. Salads make a great break-fast — they're nutrient-dense, easy to make, leftover-friendly, incredibly versa-tile, and trans-portable. Salads are your perfect twofer. You can wake up your brain, and clean out your fridge at the same time.

Fresh or Dried Herbs

Herbs are the leaves, seeds, or flowers of plants. They add GREENs, flavor, and fragrance to your bowls.

- Basil, chives, cilantro, dill, lemon balm, mint, parsley, tarragon, thyme

Sauce

Finally, tie it all together with a flavorful dressing or sauce that complements the ingredients in your bowl.

 TRY THESE REAL FOOD RECIPES!

Korean-Style Tofu Bowl pg. 259
Maple Mustard Vinaigrette pg. 249

PLAY 23 — FIRST AID FOR YOUR FOOD

Add Flavor with Antioxidants

Herbs and spices — what's the difference? A culinary herb, such as oregano, basil, or mint, is the leaf of a plant used in cooking. Any part of the plant other than the leaf, such as the buds, bark, roots, berries, seeds, and the stigma of a flower, is called a spice. Cinnamon, paprika, and cayenne, for example, are spices. Culinary herbs and spices not only add flavor to food, but impart COLOR and contain a wide range of phytonutrients.

When fresh herbs aren't available or convenient, you can use dried herbs. Buy bottled herbs and spices in small amounts because their potency lasts for only about six months to a year. Date your herbs, give them a good sniff for freshness, and clean out your herb locker periodically. If they smell flat or musty, toss them out. Whole and cut herbs retain their essential oils (flavor and aroma) longer than those that have been pulverized into powder form.

If you grow your own herbs and can't keep up with the harvest, you can dry them. You'll save money too. Store-bought herbs are not cheap, in fact, they can be quite expensive. You also don't know how long they've been on the shelf. Some herbs, like oregano, rosemary, thyme, marjoram, bay, and sage intensify in flavor when dried. Others like parsley, chives, dill weed, and cilantro lose their flavor when dried, so for those, fresh is best when possible.

How to Dry Fresh Herbs in the Oven

1. Remove the tender leaves from their stems. An herb stripper takes the tedium out of this job and makes it really fast and easy. No more picking them off one by one! Gently rinse and dry completely by spinning them dry in a salad spinner or by thoroughly pressing them between towels.

2. Place herb leaves or seeds on a baking sheet lined with parchment paper. Try to keep the leaves in one layer, so they can dry evenly and completely.

Coach Karen says

Make sure the leaves are dry because any residual moisture is a breeding ground for mold and mildew.

3. Preheat your oven to its lowest setting — 170°F. You want to dry the herbs, not bake them. Place the tray of herbs on the center rack, and leave the door slightly open to let moisture out. Ideally, the herbs should be dried at no more than 100°F. Leaving the door open will also let the leaves dry while the heat within the oven slowly dissipates. How long the leaves take to dry will depend on the plant. Parsley leaves may dry in 10 to 15 minutes, whereby others may take an hour.

4. When dried, the leaves will look shriveled, and their color will darken. Dried herbs will crumble easily.

5. When cool, store the dried herbs in a labeled, dated airtight glass jar, such as an empty spice jar or Mason jar. Use them within one year for maximum flavor as they will lose their pungency over time. For best flavor, keep the leaves whole, then crush them when you're ready to use them.

The Guide to Seasoning (use one or a combination of seasonings)

VEGETABLES	SUGGESTED SEASONINGS
Artichokes	Bay leaves, garlic, Italian seasoning (basil, marjoram, oregano, rosemary, sage, thyme), lemon juice, parsley
Asparagus	Chives, garlic, lemon juice, mustard seed, onion, sesame seed, tarragon
Beets	Allspice, basil, dill, ginger, mint
Bell peppers	Basil, oregano, rosemary
Bok choy	Sesame seed
Broccoli	Garlic, lemon juice, red pepper, savory, sesame seed, turmeric
Brussels sprouts	Basil, caraway seed, dill, mustard seed, nutmeg, savory, tarragon
Cabbage	Caraway seed, celery seed, juniper berries, tarragon
Carrots	Allspice, bay leaves, caraway seed, cinnamon, cloves, ginger, mint, sage, star anise, tarragon, thyme
Cauliflower	Chives, coriander, sage, turmeric
Corn	Basil, chives, dill, oregano
Cucumbers	Dill, mint
Eggplant	Basil, cumin, marjoram, oregano
Green beans	Basil, dill, garlic, ginger, onion, savory
Lima beans	Marjoram, oregano, sage, savory, tarragon, thyme
Mushrooms	Black peppercorns, marjoram, nutmeg, oregano, parsley, sage, tarragon, thyme

VEGETABLES	SUGGESTED SEASONINGS
Onions	Caraway seed, mustard seed, nutmeg, oregano, sage, thyme
Peas	Mint, onion, parsley, rosemary tarragon, turmeric
Polenta (cornmeal)	Basil
Potatoes	Caraway seed, chives, dill, paprika, parsley, rosemary, thyme, turmeric
Snap peas	Basil, dill, marjoram, mint, mustard seed, oregano, savory, tarragon, thyme
Spinach	Dill, nutmeg, tarragon
Sweet potatoes	Allspice, cardamon, cinnamon, cloves, nutmeg
Tomatoes	Basil, black peppercorns, cilantro, cumin, fennel seed, garlic, oregano, red pepper, rosemary, saffron, tarragon, thyme
Zucchini	Basil, oregano
Winter squash, baked	Cinnamon, ginger, nutmeg

FRUITS	SUGGESTED SEASONINGS
Apples	Cardamom, cinnamon, cloves, ginger, nutmeg
Bananas	Nutmeg
Berries	Black peppercorns, cinnamon, mint, star anise
Cranberries	Cloves, ginger
Mango	Cilantro
Melon	Lemon juice
Orange	Cardamom, fennel seed, mint, thyme
Papaya	Lime juice
Peaches	Cloves, nutmeg
Pears	Bay leaves, black peppercorns, cardamom, cinnamon, star anise
Pineapple	Cloves, ginger, lemongrass, mint, rosemary
Plums	Cinnamon, cloves, nutmeg, star anise

VARIOUS DISHES	SUGGESTED SEASONINGS
Beans	Parsley
Bean dishes	Chili powder, onion
Bulgur dishes	Mint
Casseroles	Onion
Fish	Basil, dill, ginger, lemon juice, onion, parsley, sesame seed, tarragon, thyme
Lentils	Curry
Pasta sauces	Garlic, onion, oregano
Pizza sauces	Basil, oregano
Rice	Curry, dill, nutmeg, parsley
Salad dressings	Garlic, ginger, mustard seed, poppy seed, tarragon
Salsas	Garlic, onion
Shellfish	Garlic
Soups, cold	Lemon juice, lime juice, mint
Soups	Chili powder, coriander, curry, dill, garlic, onion, oregano, parsley, thyme
Stews	Allspice, chili powder, coriander, dill, ginger, onion, rosemary, thyme
Tacos	Chili powder
Tofu	Chili powder, coriander, garlic, ginger, sesame

ETHNIC FLAVORS	SUGGESTED SEASONINGS
Cajun/Creole	Allspice, black peppercorns, cayenne, chili pepper, cloves, cinnamon, cumin, garlic, onions, oregano, paprika, parsley, red pepper flakes, thyme
Chinese	Cayenne, chili powder, cilantro, curry, fennel, five-spice powder, garlic, ginger, hot mustard, star anise
French	Basil, chervil, chives, garlic, nutmeg, lavender, marjoram, nutmeg, oregano, parsley, rosemary, sage, tarragon, thyme
German	Bay leaves, caraway seed, celery seed, dill, cinnamon, cardamom, garlic, ginger, lemon, mace, mustard seed, rosemary, paprika, savory
Greek	Basil, bay leaves, black pepper, cumin, dill, fennel seed, garlic, lemon, marjoram, mint, nutmeg, onion, oregano, paprika, parsley, rosemary, sage, thyme
Indian curries	Black peppercorns, cardamom, cayenne, cinnamon, clove, coriander, cumin, coriander, fenugreek, garlic, ginger, mace, mustard seeds, nutmeg, paprika, saffron, turmeric

ETHNIC FLAVORS	SUGGESTED SEASONINGS
Italian	Oregano, sweet basil, fennel, garlic, marjoram, parsley, rosemary, tarragon
Japanese	Garlic, ginger, sesame seed
Korean	Garlic, ginger, chili pepper (Gochugaru)
Mexican or Latin American	Chili pepper flakes, chili powder, cilantro, cumin, garlic, onion, oregano, paprika
North African/ Moroccan	Anise, cardamom, cayenne, cinnamon, cumin, ginger, hot paprika, lemon, mace, mint, nutmeg, sweet paprika, saffron, sesame seeds, turmeric
Southwestern	Black pepper, cayenne, chili powder, coriander, cumin, garlic, onion, oregano, red pepper flakes, smoked paprika
Thai	Chili peppers, cilantro, coriander, cumin, garlic, ginger, lemongrass, mint, red pepper, turmeric
Vietnamese	Aniseed, annatto seeds, bay, basil, cardamon, chili, cilantro, cinnamon, cloves, coriander, fennel seeds, green peppercorns, lemongrass, mint, star anise

 TRY THESE REAL FOOD RECIPES!

Chipotle Sauce pg. 277
Tofu Dill Dip pg. 281

PLAY 24 — SUBSTITUTIONS

From Center Court to Sideline

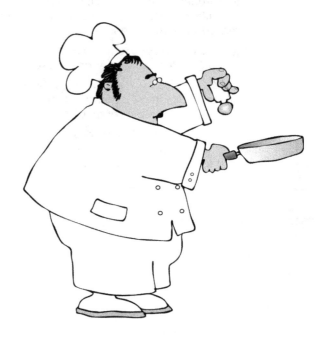

Coach Karen says

Red or "split" lentils (they're actually bright orange) cook down into a thick, porridge-like consistency, so they're perfect for thickening soups or making hummus, dips, curries, chilis, and stews.

For some brand recommendations, go to *Play 28: Stock Your Locker — The Go-To Pantry (Your Reserves)*.

SIDELINE THIS	SUB IN THAT
DAIRY	
Cream to thicken soup	• Puréed sweet potato • Red split lentils • Garbanzo bean (chickpea) flour • Konjac root (a.k.a. glucomannan, konnyaku) • Oat or barley flour • Potato flakes (dehydrated potatoes)
Mayonnaise	• Homemade tofu mayonnaise • Greek yogurt • Hummus, avocado, guacamole for sandwiches
Milk, cow's	• Organic soy milk, unsweetened

SIDELINE THIS	SUB IN THAT
Parmesan or Romano cheese	• Homemade vegan Parmesan cheese
Ricotta cheese	• Tofu 'ricotta' cheese
Sour cream	• Greek yogurt or tofu dill dip
EGGS	
1 whole egg	• Flax or chia egg
OIL/VINEGAR	
Vinegar, balsamic or distilled	• Japanese rice vinegar (a milder and more mellow distilled vinegar)
Butter or oil in baking	• Applesauce, organic, unsweetened • Flaxseeds, ground • Mashed avocado • Mashed banana • Puréed pumpkin
Butter or oil for sautéing	• Low-sodium vegetable broth
SUGAR	
Brown sugar, honey, sugar	• Applesauce, organic, unsweetened • Date sugar (ground dehydrated dates) • Homemade date paste • Mashed bananas
STARCHES	
Bread crumbs	• Almond meal/flour • Chopped pecans • Hazelnut meal/flour • Rolled oats • Sprouted whole grain bread crumbs
Cornstarch for thickening	• Konjac powder/flour (a.k.a. glucomannan powder; konnyaku) • Oat flour
Croutons (made from enriched wheat)	• Unsalted walnuts or almonds, toasted • Ground flaxseeds • Dehydrated fruits and vegetables • Sprouted whole grain bread croutons
Pasta, durum wheat or semolina	• Legume pasta (red/green lentil, soybean, edamame, black bean); quinoa pasta • Spiralized vegetables or spaghetti squash • Tofu shirataki fettuccine
White flour	• Almond meal/flour • Oat flour

Coach Karen says

Combine 1 table-spoon ground flaxseeds or chia seeds with 3 tablespoons water. Let set for five minutes, then substitute for one egg.

Coach Karen says

When swapping mashed bananas or applesauce for sugar, cut other moist ingredients like milk or water.

SIDELINE THIS	SUB IN THAT
White rice	• Quinoa • Black, brown, red, or wild rice
MEAT	
Ground beef	• Pressed extra firm tofu
SOUP	
Chicken stock	• Low-sodium vegetable broth
Tomato soup, canned	• Quick gazpacho (chilled tomato soup) — Combine two cups no-salt organic tomato juice with one container of fresh tomato salsa in a large bowl. Refrigerate for 20 minutes, then pour into serving bowl. • Quick homemade tomato vegetable soup — Combine no-salt organic strained tomatoes with chopped vegetables and simmer until veggies are tender. Season with fresh or dried herbs.
SEASONING	
Table salt (1,200 mg sodium per teaspoon)	• Herbs (concentrated source of phytochemicals) • Hot sauce • Hot yuzu sauce • Ponzu sauce • Tamari, low-sodium • Granulated celery seed, garlic, onion, parsley • Fresh garlic, onion • Lemon juice
SAUCES	
Grand Marnier® creme sauce	• Plain yogurt blended with orange juice concentrate and Mexican vanilla
Orange marmalade glaze	• Fruit salsa makes a naturally sweet substitute for sugary glazes. Slice any fresh or frozen fruits you have on hand — e.g., mango, peach, pineapple, papaya, and berries. Add chopped onions, fresh cilantro, fresh squeezed lime, and jalapeño. Pairs well with fresh fish or cinnamon chips!

In a pinch? Here are some worthy workarounds:

VEGETABLES	
Beets, fresh	• Vacuum-sealed ready-to-eat cooked beets • Organic frozen red beets
Celery, fresh chopped	• Frozen chopped celery • Canned water chestnuts
Garlic, fresh	• Granulated garlic • Freeze-dried garlic

Ginger, fresh	• Ginger powder • Freeze-dried ginger
Green bell pepper, fresh chopped	• Frozen chopped green pepper • Chopped green chiles, canned
Green onions, fresh chopped	• Frozen chopped green onions • Dried or freeze-dried chives
Onion, fresh chopped	• Frozen chopped onion • Onion flakes • Freeze-dried red onion
Parsley, fresh	• Dried or freeze-dried parsley
Red pepper, fresh chopped	• Pimentos, jarred
Tomatoes, fresh	• Organic tomatoes, no added salt. Packed in glass jars, aseptic boxes, or BPA-free cans.
Vegetables, fresh	• Frozen vegetables, no added salt • Frozen salt-free mirepoix (pronounced "meer-PWAA"). Mirepoix is a combination of onion, carrot, and celery generally cut to the same size.
FRUIT	
Fruit, fresh	• Frozen fruit without sugar added • Fruit gazpacho (fruit soup) made with fresh and frozen berries, diced melons, citrus juice, and sparkling water
Raisins	• Chopped dried dates or figs
BEANS / GRAINS / SEEDS	
Beans, dried	• Cooked canned beans in BPA-free can or aseptic box
Brown rice	• Frozen rice or quinoa, commercial or home-cooked
Flaxseeds, ground	• Chia seeds (hydrate for five minutes before eating)
Granola	• Muesli, unsweetened
Oatmeal	• Cooked barley, farro, lentils, or quinoa

 TRY THESE REAL FOOD RECIPES!

Black Rice Salmon Bento Bowl with Mellow Miso Lime Dressing pg. 258
'Creamy' Lemon Dill Vinaigrette pg. 248

PLAY 25 — YOUR AWAY GAME

Real Road Food

Eating at home often has the home team advantage. You're familiar with your kitchen and the cook (be it you or some other culinary genius), and have influence over the provisions and the menu. But when you must travel to another venue and are separated from your home fans, you're at the mercy of road food that has an infinite range of possibilities — from ultra swanky to gravely drab.

Optional Travel Gear

If you'll be staying in a hotel, consider packing a Lékué steamer case (pg. 202) in your suitcase (weighs eight ounces) some homemade room service in minutes. Pick up some veggies and lean protein at a local grocer, place them in the steamer case, then pop them in the microwave.

If you don't have access to a microwave, consider a Hot Logic® Mini (pg. 201). Basically, it's a personal "portable oven" that looks like an insulated lunchbox and can be plugged into an electrical outlet or car cigarette lighter socket. Great for on-the-go, out-in-the-field hot meals. Slow cooks and reheats your fresh or frozen meal to 165°F and keeps it warm.

Here are a few meal ideas that are between the extremes for when you're away at work, a game, or on vacation.

VISITOR'S MENU

BREAKFAST

Market or Hotel

- **Oatmeal cup with flax and chia** (no sugar added) **+ sliced banana + organic raisins + a handful of raw nuts/seeds**
- **Bean burrito + cilantro hummus + fresh salsa, and satsuma mandarin or sumo citrus orange**

- Almond milk Greek yogurt + whole grain cereal + chopped apple + a handful of raw nuts/seeds
- Muesli + soy milk, mandarin oranges, and whole grain toast or brown rice

Coffeehouse

- Oatmeal + soy milk + dried fruit + a nut medley (no brown sugar), **navel orange, and coffee**

SNACK (IF YOU'RE HUNGRY)

Market

- Baby carrots + hummus or guacamole
- Navel orange and homemade energy bar
- Apple slices + nut butter packets
- Almond butter banana roll-ups (sprouted grain tortilla smeared with almond butter, banana, hemp or chia seeds, cinnamon)
- Pear and soy nuts, roasted chickpeas, or edamame

Burger Grill

- Baked potato topped with salsa

LUNCH / DINNER

Market or Hotel

- Salad bowl with beans. Easy on the olives; no cheese. Include a cup of ready-to-eat **pomegranate seeds.**
- Lentil vegetable soup and whole grain roll
- Brown rice bowl with grilled salmon and vegetables

Sub Shop

- Whole grain veggie boat — Scoop out the bread and load up with lettuce, tomatoes, banana peppers, spinach, onions, cucumbers, and avocado or hummus. Hold the cheese.

Burger Grill

- Portobello mushroom burger (grilled portobello mushrooms, caramelized onions, crisp lettuce, fresh tomato on grilled sourdough) **and garden salad** (fresh romaine, red leaf, Roma

Coach Karen says

Instead of croutons, add some nuts, seeds, or freeze-dried fruit/veggies if you crave some crunch.

tomatoes, cucumbers, red onions, carrots) with balsamic vinegar and olive oil or red wine vinaigrette. No croutons.

Steakhouse

Sides are your mains. Order as many sides of vegetables as you desire.

- **Baked potato** topped with chives, lemon, and/or horseradish, **garden salad with balsamic dressing or non-creamy vegetable soup, and steamed or sautéed vegetables** (broccoli, corn, spinach, or mushrooms)

Mexican

- **Garden salad** with side of light balsamic dressing, fresh salsa, and spoonful of guacamole
- **Vegetarian fajita** (grilled veggies (red, orange and green bell peppers, spinach, red onions) — Enjoy with a side of fresh black beans, brown rice, and salsa.
- **Bean tacos** (corn tortillas, whole beans, salsa, shredded lettuce or cabbage) — Pair with a side of grilled veggies (red, orange and green bell peppers, spinach, red onions).
- **Bean bowl** (pinto or black beans, rice, and vegetables) — You can ask for double beans.

Indian

- **Aloo gobi** (potato-and-cauliflower combo in a flavorful sauce of turmeric, ginger, garlic, and cumin)
- **Brown basmati rice**
- **Chana masala** (chickpeas in a tomato-and-onion sauce blended with garlic, ginger, chiles, and Indian spices)
- **Dal** (deeply spiced stew made with simmered puréed cooked split lentils)

Italian

- **Bruschetta** (grilled bread rubbed with garlic and a variation of toppings, such as chopped tomatoes, vegetables, beans)
- **Cheese-less pizza** (pizza sauce topped with portobello mushrooms, artichoke hearts, tomatoes, roasted garlic, roasted red peppers, fresh basil)
- **Garden salad** with Italian dressing or olive oil and/or balsamic vinegar

- **Minestrone soup** (hearty vegetable, bean, and pasta soup) — Some contain meat or are made with an animal bone-based stock, so ask your server before ordering.
- **Pasta primavera** (pasta and fresh vegetables) — Top your pasta with a lycopene-rich marinara sauce.

Chinese

- **Braised eggplant** with spicy garlic sauce
- **Spicy tofu vegetable stir-fry** (steamed tofu with a vegetable combo, such as broccoli, bok choy, and black mushrooms)
- **Steamed brown rice**
- **Stir-fried mixed vegetables**

Japanese

- **Edamame** (steamed or grilled whole soybeans in the pod)
- **Hiyayakko** (chilled tofu salad)
- **Miso soup** (a savory miso-based broth with silky tofu and green scallions) — Miso is a fermented soybean paste and a gut-healthy probiotic.
- **Mixed green salad** with miso or citrus-ginger dressing
- **Soba (buckwheat) noodles**, hot or cold, served with a dipping sauce
- **Sushi rolls** made with veggies and tofu
- **Tofu dengaku** (tofu with miso glaze)
- **Tofu yosenabe** (variety of vegetables, noodles, and tofu prepared nabemono style in a seasoned broth) — Nabemono or simply "nabe" means "cooking pot" + "mono", which means "thing" = "things in a pot". Dip your "things" in a ponzu dipping sauce, a citrus-y soy sauce.

Korean

- **Banchan** (small side dishes of veggies, such as pickled cucumbers, spicy daikon, bean sprouts, spinach)
- **Heukmi bap** (purple rice) — Korean rice is cooked with black rice and ends up with a purple hue.
- **Japchae** (stir-fried glass noodles) — These noodles are clear cellophane noodles made from sweet potato starch.

- **Kimbab** (veggie, tofu, rice, and seaweed roll) — Can be requested without meat. Looks like a Japanese-style sushi roll.
- **Kimchee** (spicy hot fermented cabbage) — Kimchee is a gut-healthy probiotic.
- **Vegan bibimbap** (warm rice served in a super-hot stone pot with a mix of fresh sautéed vegetables) — Typically served with a fried egg, which can be omitted.

Thai

- **Brown Jasmine rice**
- **Cucumber salad** (sliced cucumbers tossed in a rice vinegar dressing)
- **Curry, vegetarian** (yellow, red, or green curry with tofu and mixed vegetables)
- **Fresh vegetarian mint rolls** (rolled with veggies and tofu, and topped with ground peanuts with garlic sauce) — Not to be confused with fried egg rolls with pork.
- **Pad Thai, vegetarian** (rice noodles, bean sprouts, tofu stir-fried in a tangy-sweet pad thai sauce)
- **Papaya salad** (fresh shredded green papaya with tomato, green beans, and peanuts in thai spicy-sour sauce)
- **Tofu satay** (grilled Thai tofu satay skewers) with peanut sauce

DESSERT

- **Fresh fruit + dark chocolate + almonds, hazelnuts, and/or pecans**

 TRY THESE REAL FOOD RECIPES!

Baked Kale Chips pg. 287
Cajun Soy Nuts pg. 288

The doctor of the future will give no medicine, but will interest his patients in the care of the human body, in diet, and in the cause and prevention of disease.

THOMAS EDISON 1847-1931

PLAY 26 — TEAM MEETING

What You and Your Doctor Should Discuss

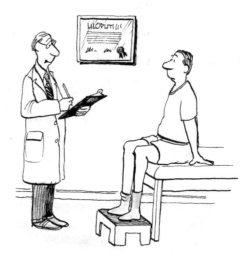

"I'll do some tests rather than give you a guess."

The results of these 11 self-tests are all things your doctor should know. The more that's known about you, the more accurately your doc can assess your health and increase your longevity. Since the signs of a medical condition are not always apparent to your physician from the standard battery of probing questions and tests, some health problems can be missed. Diagnosing diseases, such as Alzheimer's disease, atherosclerosis, and congestive heart failure, can be invasive, costly, and time-consuming. The earlier an issue can be identified, the sooner it can be diagnosed and treated, which could potentially save your life and ultimately, preserve your independence.

Just take a look at Americans receiving home health care in the U.S. today. According to a CDC report, 48% have high blood pressure, 39% have heart disease, 32% have diabetes, 15% have chronic obstructive pulmonary disease, and 13% have osteoarthritis.[1] These statistics could be clues to your functional future. Discuss the results and ramifications of the following self-assessments with your doctor:

1. You can't sit and reach your toes.
2. You can't sit on the floor and get up by yourself.
3. Your right and left nostrils can't smell peanut butter from equal distances.
4. It hurts to walk.
5. You're forgetful.
6. You get short of breath when you bend over.
7. You get migraines.
8. Your blood pressure is not the same in both arms.
9. Your BMI is 23 or over.
10. You can't balance on one leg for 20 seconds or longer.
11. You're too wide for your height.

The Eleven Clues to Your Longevity

1. You can't sit and reach your toes.

How far you can reach beyond your toes from a sitting position (normally used to define the flexibility of your body) may be an indicator of arterial stiffness. Among people 40 years old and older, performance on a "Sit-and-Reach Test" could also be used to assess flexibility of arteries.

Blood vessels should have good elasticity, or the heart has to work hard to pump blood throughout your body. Because arterial stiffness often precedes cardiovascular disease, trunk inflexibility suggests an individual's risk for early death from a heart attack or stroke. Flexibility exercises may cause physiological changes that slow down age-related arterial stiffening, so *S-T-R-E-T-C-H*. Stretching daily is not only a tactic for physical conditioning, but for anti-aging as well.[2]

Coach Karen says

Stretch your body when it's warmed up — that's when it's most 'pliable'. Hold each stretch for 30 seconds and 60 seconds if you're 60 or older.

2. You can't sit on the floor and get up by yourself.

Sitting and rising from the floor requires muscle strength, joint coordination, balance, and flexibility. Take a lesson from the traditionalists in Okinawa, Japan — a hot spot of longevity. One of the keys to their durability lies in the homes of elder Okinawans (over 70 years) and centenarians (over 100 years). Their homes are pretty stark — no cushy couches, dining sets, or Lazy Boys. They have nearly no furniture. That means, even in their 90s and 100s, the Okinawans continually get up and down from the floor, which is an excellent indicator of their musculoskeletal fitness.

Squatting and lunging (basic human movement patterns) are a natural part of their minimalist lifestyle — both of which require significant strength in the legs, calves, hips, back, abdominals, and even the feet. In addition, the elderly Okinawans are physically active throughout the day, so it's no surprise that they live independently. They're either gardening, preparing food, cleaning, or walking, which keeps them on their feet, moving, and eating well. Contrast the lifestyle of the Okinawans with Americans, whose occupational and recreational pursuits are spent sitting in a chair or car, which makes them vulnerable to life-threatening falls, compromised health, and assisted living.

In the U.S., most of those receiving home care are 65 years and older with approximately 97% requiring assistance with bathing, and 91% requiring assistance transferring in and out of bed. Of the home health patients requiring assistance, 81.1% require assistance with toileting.[3] Lowering oneself to use the toilet requires squatting — a very important motor pattern that the Okinawans do naturally multiple times a day.

Coach Karen says

Keep good posture when sitting in a chair. Pull your shoulders back and think about "pulling your belly button into your spine".

DO CHAIR STANDS DAILY

Get stronger to live longer by standing up repeatedly from a chair. Sit in the middle of the seat with your back straight and feet flat on the floor, shoulder-width apart. Cross your arms at your wrists, and hold them close to the chest. Stand up to a full stand where your back is straight (not tipping forward), and sit back down. Repeat for 30 to 60 seconds.

---

3. Your right and left nostrils can't smell peanut butter from equal distances.

The ability to smell is associated with your first cranial nerve located in the olfactory cortex, which is one of the first sites of the brain to deteriorate in Alzheimer's disease. The olfactory cortex is located in your temporal lobe, and that's also where new memories are formed. Being unable to capture new information and remember it later is characteristic of Alzheimer's disease.

According to researchers at the University of Florida, their 'peanut butter smell test' revealed dramatic differences between the left and right nostril in patients with early stage Alzheimer's disease. When smelling the peanut butter, the left nostril in the Alzheimer's patients could not detect the smell of the peanut butter until it was an average of 10 centimeters (about 4 inches) closer to the nose than the right.[4] Peanut butter was used because it's easy to access and exclusively detected by the olfactory nerve. In contrast, many smells are picked up by both your olfactory nerve and trigeminal nerve (think onions) that can cause increased tearing and a runny nose.

A normally functioning olfactory nerve can detect odors at about 20 cm (about 8 inches) from the test agent. The loss of the sense of smell may indicate the brain is losing its ability to self-repair and marks someone who needs closer monitoring and further testing. In moderate to severe Alzheimer's, nearly 100% have impaired smell. In other types of dementia, there were either no differences in odor detection between nostrils or the right nostril was worse at detecting odor than the left one.

Unrelated to Alzheimer's, a history of smoking can damage the olfactory nerve receptors permanently, so if you've smoked for a long time, the nerve endings may not regrow. Other *temporary* losses of smell include: viral infections, allergies, polyps in the nose or sinuses, cancer treatments, and medications.

"Of all human senses, smell is the most undervalued and underappreciated — until it's gone."

Prof. Jayant M. Pinto

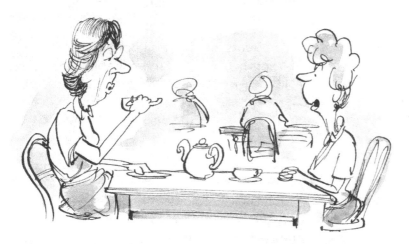

**"I hope you have new complaints,
because mine are all the same."**

4. It hurts to walk.

Excess body weight puts additional stress on weight-bearing joints, particularly your knees, hips, and ankles. The force on your knees is equivalent to three to six times your body weight per walking step. If you're carrying around an extra 20 pounds, that's 60 to 120 pounds of added pressure on each knee. Pressure multiplies when running and skyrockets when jumping. For every pound of weight that you carry, you exert 10 pounds of pressure across the knee when running; and 16 pounds when jumping. So jogging to lose weight can kill your knees in the process.

When bone starts rubbing on bone, your weight can accelerate the breakdown of cartilage and the risk of developing age-related osteo-arthritis (a.k.a. wear-and-tear arthritis). Knee osteoarthritis is one of the five leading causes of disability in older adults globally. Patients with osteoarthritis are at higher risk of death compared to the general population. Their walking disability puts them at an increased risk of death from cardiovascular causes.[5]

Coach Karen says

If you have stiff, arthritic knees, start out by going 1/4 of the way down when doing a squat or lunge. These exercises strengthen the muscles surrounding the knee joint and help keep it stable.

BEND YOUR LEGS TO STAY FUNCTIONAL

Squats and lunges are two of THE BEST exercises that'll save your back and keep you functionally independent. As the legs weaken, people often stop bending their knees, making it difficult to sit down on and get up from a chair or toilet. To pick up something off the floor, instead of squatting down, they may bend over with straight legs — a sure way to injure the back!

When done correctly, squats and lunges improve overall leg, hip, calf, and core strength, leading to more stable joints. Bend your knees to 90 degrees. Be sure to maintain good posture, and keep your knees in line with your ankles, not over your toes. Push through the heels, not the balls of your feet.

5. You're forgetful.

A study revealed that high cholesterol and high blood pressure are not only risk factors for heart disease, but for early memory loss as well. Cardiovascular risk and cognitive function were tested in nearly 5,000 middle-aged adults (average age 55). Risk assessment included age, sex, total cholesterol, HDL cholesterol, systolic blood pressure, and whether participants smoked or had diabetes.

The researchers studied the participants for 10 years and found those with a 10% higher risk of cardiovascular problems also scored poorly on cognitive tests (areas of memory, attention, and executive function). Unfortunately, these symptoms are often minimized as signs of "normal" aging, and in fact, these cognitive changes are reported as "healthy" aging. It is at this subtle stage that management is critical to prevent worsening of symptoms and prevent dementia. Cardiovascular disease risk factors, such as high blood pressure, diabetes, and obesity appear to have a significant effect on brain structure and cognitive impairment.[6]

A UC Davis study revealed a link between cholesterol levels and amyloid plaques in the brain. Deposits of amyloid plaque (detected by a brain scan) are indicative of Alzheimer's. Amyloid beta is a protein necessary for normal brain activity. In early stages of Alzheimer's, this protein forms amyloid plaques, which disrupt communication between nerve cells in the brain. Researchers found that high levels of LDL (bad) and low levels of HDL (good) cholesterol are associated with higher levels of amyloid plaque deposits.[7]

6. You get short of breath when you bend over.

Do you get short of breath when you bend forward, such as to tie your shoelaces or put on a sock? If so, this is a symptom recently coined as bendopnea ("bend-OP-nee-ah"). A study of 102 heart failure patients showed bendopnea was present in 29 out of 102 subjects (28%). The average time it took for these symptoms to appear was eight seconds. Some patients thought their bendopnea was due to being out of shape or overweight when it was more likely they had signs of advanced disease.[8]

7. You get migraines.

Studies reveal a definitive link between people who get migraines and those who get ischemic strokes (clots). An ischemic ("is-SKEEM-ik") stroke is a type of stroke caused by a blockage in an artery that supplies blood to the brain. The blockage reduces blood flow and oxygen to the brain and results in damage or death of brain cells. The majority of all stroke cases in the U.S are ischemic strokes.

According to a meta-analysis of 21 international studies, people who get migraines are twice as likely to have an ischemic stroke. The precise cause isn't fully known, but migraine pain involves constriction and swelling of brain blood vessels. One theory is that migraine sufferers may have a dysfunction in the blood vessels throughout the entire body. If you get migraines, be especially mindful of your stroke risk factors, like smoking, high blood pressure, diabetes, atrial fibrillation, physical inactivity, and poor diet.[9]

Coach Karen says

Exercise boosts HDLs and makes small dense LDL particles become larger, fluffier, and more buoyant. When they're small, they're better at burrowing into the walls of your arteries than larger LDLs.

8. Your blood pressure is not the same in both arms.

Repeated differences in readings between arms could signal an underlying problem and be a risk marker for developing heart disease and related complications in the next 10 years. A difference of 10 to 15 points (systolic, the top number) and 10 or more points (diastolic, the bottom number) could indicate vascular disease, such as possible narrowing of main arteries to that arm, diabetes, heart defects, and kidney disease.[10]

9. Your BMI is 23 or over.

BMI stands for body mass index. Your BMI is simply an estimate of your body fat and is a gauge of your risk for diseases that occur from carrying around too much body fat. The higher your BMI, the higher your risk for lifestyle diseases, such as heart disease, high blood pressure, type 2 diabetes, breathing problems, and certain cancers. A BMI of 18 to 22 is considered "lean", and if you've stayed lean throughout your life, your risk of disease is reduced.

Okinawan centenarians are lean because they've lived a physically active lifestyle, instinctively eat a low-calorie, low-glycemic diet, and control their intake of food. They stop eating when they're 80% full — known as "hara hachi bu".

10. You can't balance on one foot for 20 seconds or longer.

If standing on one leg to put on your pants is now a challenge, read on. Poor balance not only puts you at risk for falling, it can reveal more about your health status. A Japanese study found that struggling to balance on one leg for 20 seconds or longer is linked to an increased risk of small blood vessel damage in the brain and reduced cognitive function.[11]

Coach Karen says
You can work on your balance anytime and anywhere. Stand on one leg while standing in line at the grocery store, brushing your teeth, or washing dishes.

> **TAKE THE SINGLE-LEG BALANCE TEST**
>
> Cross your arms at your wrists, and hold them close to the chest. Elevate one leg until the thigh is parallel with the floor. Once stable, time how long you can hold this position. Any re-positioning of the foot or arms is considered a loss of balance.

The one-leg standing test is an easy way to determine if there are early warning signs of being at risk for a stroke and cognitive impairment and whether you need further evaluation and more attention.

The test is also designed to measure functional stability, identify muscle imbalances, and overall muscle strength. Exercise, particularly core and lower extremity strength training, can improve your postural balance.

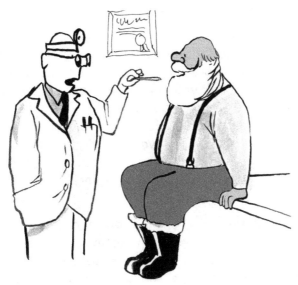

"Cut back on the Ho-Ho's."

11. You're too wide for your height.

As a general guideline, your waistline should be less than half of your height. That is, if you're 5'10" tall (or 70 inches), your waist should be a trim 35 inches or less. Waist size increases the risk of diabetes in men, and one that's over 40 inches increases risk by 12 times.

Fat accumulated below the equator (on your hips, thighs, and backside) is known as subcutaneous fat. It's the "pinchable stuff" that lies under your skin, but above your layers of muscle. On the other hand, visceral fat (a.k.a. belly fat) lies out of reach and is tucked deep within your abdominal cavity, where it pads the spaces between and around your "viscera" — your internal organs, such as your heart, lungs, liver, and digestive organs.

Excess visceral fat settles near the vein that carries blood from your intestines to your liver, which is why carrying too much cargo in the belly is so much more harmful than those lovable 'handles'. A bigger belly and higher BMI are signs linked to a **fatty liver**. Yes, even your liver can get fat! It's considered fatty if more than 5% of it is fat. A fatty liver is dangerous because it's linked with many known heart

Coach Karen says

Your waist circumference is measured at your belly button. It's not the same as the waist size in your pants size.

disease risk factors and can progress to scarring of the liver and potentially life-threatening liver failure.

Coach Karen says

If you don't need much energy to thrive (for example, you spend more time on the bench than on the court), body fat sits in long-term storage.

HOW YOUR LIVER GETS FAT

Several studies have reported that consuming too much processed sugar and fat, white bread, refined grains, sweets, soft drinks, saturated fats, and red meats and not enough whole grains, fruits and vegetables can pack on liver fat.[12] Here's how it works. When you overindulge in these types of foods, triglycerides (a type of fat in your blood) rise, and your liver has to make VLDLs to move them along. Think of VLDLs as buses that ferry big busloads of triglycerides to the blood vessels in your fat and muscle tissue, where they're stored until you need to produce energy.

Once the VLDL buses deliver the triglycerides, they don't go away. They transform into LDL cholesterol and contribute to plaque buildup that narrows your arteries and blocks blood flow. This is where the HDLs (the 'good' cholesterol) come in for the big save. HDLs help your body get rid of excess LDLs, so they're less likely to burrow into the walls of your arteries. But if your HDL levels are low, they have less impact on the LDL overload.

Diabetes

It's common for patients with type 2 diabetes to have elevated VLDLs (and thus, high LDLs) since being overweight is a main risk factor for the disease. People with diabetes are twice as likely to have heart disease or a stroke, and 70% of them have fatty liver disease.[13]

Triglycerides + Belly Fat

Middle-aged men with high triglycerides who sport a pot belly have nearly twice as much fat stored in their livers as men with normal triglyceride levels. Researchers showed that belly fat and liver fat carry an increased risk of heart disease and premature death:

(continued on next page)

(continued from previous page)

- Overweight* men with elevated triglycerides had livers that were 13% fat.

- Overweight* men with normal triglycerides had livers that were 6.9% fat.

- Non-overweight men had livers that were 2.9% fat.[14]

*Overweight subjects had a BMI of 27 or higher and waist circumference of 38" or more. Elevated triglyceride levels were over 150 mg/dL.

The Fatty Liver Link to Aging

Liver fat is an emerging powerful predictor of aortic stiffness. The aorta is the largest artery in the body and pumps oxygen-rich blood from the heart to other parts of the body. A healthy aorta is very 'stretchy', so it can contract and expand maximally and pump lots of blood through it.

Increasing age, liver fat, and high triglycerides are all related to increased aortic stiffness in adults. It occurs early in the obesity process and is seen in children as young as 10 to 15 years old.[15] Aortic stiffness is a risk factor for high blood pressure, stroke, heart disease, and cardiovascular death, and it's associated with age-related physical and cognitive decline.[16]

Lifestyle modifications that involve losing just 3% to 5% of your body weight can lower fat in your liver. You may need to lose 7% to 10% of your body weight to reduce liver inflammation, which can stop the fibrosis (formation of excessive amounts of scar tissue in the liver), and allow the liver to heal. Liver damage is usually reversible in the early stages with a well-managed exercise and nutrition plan, but rapid weight loss (losing more than 2 pounds a week) can worsen the disease.[17]

Coach Karen says

High triglycerides are a consequence of how much food and the quality of the food you eat.

 TRY THESE REAL FOOD RECIPES!

Citrus Mango Cooler pg. 242
Mellow Miso Lime Dressing pg. 249

*The only real stumbling block
is fear of failure. In cooking you've got
to have a what-the-hell attitude.*

JULIA CHILD

PLAY 27 — THE EQUIPMENT ROOM

Tools to Fire Up Fast Food

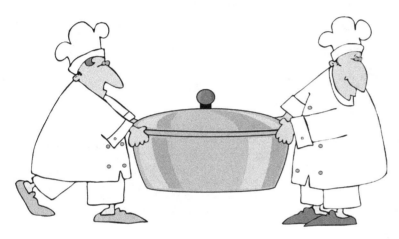

Breaking the culture of convenience starts at home and means stocking up on healthy food and working faster than Burger King. To improve your cooking speed, stamina, and techniques, you'll need the right tools. Would it ever cross your mind to play a round of golf without your favorite driver, irons, and putter? Would you ever play tennis with just one ball? Well, it's no different when it comes to preparing your own meals. If you're a rookie cook, approach the kitchen like you're taking up a new sport. First, invest in some decent equipment. You'll save time and aggravation. When you have the essential gear, you'll be a more efficient cook.

Here's a full list of equipment from essential to optional. The bare minimum tools every cook should own are marked with a check.

Prepping

PREPPING

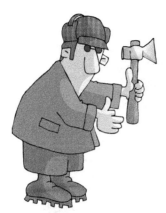

1. Knives and Cutting Accessories

Razor-sharp knives can revolutionize your daily meal prep. You can chop, dice, and mince ingredients faster and with more control. High quality knives can make cooking feel like less work, not to mention make it safer. But there's no need to buy a full set of knives. It's like a beginner golfer going out and buying a 12-club set. You just need the essentials: a chef's knife, paring knife, and serrated knife. These three would basically cover anything you need to cut. Learn basic knife skills. Take a lesson. Search "Basic Knife Skills" on the Internet and watch some videos, then practice, practice, practice. Cooking without mastering the basic strokes is like trying to keep score without knowing how to count.

☑ **Chef's knife, 8"-10"** — A general utility knife and usually eight inches in length, but can vary from six to 14 inches. Use this knife for slicing and chopping herbs and vegetables. The 8" is the most versatile and easy to handle for most home cooks, so if you only get one knife, pick the 8". It should feel like an extension of your arm (much like your favorite tennis racquet or putter) and feel neither too big nor too small in your hand.

☑ **Paring knife** — A thin-bladed knife for more precise cutting, such as coring and peeling fruit, and slicing smaller soft fruit like strawberries.

☑ **Serrated knife** — A serrated blade slices through bread and tomatoes without smushing them.

☑ **Sharpening steel** — A dull knife is more dangerous than a sharp one. When your blade is dull, it requires more pressure to cut. This increases the chance that the knife will slip with a lot of force behind it!

☑ **Wood or plastic (high density polypropylene) cutting board** — To chop at high speeds, you need a solid, stable cutting surface. Glass or stone cutting boards look pretty, but NEVER cut on one. They were designed to roll out pastries because they're cooler and dough will be less likely to stick, but that's it. These surfaces are going to dull your knives. As far as size, a medium-sized board is great for smaller jobs, but if you only buy one, get the biggest board you have room for, so you have plenty of space. When chopped veggies are falling off your board, or you have to constantly transfer them to a bowl, it's going to slow you down.

☑ **Bench scraper (a.k.a. bench knife, dough scraper), 6"x4" stainless steel** — A bench scraper is a flat, rectangular piece of steel with a handle along one edge. This versatile tool is super handy for scooping up and moving sliced or chopped vegetables to a bowl or pan as well as removing anything sticky from your cutting board. Never use the sharp side of the knife as a scraper. Dragging food across a cutting board will dull the edge of the blade. A bench scraper will shave many minutes off your prep time! It's like the difference between moving a mound of dirt with a bulldozer vs a little shovel. Also, because it has a straight edge that lets you cut straight down, you can quickly slice a lasagna or casserole and cut a pan of Fudgy Oatmeal Bars (pg. 292) into perfect squares. Get one with one-inch measurement marks along the blade edge for perfect portions.

Coach Karen says

If you go wild and chop too many onions, chives, green onions, tomatoes, peppers, or celery, you can freeze them for later use.

☑ **Non-slip matting [Dycem®]** — A must-have for faster prepping! Dycem is a multipurpose, rubber-like non-slip material used to help stabilize objects or improve grip. (It's widely used by physical and occupational therapists.) Comes in a roll or in pre-cut shapes and sizes. Cut a piece the size of your cutting board, and slip it under your board and bowls to hold them in place. A stable surface will speed up chopping, grating, and mixing! Also use it under blenders, serving trays, food, drinks — anything you want to make slip-proof.

☐ **Mandoline slicer** — A razor-sharp hand tool for evenly and effortlessly slicing vegetables like cucumbers, zucchini, carrots, and potatoes. Don't multitask when using this tool. WATCH YOUR FINGERS!!! Better yet, wear a cut-resistant glove.

☐ **Cut-resistant gloves** — These gloves are designed to protect your sporting hands from cuts while working with sharp tools.

☑ **Vegetable peeler, "Stainless Steel Universal Magic Peeler" [GEFU]** — Watch out. This is NOT your run-of-the-mill vegetable peeler. It has a very sharp Japanese steel blade that swivels. That means you can peel in both directions and literally skin a carrot in seconds! Works for lefties as well.

☑ **Zester-grater [Microplane®]** — Razor-sharp stainless steel teeth grate in both directions. Cooking with fresh citrus can up your game in the kitchen. Start with some "Cilantro Lime Farro" (pg. 279).

2. Food Prep Gadgets

☐ **Basting brush** — For basting big pieces of fish, tofu, or vegetables with thicker sauces, a silicone brush is durable (strands are less likely to fall out) and washes easily. A pastry brush with natural boar bristles is better for delicate baking tasks.

☑ **Box grater, stainless steel** — This four- or six-sided ultra-sharp metal tool shreds hard and soft fruits and vegetables.

☑ **Can opener, manual**

☐ **Citrus juicer, "Fresh Force" [Chef'n®]** — Love this hand-held juicer. It's an inverted press and can extract every last drop of juice from any lemon or lime while retaining all of the pulp.

☑ **Kale and herb stripper [Talisman Designs]** — A true timesaver! No more picking off leaves one by one. Strip them right on your cutting board.

☑ **Kitchen shears** — Not only are they a good utility tool, they're a must-have for chopping leafy greens in your bowls (pg. 160).

☐ **Meat tenderizer (as a 'garlic crusher'), 3" flat round head, 4-1/4" high, heavy stainless steel with perpendicular handle** — Peel and crush garlic cloves with this heavy flat pounder. This 'hack' peels garlic cloves fast! Smash a garlic clove with the pounder, and the skin will easily detach from the clove. It's a great way to take out your frustration. Weighs one pound.

☐ **Melon baller**

☑ **Non-slip lid opener, 4.5" diameter [Dycem®]** — Opening jars with super-tight seals can be tough for even the strongest athletes in aprons. This dome-shaped gripper fits right in the palm of your hand and helps grasp slippery lids, faucets, door knobs, and stubborn bottles.

☑ **Potato masher, double-action stainless steel** — Has spring-loaded top wires that slide down for a second stroke every time you mash. The double action mashes in half the time. Ideal for potatoes, tofu, avocados, or baby food.

☑ **Salt and pepper grinder set, "Mess-Free" [OXO Good Grips®]** — Tired of messy grinds on your counter or table? These grinders are the best. That's because they ingeniously dispense from the top (not the bottom).

☐ **Strawberry huller, stainless steel** — Works great for tomatoes too.

☑ **Vegetable brushes** — The mechanical action of scrubbing your fruits and vegetables with a vegetable brush under tap water helps remove pesticide residues. Rubbing with just your fingers won't do the job. Use a softer brush for delicate produce and a stiffer one for potatoes, carrots, and other root vegetables.

☐ **Whisk, stainless steel, 10" or 11.5"**

☐ **Whisk, flat (or roux), stainless steel** — The perfect shoehorn-like shape for blending sauces and dressings.

3. Tofu Press

☑ **Tofu press [TofuXpress®]** — An absolute must-have for making a plethora of tofu dishes that grill, bake, marinate, and crumble tofu! Makes pressing the water out of tofu incredibly easy and mess-free. No more plates, weights, cutting boards, and paper towels. Comes with a lid for marinating tofu. Use with a 12- to

14-oz block of tofu and to make Tofu Tacos with Citrus Salsa (pg. 274).

4. Oil Sprayer

☑ **Non-aerosol oil sprayer [Evo™]** — No more hard-to-clean misters that clog, aerosol cooking sprays laced with petroleum-derived propellants, or using too much oil. Evo is a trigger sprayer that dispenses oil (and vinegar) in what they call a "fan spray pattern", so it dispenses the exact amount you want and where you want it. When you squeeze the trigger, 1/4 teaspoon of oil is dispensed. Great for portion control. Get a pair for your favorite oil and balsamic vinegar, and spray your salad greens instead of pouring on the salad dressing. Perfect for taking on picnics, tailgates, or camping trips. Just be sure to lock the trigger sprayer before packing it up.

5. Electric Prep Tools

☑ **Stick blender (a.k.a. immersion or hand blender)** — Purée in the pot! This kitchen hand tool was named for what it is. It's a stick with blender blades at the end of it. Great for blending soups, sauces, gravies, salad dressings, salsas, baby food, batters, and more. You can immerse the stick in any pot or container. Don't be surprised if you start looking for things to stick it in and blend — e.g., peanut butter that has separated, whole tomatoes in a can to make tomato sauce, ripe avocados to make guacamole. Just don't go overboard. Most blades can't handle hard things like coffee beans, frozen fruit, or ice.

☐ **Blender, 6- or 8-cup [Vitamix®]** — A high-performance, pricey machine, but if you want to splurge, it's well worth the investment. It can grind frozen fruit, ice cubes, and the most fibrous tubers into a smooth velvety purée or smoothie. Brace yourself before jamming it into high gear though. It's not your grandma's blender. The speed of the blades creates enough friction to heat raw ingredients. That is, it can purée and heat your veggies in one step. You'll have steaming hot soup in about six minutes!

☑ **Blender, 6- or 8-cup** — If you nix the Vitamix, consider another blender for making fruit and vegetable smoothies, shakes, and soups (as long as they're not hot). Unlike the Vitamix, other blenders can't handle hot ingredients.

☑ **Food processor, mini 3-cup** — A blender is typically better for foods that will end up being liquid (like smoothies and soups), whereas a food processor is better for foods that will end up being mostly solid. If your knife skills aren't up to par, and you're deathly afraid of mandolines and box graters for fear of shaving off your knuckles or fingertips, this handy tool is for you. But more than that, it can chop herbs and garlic; emulsify pesto, hummus, and sauces; transform crunchy nuts into creamy nut butter; and amazingly slice, shave, grate, and shred a hockey puck…in seconds.

☐ **Hand mixer** — If you're not a serious baker making big batches of dough or batter, a stand mixer is overkill and not something you'd want to lug out for short, small projects. The good ol' hand mixer is much less expensive, small, light, portable, and easy to store.

6. Measuring Devices

☑ **Kitchen scale, digital** — If you want to achieve more consistent results in your cooking, use a kitchen scale. Weighing food is not only more accurate than simply measuring by volume, that is, filling a measuring cup or spoon, it's faster! There's also less mess and fewer dirty dishes that slow down food prep.

☐ **Kitchen timer**

☑ **Measuring spoons, spice jar** — These spoons are designed to fit in spice jars.

☑ **Measuring cups, dry, set of 6** — Used for measuring dry (solid) ingredients like flour, sugar, grains, and powders.

☑ **Measuring cups, liquid, glass** — Designed to measure and pour liquids like water, oil, and vinegar, so it's ideal for making salad dressing. Microwave- and oven-safe. Glass is convenient for heating liquids…as well as melting chocolate! A spout makes for easy, drip-free pouring. 1-cup, 2-cup, 4-cup sizes.

☑ **Thermometer, cooking, digital turbo-read, "Taylor 9867" [Taylor®]** — Plant-eaters need a meat thermometer too. Leafy greens and other produce can be high-risk foods. A food thermometer is the only way to be sure your food is cooked, cooled, maintained, and reheated to the proper temperature, so dangerous microorganisms don't multiply or are killed. A thermometer is a must-have — particularly at tailgate parties, picnics, and potlucks where food sits out and for making incredibly moist salmon (pg. 271). What's to love about it: ultra fast (5 seconds or less), ultra-thin 1-1/2-mm tip, professional-grade accuracy, 4" probe that folds into the thermometer casing, and a large, backlit easy-to-read display.

Coach Karen says

The danger zone is 40°F to 140°F, that is, germs that make you sick grow quickly when food is lukewarm.

☑ **Thermometer, refrigerator** — Check your fridge's temperature with a thermometer to make sure it's staying as cool as it should. You want to avoid the "danger zone", where bacteria can grow rapidly. Freezers should be kept at or below 0°F. After a power outage, it's especially important to check fridge and freezer temperatures to determine if the food is safe to eat.

7. Prep-and-serve Bowls and Colanders

☐ **Batter bowl, 2.5-quart [Nordic Ware®]** — Looks like a bowl with a pour spout and handle attached to it. It's the perfect mixing and pouring bowl for pancake, waffle, muffin, and cupcake batters. Lightweight material, so it's easy to pour when full. Non-skid bottom. BPA-free and melamine-free plastic.

☑ **Mixing bowls, 2-, 3.5-, 5-, 7-quart with lids [Nordic Ware®]** — Lightweight with slip-free silicone bottoms. Perfect for mixing, prepping, serving, and storing. Great for serving food at potlucks, picnics, and tailgate parties. All bowls and lids nest neatly together for compact storage. BPA-free and melamine-free plastic.

☐ **Mixing bowl, 3-quart, MixerMate™ [New Metro Design®]** — This bowl is designed specifically for hand mixers. At 8" high, it has tall (not wide) sides with a funnel shape design that prevents spatter. Love this as a sleek compact garbage bowl (a.k.a., dump bowl) to keep on the countertop during food prep because it doesn't take up much space like a wide-mouth bowl. This collector of food scraps, wrappers, odds, and ends will keep your work space tidy, but most of all, it'll save steps from having to move to and from the trash, compost, or recycling bin while cooking. Saving time means more play time!

☑ **Salad spinner, large, 6.22 quart [OXO®]** — A spinner is like the spin cycle of your washing machine. It's indispensable for quickly and efficiently removing excess water from leafy greens, microgreens, and herbs after they've been washed. Remember, oil and water don't mix, so salad dressing won't stick to wet leaves. And there's more! Use the clear bowl for serving, the basket separately as a colander, or both the bowl and basket to wash, soak, and drain fruits and veggies. Spinners do take up valuable cabinet space, but love that this one has a flat lid for better storage and stacking.

☑ **Colander, 5-quart**

☐ **3-in-1 berry bowl, 1-quart [Hutzler®]**— This is basically a small 4-cup colander-covered bowl. Use to wash, serve, and store berries. Fruit doesn't sit in water and berries stay fresh. See "Keep the Fuzz Off Fresh Berries" (pg. 294).

☐ **Japanese rice washing bowl** — A handy inexpensive bowl for washing and draining rice as well as beans and lentils. These are available at Japanese grocery stores.

☑ **Sieve, stainless steel mesh, large and small** — Colanders drain and sieves strain. Use for rinsing quinoa, straining liquid, such as broth for stock, liquid from canned beans, and rice after cooking. See "Cooking Tips to Reduce Arsenic in Rice" (pg. 257).

COOKING

8. Cookware

Pans (a.k.a. Skillets, Frying pans, or Frypans)

☑ **Small nonstick, 8"** — Ideal size when cooking for one or making small amounts. It's tortilla-sized diameter (6") is perfect for warming a tortilla; making a crepe, omelet, sandwich, or tofu scramble; cooking a salmon fillet or plant burger; and toasting some nuts, seeds, and spices.

☑ **Medium cast iron, 10.25" [Lodge®]** — Once it's seasoned, cast-iron cookware is naturally nonstick, so you end up using less oil than a standard stainless steel pan. Cast iron is a chemical-free alternative to nonstick pans. And the more you use it, the more seasoned it becomes. Use in the oven, on the stove, on the grill, and over the campfire. It's great for portable induction cooktops too. Cast-iron cookware retains heat well, so if you bring it to the table, it'll keep your food warm. (Be sure to put a hot pad underneath.) Cast iron is extremely durable and will last for decades. So when you break 100, it'll still be around and as seasoned as you.

☐ **Large cast iron, 12" [Lodge®]** — This is the perfect size for family dinners.

☑ **Glass lid, 10.25" [Lodge®]** — Keep moisture and flavor in the pan while keeping an eye on what's cookin'. Also available in 8", 12", and 15" sizes.

☑ **Pot holder, silicone handle holder or grips** — Cast-iron handles get hot, so be sure to have an oven mitt or pot holder to grab the handle.

Coach Karen says

Seasoning is a thin layer of "polymerized" oil, which gives cast iron its nonstick properties. A properly seasoned cast iron pan is one that has been rubbed with oil and heated repeatedly. The oil breaks down into a plastic-like substance and bonds to the surface of the metal.

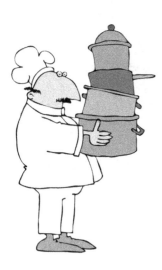

Pots (a.k.a. Saucepans) with Covers

Saucepans are good for heating up liquids and stainless steel conducts heat better. Get heavier gauge steel pots, and they'll last as long as you.

- ☑ **1.5 to 2.5-quart, stainless steel** — Perfect for sauces and portions of soup, oatmeal, and grains. Easy to handle and wash. Good for single cooks and small families.

- ☑ **3- to 4-quart, stainless steel** — Super versatile pot for everyday use. Couple with a smaller pot for a great multipurpose combo.

Stockpots (a.k.a. Pasta Pot) with Covers

- ☑ **5-quart, stainless steel** — Stockpots are larger than saucepans (5 quarts or bigger typically). Good for small batches of pasta and family-size pots of stew, chili, and soup.

- ☐ **8-quart, stainless steel** — You'll need a pretty beefy pot to cook a full pound of pasta or party-size tanks of chili. If you make your own soup stock, this is a great size, but if you like to really stock up (pun intended), consider the 10- to 12-qt stockpots.

- ☐ **Wok, 14"** — A wok is one of the most versatile vessels in the kitchen. Its deep bowl shape can handle steaming and stir-frying big mounds of veggies.

- ☐ **Griddle, 11" square, nonstick** — A must-have for pancakes, but also great for grilling vegetables and sandwiches. Offers more surface area than a round pan.

- ☐ **Grilling basket, outdoor roasting pan, or outdoor griddle, stainless steel** — Ideal for cooking fish and veggies on the grill. It's perforated to circulate heat and keep your food from falling into the grill.

9. Bakeware

- ☑ **Glass baking dish with airtight lid, 9" x 13" (3 quart)** — Glass will not warp, stain, retain odors, or leach chemicals into your food. Prep your dish the night before, cover it, store it in the fridge, then pop it in the oven the next day. For leftovers, cover and store them in the same dish. No more foil and plastic wrap.

- ☑ **Glass baking dish with airtight lid, 8" x 8"** — A versatile size for making casseroles, veggies, brownies, and desserts, like Spiced Apples with Cinnamon Crunch (pg. 297).

- ☑ **Rimmed baking sheet, 11.5" x 17" x 1" (half-sheet), nonstick** — A versatile piece for baking cookies, roasting veggies, and catching drips. The thick gauge metal ones are durable and won't warp or dent. Pair with a half-sheet cooling rack. Line with parchment paper for easy clean-up.

☐ **Cooling rack, 11" x 16.5" x 1" (half-sheet), nonstick, stainless steel wire** — Cooling racks not only cool your freshly baked goodies, but can double as a roasting rack for vegetables. Fits perfectly inside a half-sheet baking pan.

☐ **Cookie sheets, insulated (2)** — Insulated cookie sheets have a central air chamber that insulates food from excessive heat. That means, you end up with more evenly baked cookies (not burnt ones from excessive or uneven heat).

☐ **Loaf pan, 8.5" x 4.5" x 2.5", 6 cups**

☐ **Muffin pan, 12-cup or 24-cup (mini)**

☐ **Pie pan, 8"** — Perfect for making a Pear and Blueberry Crumble (pg. 295).

☐ **Pizza pan**

☑ **Parchment paper (a.k.a. baking paper), unbleached** — Makes clean-up fast and easy. Parchment paper provides a heat-resistant, nonstick surface for baking or roasting. Grease-proof and moisture-resistant.

10. Electric Cookware

☐ **Lunchbox [Hot Logic® Mini]** — If you're tired of cold sandwiches for lunch, this electric insulated lunchbox cooks your food. Basically, it's a personal "portable oven" that you can plug into the electrical outlet or cigarette lighter in your vehicle. It slow cooks and reheats your fresh or frozen meal to 165°F, and keeps it warm. Great for on-the-go, out-in-the-field hot meals. Remove the heatable base unit, and use it to keep your artichoke dip warm at your next Super Bowl or tailgate party.

☐ **Multi-cooker** — This is the latest in multifunctional, space-saving appliances. It's a pressure cooker, steamer, rice cooker, warmer, and slow-cooker rolled into one. Stainless steel inner pot.

Slow Cookers

Toss five to ten COLOR-ful ingredients into the crockery, turn it on low, and romp out for a round of golf — or even two! When you get back, you'll have a home-cooked meal waiting for you. The advantage of slow cooking is the low temperature. The low setting cooks at 190°F, while the high setting cooks at 300°F. It's slow enough for unattended cooking, yet fast enough to keep food above the danger zone (40°F to 140°F).

☐ **2-quart** — Perfect for feeding two adults with little or no leftovers.

☐ **3-quart** — Good for two people and if you or the second person has a hefty appetite.

☐ **4-quart** — Good size for a family where there are two adults and two kids under 12. If you want leftovers for another meal or for freezing, go for the 5- or 6-quart size.

☐ **6-quart** — Great for making stock.

11. Steamers

Steam some veggies, then drop them in a Vitamix, and you can eat soup right out of the blender in minutes. Using moist heat like steaming reduces the formation of aging AGEs and acrylamide.

☐ **Steamer basket, stainless steel**

☑ **Steam case / microwave cooker [Lékué]** — This platinum silicone steam case steams ingredients in their own juices and preserves all their nutrients. The perforated steam tray ensures your food doesn't sit in water. Uses only 1-2 tablespoons of water for steaming. There are no petroleum-based chemical materials that can leach into your food. Steam a stack of veggies together with some frozen grains. Make a hearty veggie stew. If you travel, pack one in your suitcase, pick up some ingredients at the local grocer, and make your own home-cooked meal in minutes. Say goodbye to having to boil water in a large covered pot with a steamer basket. Comes with a Lékué cookbook, "From the Kitchen to the Table in 10 Minutes".

12. Spoons and Spatulas

☐ **Cooking spoon, slotted**

☑ **Cooking spoon, silicone with stainless steel inner core, nylon, or wood**

☑ **Ladle** — If you've ever tried to scoop up soup with a spoon, you'll know why a ladle makes the essential list.

☑ **Tongs, stainless steel serving tongs, silicone tips with ring and pull locking mechanism, 7" and 9"** — Perfect for flipping and grilling as well as serving salad. The ring and pull locks the tongs closed.

Cooking Spatulas

Essential for all types of cooking. They're needed for lifting, flipping, scooping, and spreading.

☐ **Flexible slotted spatula (a.k.a. flex or fish turner), stainless steel or nylon** — The head of a flex turner is thin, flexible, and angled making it perfect for lifting and turning delicate foods, like fish. The slots help drain away any excess fat or sauces.

☑ **Sturdy slotted spatula (a.k.a. turner), nylon [Berndes®]** — The BEST all-purpose cooking spatula! Made in Sweden. This angled spatula has a nice thin blade, is not too big and not too small, and has just the right amount of flex. The slotted blade is 2-3/8" x 4". Unlike a flex turner, this type of spatula is less flexible and sturdy enough to flip a hunky burger or hold a stack of pancakes. However, if you'll be doing some outdoor grilling, you'll need a metal turner, or you'll be serving up molten spatula with your culinary masterpiece.

☐ **Icing spatula (a.k.a. icing spreader), stainless steel** — This sturdy yet flexible spatula is made for icing cakes, brownies, and other baked goods, but it's straight edge is also handy for leveling off dry ingredients like flour when you need to measure accurately.

Silicone Spatulas

The following heat-resistant spatulas are useful for folding, mixing, stirring, and scraping bowls, jars, pots, and pans. They come in various sizes, shapes, and lengths to serve your immediate needs.

☑ **All-purpose spatula, 11" and 8" (mini)**

☑ **Blender spatula, 12.5"** — This spatula is long and narrow for getting around the blades and sides of the container. You'll need the perfect combination of flexibility, hardness, and length for getting every last bit out of the blender, particularly thicker frozen drinks and nut butters.

☑ **Narrow spatula, 10"** — The narrow flexible silicone blade is designed to fit inside narrow bottles to easily stir and remove every last bit of what's inside.

☑ **Omelet turner, "Flip and Fold" [OXO®]** — This silicone turner is soft, flexible, and conforms to rounded pan edges making it *the* best bowl scraper! It's also good for what it was designed to do too, i.e., flipping and folding delicate omelets as well as quesadillas.

☑ **Spoonula, 11" and 8" (mini)** — A spoonula is a cross between a spatula and a spoon. Rather than having a flat end, it has a spoon-shaped end, which is ideal for mixing batters, doughs, fruit salads, grains, just about anything.

STORING

13. Storage Containers

☐ **Containers with airtight lids, BPA-free, "POP" [OXO®]** —Super useful for storing grains, cereals, flour, beans, pastas, and rice, and stacking them for compact, organized storage.

☑ **Glass containers, rectangular with airtight locking lids** — Great for storing leftovers in the fridge or freezer. Glass doesn't stain, absorb odors, or harbor flavors. Microwave, freezer, fridge, and oven safe.

☑ **Glass baby food containers, locking lids, 5-oz [Lunchley™]** — Perfect size for storing, freezing, reheating, packing, and stacking leftover sauces, dressings, dips, spices, and snacks. Set of 12.

☐ **Glass Mason jars, wide-mouth** — Wide-mouth jars are the solution when you need an airtight vessel with a wide enough mouth to fill, stir, and scoop. The quart-size (32-oz) airtight jars are handy for storing and freezing homemade soup stock, sauces, and cut fruits or veggies. The 'pint' jars (16-oz size) are perfect for Overnight Oats (pg. 237).

☐ **Glass spice jars** — Reuse empty spice jars, and store your own homemade spices and dried herbs in them (pg. 165).

☐ **Pitcher, 2-quart Airtight [Takeya®]** — This pitcher is airtight and leakproof, so it can be stored upright or on its side. Optional accessories include a fruit infuser, tea infuser, and ultra-fine mesh coffee filter.

14. Produce Keepers

☑ **Produce keeper (a.k.a. ethylene absorber) [BluApple®]** — What's the most expensive food you buy? It's the food you throw away. The culprit is ethylene gas. This gas triggers cells to degrade, which causes fruit to ripen faster, leaves to go limp, and tubers to sprout. These ethylene gas absorbers (activated carbon) extend the life of your produce and ensure what you put in your grocery cart ends up in you.

☑ **Produce bags, reusable mesh [SPLF/Simple Life]** — These see-through mesh bags allow your fruits and veggies to breathe while stored in your produce bins. The thin single-use plastic produce bags from the supermarket don't allow fresh air in nor do they allow ethylene gas to escape.

DISHING UP

15. Bowls

☑ **Donburi bowls [Zen Table Japan]** — Donburi ("DOHN-boo-ree") is a traditional rice bowl meal and considered Japan's ultimate comfort food. The oversized bowls are deep enough to contain your BASIC and toppings (pg. 163). Authentic Japanese donburi bowls are about 6.25" in diameter and 3.25" high and hold 32-ounces. They're smaller than the wider-mouth ramen noodle bowls (8.5" x 3.5"), which are large (45-50 oz) since they're made to accommodate a lot of noodles, toppings, and broth. Donburi bowls make great vessels for leafy green salads, popcorn, soupy pastas, stews, and more! Try "Black Rice Salmon Bento Bowl with Mellow Miso Lime Dressing" (pg. 258).

16. Tea Needs

☑ **Tea mug with infuser and lid, 16 oz** — Steep your antioxidant-rich tea leaves in a removable stainless steel infuser. The lid keeps your tea hot while it steeps, then doubles as a coaster for the infuser.

☐ **Kettle, gooseneck electric temperature control, stainless steel [Kiket]** — Precisely heat water for the perfect cup of green tea (140°F to 190°F depending on the type of tea) or coffee (195°F to 205°F). Why does water temperature matter? Green tea prepared with water that's too hot can scorch the leaves and reduce their antioxidant activity.[1] Brewing or pressing coffee grounds with water that's too hot can result in a bitter taste from extracting too many coffee grounds too early.

 TRY THESE REAL FOOD RECIPES!

BLT — Barbecue-seasoned tofu, Lettuce, and Tomato pg. 265
Tofu 'Ricotta' pg. 283

PLAY 28 — STOCK YOUR LOCKER

The Go-To Pantry (Your Reserves)

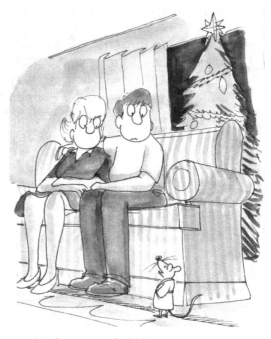

"In the course of nibbling in your pantry
I have discovered I have several food allergies."

Breaking 100 starts with a healthy pantry. But not sure where to start and what to buy? No worries! First, clear out your locker, and start anew. Get rid of everything that's refined, over-processed, over-salted, over-sweetened, and artificially colored. Refer back to the foods to ditch (pg. 15) and those that inflame (pg. 26). Next, stock your shelves and your fridge using the "Sample Shopping List" as a guide and "Coach Karen's First Round Picks" (approved brands and sources). This is where you start putting this nutrition playbook into practice.

Sample Shopping List

BUILD YOUR PANTRY, FRIDGE, AND FREEZER AROUND THESE COLOR-FUL ANTI-AGING STAPLES

☐ **Fresh fruits** e.g., apples, bananas, cantaloupe, grapefruit, oranges, peaches, plums, strawberries, watermelon

☐ **Fresh vegetables** e.g., artichokes, avocado, bell peppers, broccoli, carrots, celery, cucumbers, Romaine lettuce, tomatoes, zucchini

☐ **Starchy vegetables** corn, orange and purple sweet potatoes (a.k.a. Hawaiian or Okinawa sweet potatoes), peas, taro, winter squash

☐ **Frozen and dried fruits/vegetables** e.g., berries. cherries, green beans, mango, peas, pineapple

☐ **Intact grains and pseudo-grains** e.g., barley, buckwheat, bulgur, farro, oats, quinoa, rice (black, brown, red, or wild)

☐ **Sprouted whole grain products** e.g., Ezekiel 4:9® bread, cereal, English muffins, tortillas

☐ **Legumes** e.g., beans (canned or dried), edamame, lentils (all colors), soybeans, tofu

☐ **Protein pasta** e.g., black bean, edamame, lentil, or soybean pasta

☐ **Plant-based dairy** e.g., soy milk, almond milk Greek yogurt

☐ **Nuts and seeds** e.g., almonds, pistachios, walnuts; flax, chia, hemp seeds, pepitas

☐ **Low-mercury fish rich in omega-3s** SMASH: Salmon, Mackerel, Anchovies, Sardines, Herring (fresh, frozen, or canned)

☐ **Tea** green, black, and hibiscus

COACH KAREN'S FIRST-ROUND PICKS

These top picks aren't influenced by any affiliate partnerships — they're just products that are truly loved for their taste, health benefits, and nutrition! Start with the staples, then fill in with the extras.

Staples

Extras

Shopping Tips

STAPLES

1. Produce

- **Dried fruits, unsweetened, organic [North Bay Trading Co.®, Nuts.com]**— e.g., apples; blueberries; cherries; dragon fruit; mango; Black Mission figs; persimmons; pineapple

- **Dates, Fancy Medjool [Hadley®]** — Compared to some other Fancy Medjools, Hadley's aren't overly dried — they're plump (bigger and softer than the average date) with a jammier, more caramel-y flesh. Medjools, referred to as the "crown jewel of dates" are a natural sweetener with lots of BROWNs, calcium, potassium, and fiber. "Fancy" is the grade and identifies the quality of the date (also called U.S. Grade A), whereas "Choice" is a lower quality (U.S. Grade B). Its cousin, the Deglet Noor date, is smaller, firm, drier, and less intensely sweet, so Medjools are the best type to use to naturally sweeten up your recipes.

- ☐ **Freeze-dried produce, organic [Natierra®, North Bay Trading Co.®, Nuts.com]** — e.g., apples; blackberries; raspberries, cherries; mangos; strawberries; green peas; sweet corn; kale powder. Toss them in soups, smoothies, oatmeal, and puddings. Unlike dehydrated foods, several studies show that the antioxidant-rich phytochemicals found in freeze-dried fruits were almost as high as fresh (pg. 48).

- ☐ **Kabocha squash, frozen [Earthbound Farm®]** — Kabocha is a naturally sweet Japanese variety of winter squash. Eat it mashed, add it to soups, smoothies, stews, or mix it in with a variety of veggie dishes.

- ☐ **Live leafy greens [Pete's®]** — Finally, leafy greens that last! When stocking your fridge with healthy crisp greens at the beginning of the week, who wants yellowed, limp leaves by the end of the week. Live lettuce is grown hydroponically and sold living with the "root ball" still intact. You harvest when you're hungry and eat 'fresh-picked' organic leaves that retain their GREENs, vitamins, and crunch even after 7+ days in your fridge.

- ☐ **Shiitake mushrooms, dried [Eden®]** — Shiitake ("SHEE-tah-keh") mushrooms are a staple in Japanese cuisine and prized for their health benefits and rich, distinctive flavor. Like humans, mushrooms can synthesize vitamin D when exposed to UV light. These mushrooms aren't grown in the dark like many commercially grown mushrooms, but outdoors on logs of the 'shii'

Coach Karen says

Black Mission figs are a powerhouse of fiber with 7 gm per serving (2 medium figs). One medium apple contains 4.4 gm fiber.

Coach Karen says

Baby greens are miniature leafy greens, e.g., arugula, kale, lettuces, spinach, and more, that are harvested when they're just a few weeks old. These babies are more tender (and perishable) than their grown-up counterparts.

Coach Karen says

Vitamin D is now considered a nutrient of "public health significance" and must be listed on the label. For commercially grown mush-rooms, check for its amount of this sunshine vitamin.

Coach Karen says

You can cook up larger batches of grains, and freeze them. They make a nutritious timesaver.

Coach Karen says

Cooked grains that freeze well: barley, buckwheat, bulgur wheat, farro, millet, quinoa, rice and rice medleys, rye berries, wheat berries.

tree in Japan (not artificial logs) without fungicides. Use in soups, stews, stir-frys, pasta dishes, lettuce wraps, and sushi rolls.

☐ **Tomatoes, strained, organic, no added salt [Bionaturae®]** — Every anti-aging pantry needs plenty of REDs. These organic strained tomatoes from Italy are naturally sweet with no added sugar, salt, or citric acid added. Make a flavorful Italian tomato sauce in 10 minutes (recipe on the jar) or a COLOR-ful tomato vegetable soup. Bionaturae states that their tomatoes are hand-harvested and packed within 24 hours — probably why it has such great flavor. Love that it comes in 24-oz glass bottle (no tin), and you can use what you need, then easily store the rest.

2. Intact Grains and Pseudo-Grains

☐ **Hulled, Hulless, or Heirloom Purple Hulless Barley [Shiloh Farms®]** — When buying barley, be sure to buy hulless, hull-less, or hulled (sometimes called dehulled) barley. Just one 1/4-cup (dry) contains a colossal 8 gm fiber and 6 gm protein. Barley has a rich, nut-like flavor that ramps up your intake of beta-glucans, making it perfect as a hearty side, breakfast, stew, or soup. Just be sure it's not pearled barley, which is the most popular type sold in stores.

☐ **Black rice, a.k.a. purple rice, "Black Pearl" [Lundberg®]** — Due to its low yield, black rice was referred to as "Forbidden Rice" or "Emperor's Rice" in ancient China because it was once reserved for the Chinese emperor to ensure his health and longevity, and it was forbidden to anyone else. Always check where the black rice is grown before purchasing. See "How to Select the Healthiest Rice" (pg. 226).

☐ **Brown basmati, California [Lundberg®]** — Basmati grains are extra long and thin. Brown basmati is lighter, more delicate, aromatic, and has a nuttier flavor than regular brown rice. Brown basmati grown in California has 33% less arsenic that other brown rices.[1]

☐ **Farro, organic emmer farro [Shiloh Farms®]** — This farro is whole, not pearled. See "How to Cook No-Fail Farro" (pg. 278).

☐ **Muesli, old country style [Bob's Red Mill®]** — This tasty traditional European-inspired cereal is great eaten cold or cooked liked oatmeal. Use it as a topping for yogurt or for Overnight Oats (pg. 237). Whole grains (wheat, rye, barley, oats, and triticale), almonds, flaxseed, and walnuts are sweetened naturally with dates and raisins. No added sugar.

☐ **Popcorn crimson kernels [Black Jewell®]** — One 4-cup serving of these popped non-GMO crimson kernels are a great source of fiber (5 gm), protein (4 gm), and BLUEs. Crimson kernels have a slightly nutty flavor and pop bright white. Available in heirloom black corn kernels too.

☐ **Sprouted rices and sprouted legumes, quinoa, and blends [Lundberg®, TruRoots™]** — Sprouting a grain, bean, or seed breaks down the protective exterior coatings, which unlocks more of its nutrients.

3. Sprouted Whole Grain Products

☐ **Breads, Ezekiel 4:9® and Genesis 1:29® [Food for Life®]**

☐ **Burger buns, Ezekiel 4:9® [Food for Life®]**

☐ **English muffins, Ezekiel 4:9® and Genesis 1:29® [Food for Life®]**

☐ **Pocket breads, Ezekiel 4:9® [Food for Life®]**

☐ **Cereals, Ezekiel 4:9® [Food for Life®]** — Ingredients in this crunchy cereal are sprouted and flourless. It's made with Ezekiel 4:9 bread that's dehydrated, cooled, broken up, and dried. If you've been a long-time Grape-Nuts fan, this cereal may remind you of it, but with less sodium and no flour or yeast.

☐ **Tortillas, Ezekiel 4:9® [Food for Life®]**

☐ **Tortillas, corn [Food for Life®]** — This tortilla has a 7.5-to-1 carbohydrate to fiber ratio, but it's made with sprouted whole kernel corn. It's a much better alternative to other corn tortillas made with corn flour or corn meal, gums, and phosphoric acid.

☐ **Flatbread crust, "Flatzza®" [Angelic Bakehouse®]** — This flatbread pizza crust contains sprouted ingredients, but also whole wheat flour, sunflower oil, and sweetener (agave syrup). However, sometimes you crave a pizza and need a big round platform for all your favorite toppings. Sprouted grains include red wheat berries, quinoa, millet, oat groats, barley, rye berries, and amaranth. Non-GMO, but not organic.

4. Beans

☐ **Azuki beans, a.k.a. adzuki, aduki [Eden®]** — These small red beans are one of Japan's most popular beans. They're mashed into a sweet red bean paste and used as a filling in many sweet treats, including ice cream and Hawaiian shave ice. Azuki beans have

Coach Karen says

Due to varying antioxidant and arsenic levels in grains, vary the types of grains you eat. Make a point to include more varieties in your rotation.

Coach Karen says

Sprouted grain breads get moldy faster since they don't contain preservatives. Don't buy sprouted grain bread that's been sitting on a store shelf at room temperature.

Coach Karen says

Heat, humidity, and light are bad for bread, but good for fungi and mold. At home, push the air out of the bag, tie tightly, and double bag to stay fresher longer. Then freeze or refrigerate.

a mild, slightly sweet flavor and pair well with grains and are a great addition to any dish.

☐ **Black soybeans [Eden®]** — Black soybeans ("kuromame" in Japanese) are considered the 'Crown Prince' of beans in Japan. They're low in carbohydrates (11 gm), high in fiber (6 gm), and high in protein (11 gm) — nearly half the carbs and twice the amount of protein as regular black beans.

☐ **Caribbean Rice & Beans, Cajun Rice & Beans, Brown Rice & Green Lentils [Eden®]** — These three combos are made with organic short grain brown rice from Lundberg® and contain between about 210 calories and 190 to 220 mg sodium per cup.

Dried beans are an inexpensive source of protein and fiber. When you soak and cook your own, you're not paying for the can and the production process, but you're paying for the actual food. Roasted dried legumes make nutritious "nuts" for snacks, salads, and bowls (pg. 160).

☐ **Black or yellow soybeans. dried [Shiloh Farms®]** — Black soybeans contain more vitamin C and nearly twice the iron as the yellow soybeans.

☐ **13-Bean Soup Mix, dried [Bob's Red Mill®]** — No seasonings added, just 13 different dried beans, lentils, and split peas. Great for whipping up a 13-bean chili or vegetable soup.

5. Tofu

☐ **Tofu** — e.g., silken; soft; medium firm; firm; extra firm; super firm. Per the FDA, 94% of all soy grown in the U.S. is genetically engineered to be tolerant to herbicides and pesticides. GMO soy is predominantly used to make soybean oil and feed animals, so be sure to buy organic tofu.[2]

You'll find there are many brands and textures in your search for this nutritious, yet inexpensive, curd. **House Foods** and **365 Everyday Value®** are great places to start for making Eggless 'Egg' Salad (pg. 266). Tofu comes in solid white blocks of varying softness. If you're new to the tofu space and completely confused by all these options, choose firm — it's a good 'all-purpose' tofu. Firm soaks up flavors and holds up well when cooked. Also, the firmer the tofu, the more protein it contains. Check the expiration date to get the freshest tofu.

For making creamy Tofu Mayonnaise (pg. 281) and sauces, use **Mori-Nu®**. It's packaged in a 4" x 3" aseptic carton without water and needs no refrigeration until opened. **Azumaya®** makes a

16-oz "square" block of tofu, which makes 4 square servings of tofu that fit perfectly on a BLT (pg. 265). Other tofu brands are more rectangular in shape. House Foods makes a 16-oz size, but stores usually sell the 14-oz block.

6. Pasta

☐ **Protein pasta [Liviva™, Explore Cuisine®]** — These plant-based protein pasta brands contain 22 gm and 25 gm protein per 2-oz serving and have stellar carbohydrate to fiber ratios of 1.3-to-1 (17 gm fiber) and 1.7-to-1 (11 gm fiber) respectively.

7. Plant-Based Dairy

☐ **Cream cheese alternative, plain [Kite Hill®]** — This velvety non-dairy cream cheese is a plant-based option that contains 6 gm of fat (from almonds), no saturated fat, and no cholesterol per two tablespoons. Tastes great with Summer Fruit Bruschetta (pg. 235). It's not low in sodium though (200 mg per serving), so use lightly. Two tablespoons of regular dairy cream cheese is high in fat from milk and cream (12 gm), high in saturated fat (7 gm), and a source of cholesterol (35 mg) and sodium (130 mg).

☐ **Soy milk, unsweetened [Silk®]** — Unlike nut and oat milks, soy milk's protein content is similar to cow's milk with 7 gm of protein per cup. Non-GMO. Fortified with a vitamin and mineral blend. No added phosphates. Comes in unsweetened vanilla too.

☐ **Yogurt, almond milk Greek-style, plain or vanilla bean, unsweetened [Kite Hill®]** — Due to its live active cultures, this yogurt is a gut-healthy probiotic and doesn't fall short on protein like other plant-based types and brands. Has a healthy nutritional profile with 11 gm protein, 8 gm carbs, 4 gm fiber, and no added sugar or phosphates. Vanilla unsweetened is also available.

8. Seeds

☐ **Chia seeds, ground, organic [Spectrum®]**

☐ **Flaxseed, ground, organic, cold milled [Spectrum®]**

☐ **Hemp protein powder, "Hemp Yeah! Max Fiber" [Manitoba Harvest®]** — No sweeteners, sodium, oils, or fillers added! 130 calories, 14 gm carbs, 13 gm fiber, 13 gm protein.

☐ **Hemp seeds, a.k.a. hemp hearts, organic [Manitoba Harvest®]** — Manitoba Harvest tightly controls the planting, cultivation, packaging, and distribution of their hemp seeds.

Coach Karen says

Chia, flax, and hemp seeds are rich in omega-3 fats, which are prone to damage from heat, light, and air. Don't buy seeds sold in bulk or seeds packed from bulk bins. Store in your fridge or freezer.

Coach Karen says

Hemp seeds become darker in color as they age. They should be mostly white (less than 50% green on the seed), have a fresh nutty aroma, and taste nutty, somewhat herbal or grassy, not bitter. If they don't taste like much or smell like anything, that's a sign the seeds are old.

☐ **Sesame seeds, hulled, white or black, lightly toasted or raw** — Black sesame seeds are unhulled, while white sesame seeds (the inner part of the seed) have their hulls removed. Black sesame seeds are rich in BLUEs, lignans, and flavor. Available at Japanese grocery stores or in the Asian section of the supermarket.

☐ **Flax Seed Crackers [The Organic Pantry Co.]** — Imagine, a cracker that's healthy, tastes good, and meets the 5-to-1 ratio of carbs to fiber. In fact, its ratio is just over 2-to-1, which means nearly half the carbs are from fiber. Minimal sodium, no flour, and no oil. Ingredients: organic flax seeds, organic quinoa flakes, organic pumpkin seeds, organic sunflower seeds, pink Himalayan sea salt. Varieties include: Turmeric; Rosemary; Mexican Chili; and Sunflower that are handmade in small batches.

9. Nuts

☐ **Almond butter, organic, raw [MaraNatha®]** — Due to a string of salmonella outbreaks, a law was passed in 2007 requiring all almonds sold in the U.S. (both organic and conventionally grown) undergo pasteurization. Organic almonds sold as raw are 'washed' with steam, so technically, they're not "raw". The conventional method is chemical fumigation, where the almond surface is sprayed with a petrochemical called propylene oxide (PPO). The National Toxicology Program determined PPO as "reasonably anticipated to be a human carcinogen".[3] The use of PPO is prohibited on organic almonds, so opt for organic. The healthy fats in nuts are sensitive to heat. Roasting nuts at high temperatures also increases the formation of harmful levels of acrylamide, so raw almonds are best.

☐ **Black sesame seed butter, unhulled [Eden®]** — In Japan, black sesame is called 'kuro goma' and highly valued for its flavor and health benefits. Rich in BLUEs and lignans. Spread this seed butter on toast or crackers. Drizzle it on oatmeal and in smoothies or sauces.

☐ **Nut/seed butter, organic, "Power Fuel 7 Nut & Seed Butter" [Nuttzo®]** — Upgrade your stock of nut butters with this nut and seed combo.

☐ **Peanut butter, organic, light roasted [Santa Cruz Organic®]** — Contains 55 mg of sodium per two tablespoons. Choose light roasted over dark roasted. The healthy fats are sensitive to heat.

☐ **Tahini, unsweetened, salt free [Trader Joe's Organics]** — Creamy purée of roasted hulled sesame seeds.

10. Tea

☐ **Black iced tea, original, unsweetened [Tejava®]** — Green tea and hibiscus have more antioxidants than black tea, but to switch it up occasionally, here's one to try. This "Tea from Java" contains no sweeteners, but you won't feel the need to dump a packet of sugar in your glass. This ready-to-drink brewed black tea isn't bitter or strongly astringent like many black teas. Sold in 1-liter glass bottles.

☐ **Green tea, loose-leaf [Ippodo]** — These tea leaves are used to make freshly brewed tea. There is a wide variety of Japanese tea (about 20 different types), and there are literally hundreds of reputable Japanese green tea brands in Japan. One to try is Ippodo (Kyoto), which has been providing high quality tea since 1717. It is one of the most respected, prestigious tea producers in Japan, particularly appreciated by professional tea masters. China is one of the biggest exporters of tea producing nearly 85% of the green tea in the world. However, China's tea plants are grown in an area contaminated by heavy metals due to their excessive industrial pollution.[4] Consequently, their tea plants (even their "organic" teas) are contaminated with high amounts of lead as well as aluminum and manganese.[5]

Traditional Green Teas:

Gyokuro — Smoother, richer, mildly astringent. Literally means "Jewel/Jade Dew". Prized for its delicate flavor. Premium quality.

Sencha — Most popular (first harvest)

Bancha — Lower grade sencha (later/last harvests). Literally means "last tea".

Genmaicha — Bancha leaves + roasted popped brown rice

Hojicha — Roasted bancha leaves

Kukicha — Twig tea

Coach Karen says
A 100-gm bag of tea leaves (3.53 oz) makes 30-40 cups of tea.

☐ **Hibiscus berry herbal tea, organic [Whole Foods® Market]** — Hibiscus is abundant in REDs and BLUEs, specifically anthocyanins *(polyphenols)*. One six-week study found that drinking three cups of hibiscus tea daily significantly lowered blood pressure and had anti-cholesterol effects.[6, 7] In addition to organic hibiscus, ingredients include organic rose hip, licorice, dried orange peel, apple, strawberry, and raspberry.

☐ **Matcha [Ippodo, Marukyu Koyamaen]** — These two companies have been highly regarded tea growers in Kyoto, Japan for over 300 years. Matcha is literally 'powdered green tea'. It's a fine powder made from ground high-quality green tea leaves and is vibrant jewel green in color. When drinking matcha, in contrast to drinking steeped green tea, you are drinking the whole leaf and not just the brewed water from the leaves. Therefore, when drinking matcha, you're consuming 10 times the antioxidants, i.e., the health benefits in one cup of matcha is equivalent to 10 cups of green tea!

Matcha comes in three grades: *Ceremonial; Premium or In-Between; and Culinary, Cooking or Kitchen Grade.* A culinary grade matcha is too strong for drinking. It uses less delicate tea leaves since they're meant to be mixed with other ingredients to make desserts, cookies, cakes, smoothies, and lattes. In general, unopened matcha lasts for six months, but once opened, it's best used within one to two months as the flavor and aroma will deteriorate with time.

Matcha + Milk Hot and iced matcha lattes are the new stars alongside their brewed counterparts in popular coffeehouses. But a small study found that the dietary proteins in cow's milk (casein) and soy milk (soy protein) blunted the protective cardiovascular effects of the antioxidants (catechins), so it's best to drink your tea straight.[8]

EXTRAS

11. Spices, Herbs, and Flavorings

☐ **Cinnamon, Vietnamese (a.k.a. Saigon cinnamon)** — Vietnamese cinnamon is considered the very best cinnamon in the world in terms of flavor. Cassia (a.k.a. Chinese cinnamon), the All-American classic spice found in supermarkets, is more mellow. Sprinkle Vietnamese cinnamon on oatmeal or toast, bake with it, and add it to smoothies. It's rich in anti-inflammatory compounds, but don't eat it in large doses. In general, limit the consumption of cinnamon to no more than one teaspoon a day since it contains up to 1% of a blood thinner (coumarin), which is considered a relatively high concentration.[9]

☐ **Cocoa powder, 100% cocoa, unsweetened, natural, non-alkalized [Ghirardelli®]** — Cocoa processed with alkali (a.k.a. Dutch-processed) reduces its antioxidant content. See "Chocolate 101" (pg. 289).

☐ **Gochugaru, a.k.a. Korean-style red pepper [McCormick Gourmet™]** — Medium-hot Korean crushed chili pepper is ideal for kimchi-style vegetables as well as soups, stews, and spaghetti sauces. It's coarsely ground (kind of a cross between flakes and powder). Other brands are available at Asian grocery stores.

☐ **Herbs, freeze-dried [Litehouse®]**, e.g., basil; chives; cilantro; dill; garlic; ginger; jalapeño; mint; oregano; parsley; red onion; sage; spring onion; thyme

☐ **Herb blends, freeze-dried [Litehouse®]**, e.g., guacamole herb and spice; Italian herb; salad herb — The Italian herb blend (basil, oregano, garlic, red onions, red pepper, marjoram, rosemary, sage) is perfect for making a quick pasta sauce. Add the salad herb blend (parsley, red onion, chives, shallots, garlic, dill) to your favorite olive oil and balsamic for a fast and flavorful salad dressing.

Note: Litehouse bottled freeze-dried herbs can generally be found in the produce section.

☐ **Kala namak, a.k.a. Indian black salt** — Kala namak is an Indian volcanic rock salt that has a very distinctive sulfurous mineral taste. In eggless vegan dishes, Indian black salt adds an 'eggy' taste and aroma. Available at Indian grocery stores.

☐ **New Mexico ground chile** — This flavorful spice is a must-have for your favorite chili recipes. It's pure ground New Mexico chiles (seeds and pod), whereas chili powder contains other ingredients like oregano, paprika, pepper, cumin, garlic powder, onion powder, and/or salt.

☐ **Nutritional yeast seasoning [Bragg®]** — This nutritional yeast (nicknamed "nooch") comes in a convenient, 4.5-oz jar with a shaker top (pg. 282).

☐ **Vanilla, Mexican [Blue Cattle Truck Trading Co.®]** — This traditional Mexican Vanilla really stands out in the vanilla extract space. Take a whiff and compare!

Coach Karen says

Bragg's nutritional yeast is usually in the spice aisle of most grocery stores. Look on the bottom shelf.

12. Soup Stock

☐ **Vegetable broth, low-sodium, organic [Pacific Foods®]** — 120 mg sodium per cup. No added sugar or starches.

13. Sweeteners

☐ **Dates, Fancy Medjool** (pg. 47)

☐ **Date sugar, organic [Date Lady]** — Just pure dehydrated organic dates and no added oat flour. Sprinkle it on oatmeal with nuts or scatter it on muffins and baked apples.

☐ **Date syrup, organic [Date Lady]** — Date syrup (a.k.a. date honey, date molasses, and silan) has just one ingredient: organic dates. It's a concentrated source of nutrients and BROWNs. Squirt it in your homemade dressings, post-exercise drinks, cocoa, coffee, baked goods, and over pancakes instead of sugar or brown sugar.

14. Condiments

☐ **Ketchup, spicy, unsweetened, organic [Primal Kitchen®]** — Did you know that ketchup, the classic American condiment, is loaded with sugar? Yep, just one tablespoon of this concoction of puréed tomatoes contains one full teaspoon of sugar, not to mention 190 mg of sodium! That means, if you squirt a blob of ketchup next to your fries, one-third of it is refined sugar. But no worries, this ketchup is a healthier, zippy alternative that tastes great with zero added sugar and less salt (105 mg sodium).

☐ **Mustard powder, double superfine [Colman's®]** — Mix with a little water to make a fresh batch of prepared hot mustard. Great for spicing up potato salads, vinaigrettes, and your favorite dishes. Adds a kick! Ingredients: mustard flour.

☐ **Mustard, stoneground, organic, no salt added [Westbrae Natural®]** — Add zip to your sandwiches, dressings, and sauces without adding more sodium. Ingredients: organic grain vinegar, water, organic mustard seeds, organic spices.

☐ **Tabasco® sauce** — Hot sauces often contain sugar and salt, but good ol' Tabasco sauce contains just 35 mg sodium per teaspoon with no artificial ingredients.

15. Japanese Condiments and Flavorings

☐ **Curry powder [S&B®]** — Pure spice. Very authentic for making Japanese curry roux. Mild. No preservatives. Comes in a tin can, but put some in a glass spice jar to easily sprinkle on everything! Ingredients: **turmeric**, coriander, fenugreek, cumin, red pepper, black pepper, cinnamon, ginger, star anise, cloves, cardamon, fennel, nutmeg, laurel leaves, allspice, and garlic. Product of Japan.

☐ **Hoisin sauce, gluten-free [Premier Japan®]** — Hoisin ("HOY-sin") sauce is a staple in Chinese cuisine. It's a thick dark sauce made primarily with hefty amounts of sugar (up to 9 gm per tablespoon), soybean paste, salt (up to 545 mg sodium per tablespoon), sweet potato powder, corn starch, garlic, chili peppers, and coloring. But this sweet Asian sauce is a healthier version with 160 mg sodium and 2 gm sugar per tablespoon.

☐ **Kombu, sea vegetable [Eden®]** — Add a piece of this sea vegetable to beans or root vegetables for improved flavor (umami) and a softer texture. In many Japanese dishes, kombu ("KOHM-boo") is the key fundamental ingredient as well as the base of soup stock. According to Eden, all sea vegetables imported from Japan are multi-radionuclide tested both in the USA and in Japan.

☐ **Matcha, culinary grade [Maeda-en]** — Matcha ["maht-CHAH"] is literally 'powdered green tea'. It's a fine powder made from ground high-quality green tea leaves and is vibrant jewel green in color. This culinary grade matcha is used for adding a "green tea" flavor to your food. It uses less delicate tea leaves since they're meant to be mixed with other ingredients to make desserts, cookies, cakes, smoothies, and lattes. In general, unopened matcha lasts for six months, but once opened, it's best used within 2 to 3 weeks.

Coach Karen says

Matcha comes in three grades:

1) Ceremonial

2) Premium or

3) In-Between; and Culinary, Cooking or Kitchen Grade.

☐ **Mirin, rice cooking wine [Eden®]** —- This traditional Japanese-brewed cooking wine originated during the 15th century. Mirin ("mee-REEN") is an essential ingredient in Japanese cuisine, such as broths, marinades, sushi rice, and sauces. It's sweet and savory, but contains no sugar, corn syrup, molasses, or preservatives that are added to other brands. Eden mirin is made with California-grown Lundberg® organic short-grain brown rice. Product of Japan.

☐ **Miso, mellow white, organic [Miso Master®]** — Miso ("MEE-soh") is a probiotic paste made from fermented soybeans. White miso has a sweeter, milder taste compared to its yellow and red cousins. Use it to make light miso soups, sauces, and dressings (pg. 247) and to add a unique flavor to dishes. Less sodium per serving (310 mg per 2 tsp) compared to other brands. Non-GMO.

☐ **Ponzu sauce, five flavor seasoning [Eden®]** — Ponzu ("POHN-zoo") is a Japanese citrus-based soy dipping sauce with a medley of sweet, sour, tangy, salty, and savory flavors. A tasty alternative to traditional soy sauce or tamari as it contains less sodium per serving (340 mg sodium per tablespoon; 113 mg sodium per teaspoon). Use it for dipping noodles, cooked vegetables, tofu, and fish. Also add it to salad dressings.

□ **Sansho [S&B®]** — Sansho ("SAHN-sho"] is a Japanese citrus-y black pepper. Use this peppery-lemon flavor on sushi, noodles, and as you would black pepper.

□ **Shichimi togarashi [Yawataya Isogoro]** — Shichimi togarashi ("shee-CHEE-mee toh-gah-RAH-shee") literally means "seven-flavor chili pepper" in Japanese. It's a seasoning blend that commonly contains ground red chili pepper, sansho (ground Japanese citrusy pepper), roasted orange or mandarin peel, black and white sesame seeds, hemp seed, ground ginger, shiso (perilla), and nori (seaweed). It's usually sprinkled on hot noodle soup (udon or ramen) to add flavor, spiciness, and aroma, but can also be sprinkled on rice, sushi, grilled fish, and your favorite stir-fry.

□ **Tamari (Japanese soy sauce), 50% less sodium, "Tamari Lite" [San-J]** — Soy sauce and tamari ("tah-MAH-ree") are similar in color and flavor, but soy sauce is traditionally made with wheat, whereas tamari (which is specifically Japanese) is made with no wheat and has a smoother taste than soy sauce. Use a limited amount on occasion. Contains 490 mg sodium per tablespoon; 163 mg sodium per teaspoon. Non-GMO. When comparing with other soy sauces and liquid amino acids, be sure to check the serving size, so you're comparing apples to apples. Ponzu sauce is a less salty, yet flavorful, alternative to soy sauce.

□ **Wasabi powder [Dualspices]** — This wasabi ("wah-SAH-bee") is 100% pure Wasabia japonica (wasabi powder). Product of Japan. No artificial colorants and flavors, food starch, oil, sugar, sugar alcohol, salt, gum, or other fillers that are typically found in prepared wasabi pastes and powders. Just mix a couple teaspoons of wasabi powder with a teaspoon of water, mix, wait 15 minutes, and you have pure spicy wasabi. Japanese horseradish contains ally isothiocyanate (a.k.a. mustard oil), a phytochemical, that's responsible for the fiery heat that makes your sinuses explode and eyes water. Ally isothiocyanate, which is found in many cruciferous vegetables, is being examined as a cancer chemopreventive agent.[10]

□ **Yuzu sauce, hot [From Japan™]** — This yuzu ("YOO-zoo") sauce is a bright, lively hot, and fragrant Japanese condiment (150 mg sodium per teaspoon). The yuzu doesn't yield a lot of juice, that's why it's fairly expensive — but so worth it! Contains 150 mg sodium per teaspoon, so another reason to use sparingly, and savor every drop. Drizzle it on cold or steamed tofu, vegetables, seafood, you name it. It'll brighten and liven up any dish. Ingredients:

Coach Karen says

Yuzu is a unique, refreshing Asian citrus fruit that's tastes like a cross between a mandarin orange, Meyer lemon, and lime.

distilled vinegar, yuzu citrus pepper (yuzu zest, chili pepper, and salt), chili pepper, and sea salt.

☐ **Yuzu furikake, organic [From Japan™]** — Yuzu furikake ("foo-ree-KAH-keh") is a mixture of plant-based ingredients that include toasted white and black sesame seeds, dried yuzu citrus zest, nori flakes, and sea salt. Free of additives, sugar, MSG, and artificial flavors that are in traditional furikake. Lightly dust tofu, rice, grilled fish, noodle dishes, grilled veggies, and even salads lightly with this condiment. It adds a clean, light flavor. Contains some sodium (12 calories, 35 mg sodium per teaspoon).

16. Vinegars

☐ **"Sonomic Gold Almost Vinegar" [Sonoma Portworks]** — This "almost vinegar" is made with Muscat grapes and is sweet, tart, and rich. Sprinkle it on your salad, splash it in sparkling water, drizzle it on your vegetables, yogurt, and on fresh fruit for a refreshing dessert.

Coach Karen says

Authentic brown rice vinegar is considered a healthful food in Japan and served with almost every meal.

☐ **Balsamic, sweet cherry artisan vinegar [Lucini®]** — Love, love, love this balsamic. Infused with the juice of summer cherries. No sugar added. Rich in REDs and BLUEs (anthocyanins). Great on roasted Brussels sprouts and dark leafy greens — spinach, arugula, romaine, and kale! Lucini makes a savory fig version that's also naturally sweet. Drizzle it on grilled veggies, salmon, and salads.

☐ **Balsamic vinegar, white** — Unlike balsamic vinegar, white balsamic has a sweet, fruity, and subtle flavor. It has a clean color, so it won't turn your salad dressing or sauce brown. Great for brightening up vegetable dishes, roasted veggies (such as roasted Brussels sprouts), grilled fish, and salads.

☐ **Rice vinegar, brown, organic [Eden®]** — This vinegar is an excellent condiment sprinkled over vegetables and whole grains. It's sweet, smooth, and mellow in contrast to the sharpness associated with vinegar. Perfect on salads, for vinegar-ing sushi rice, and making dressings and sauces. Eden brown rice vinegar is made with California-grown Lundberg® organic short grain brown rice. Product of Japan.

☐ **Rice vinegar, organic [Marukan®]** — Not to be confused with "seasoned" Japanese rice vinegar, which contains sugar and salt. This brand does not contain added sugar and is made with organic rice from Lundberg®.

Coach Karen says

Konnyaku ("KOHN-yah-koo"), often referred to as a "yam", is a high-fiber Japanese root vegetable. It has a rubbery jelly-like texture, no flavor, and is usually cooked in a flavorful broth or used to make translucent, gelatinous noodles.

17. Flours

☐ **Glucomannan powder [Herbal Island]** — Glucomannan ("gloo-KOH-muh-nuhn") comes from the starchy root of the Asian konjac ("KOHN-jak") plant and is a healthy substitute for cornstarch. Glucomannan is a soluble dietary fiber, which makes it a natural thickener in soups, sauces, jams, and smoothies. Whisk it first in cold water, then combine with other ingredients. Use 1/2 to 1 teaspoon per one cup liquid. It's tasteless, odorless with 10 times the viscosity of cornstarch. Contains 4 gm carbs and 4 gm fiber per teaspoon. Cornstarch is pure starch with no fiber.

☐ **Almond flour, whole almonds with skins*, organic [Nuts. com]** — Not to be confused with almond flour ground from blanched, skinless almonds. The skins contain a variety of phytochemicals that have been associated with health benefits, including antioxidant, anti-microbial, anti-viral, neuroprotective, photoprotective, and prebiotic activities.[11, 12] Here's why you should always buy organic almonds and almond products (pg. 214).

☐ **Garbanzo bean (chickpea) flour [Bob's Red Mill®]**

☐ **Hazelnut flour [Bob's Red Mill®]**

☐ **Oat flour** — You can make your own oat flour by blending rolled oats in a food processor (1-1/4 cups of rolled oats will yield 1 cup of oat flour).

☐ **Walnut flour/meal* [Nuts.com]**

*Almond and walnut flours are especially low in carbohydrates and a good source of healthy fat, fiber and protein. These properties mean it won't spike your blood sugar and will keep you satisfied longer.

Flour Rankings

Flours with the lowest glycemic index (cause a slower and smaller rise in blood sugar levels.[13]

#1 - Walnut (lowest)

#2 - Almond

#3 - Ground flaxseed

#4 - Hazelnut

#5 - Soy

#6 - Chickpea, Oat (tied)

18. 100% Fruit Juice and Spreads

☐ **Fruit butters, Concord Grape and Tart Cherry [Eden®]**
— These organic fruit spreads are made with just the pure fruit
and nothing else. These deep-colored fruits are simmered with no
water, sugar, or additives, so they're loaded with concentrated doses
of REDs and BLUEs. Smear it on your toast, muffins, pancakes,
waffles, cookies (thumbprint-style), PB&Js, and add a dollop to
your oatmeal!

☐ **Fruit spread, organic, "Fiordifrutta" [Rigoni di Asiago®]** —
e.g., Wild Blueberries; Strawberries & Wild Strawberries. These
fruit spreads contain just organic berries, apple juice, and pectin.

☐ **Fruit juice [Lakewood®]** — These 100% organic vegetable
and fruit juices offer a variety of COLORS, e.g., pure cranberry,
Concord grape, pineapple, and pomegranate.[14] Bottled in glass, not
plastic. If you drink cranberry juice regularly or on occasion to help
ward off infections, avoid popular brands of cranberry juice that
add sugar, water, colorants, and/or contain a mix of different fruit
concentrates.

19. Extra Virgin Oils

☐ **Avocado oil, extra virgin [Avohass®]** — This rich, buttery,
emerald green oil is made from Grade A California organic
avocados. Whisk it with freshly squeezed citrus juices for a bright,
refreshing vinaigrette (pg. 253). Great for your hair and skin too!

☐ **Olive oil, extra virgin** — Select a high-quality olive oil that's
been tested and certified by the California Olive Oil Council
(COOC) at www.cooc.com or look for the NAOOA, USDA QMP,
PDO, or DOP seal. When it comes to olive oil, organic is best.

Coach Karen says

The avocado,
sometimes
referred to as
'vegetable butter'
or 'butter pear',
can contain up
to 30% oil. It
was originally
extracted for
cosmetic use
because it rapidly
absorbs and
penetrates into
the skin.

Coach Karen says

Unless an oil is
explicitly labeled
"extra virgin", it's
safe to assume is
it not extra virgin.

SHOPPING TIPS

HOW TO SELECT
THE BEST COOKING OIL

"Cold pressed", "first pressed", "first cold pressed", "expeller-pressed",
and "extra virgin" — what do these terms mean?! Unfortunately, these
buzzwords are often used for marketing and are enough to make your
head spin.

There are two factors that determine the quality of oil: 1) The method used to extract the oil and 2) How many times the fruit is pressed.

First pressed — This term means the fruit was pressed only once and yields oil of the highest quality and purity, but an oil labeled "first pressed" doesn't tell you if any heat was applied during the extraction process.

Cold pressed — This term means that no heat was applied to extract the oils. The fruit was crushed at temperatures that didn't exceed 80.6°F (so it's not actually cold). Even so, "cold pressed" doesn't tell you if the fruit was pressed more than once. Crushing the fruit multiple times and using heat are often used to extract more oil, but results in a lower quality oil because healthy fats are very sensitive to heat, light, and air. These elements can alter and destroy the oil's flavors and aromas.

Coach Karen says

A cooking oil cannot be "extra virgin" if it is not first cold pressed.

First cold pressed (not an official designation for oil) — First cold pressed oils have the most flavor, aroma, nutrition, and antioxidants, so they are more expensive. The term means the fruit was crushed just one time at a temperature that didn't exceed 80.6°F. Use these oils as a finishing oil, such as over a salad or cooked vegetables.

Expeller-pressed — This term means the oil was squeezed from the fruit through a barrel-like cavity by using friction and continuous pressure. No chemical solvents are used. This process can produce higher temperatures (140°F to 210°F), even if there isn't any direct heat applied during the processing.

Refined — Refined oils are subjected to high heat and/or chemicals to extract the oil. Agents that bleach and deodorize the oils may also be used. In the edible oil industry, hexane (a chemical extracted from petroleum and crude oil) is one of the most commonly used solvents to extract oils from plants. Avoid "RBD oils" (Refined, Bleached, Deodorized).

Pure — Pure is the code word for refined. For example, refined avocado oil is often marketed as "100% pure" or simply as "avocado oil".

Extra virgin — For an olive oil to be "officially" certified extra virgin, it must be extracted using first cold pressing in accordance to the standards established by the International Olive Council or the California Olive Oil Council.

Blend — Many oils on the market are a blend of extra virgin oil and refined oil. Blending the two oils is an inexpensive way to add a little flavor and color to an otherwise flavorless oil.

Organic — Organic oils are not genetically modified or subject to pesticides. Pests, diseases, and the presence of weeds make it necessary to apply pesticides, fungicides, and herbicides. But residues can persist on **olives** and make their way into the oil. Widely used fat-soluble pesticides (organophosphates) tend to concentrate in the oil and contaminate the oil produced.[15] **Avocados** contain the least pesticides of any common produce item due to their thick peel.

Ensuring Extra Virginity

Unfortunately, being **extra virgin (first cold pressed) does not ensure high quality**. For example, some producers may use poor quality olives, use chemicals or extreme heat during the extraction process, or dilute the oil with lower grade oils and/or refined olive oil. Also, the olives used may have been damaged by poor handling, mold, frost, or by not being milled within 24 hours of being harvested. Poor quality oils might taste greasy, bland (totally flat), unpleasant, or smell rancid.

The Olive Oil Police

By purchasing olive oil with the California Olive Oil Council (COOC) seal, you can be assured that the oil has undergone rigorous testing, and the oil is a top quality% extra virgin olive oil that's made in California. Also look for the North American Olive Oil Association (NAOOA) and the USDA Quality Monitoring Program (QMP) seal for assurance that the oil is pure and authentic. Like European oils? Look for the Protected Designation of Origin (PDO, or DOP in Italian) seal.

> **Coach Karen says**
>
> Organophosphates include glyphosate, an active ingredient in Roundup® branded herbicides, which IARC upgraded to a 2A carcinogen (a probable carcinogen).

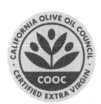
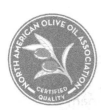
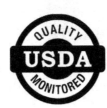
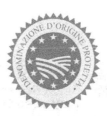

THE BEST (AND WORST) OILS TO BUY

★ ★ ★ ★ Organic 3-Star oil
(Organic oils are
not genetically
modified or subject
to pesticides.)

★ ★ ★ ☆ Extra virgin oil (Olive
oils with the COOC,
NAOOA, or QMP, PDO,
or DOP seal.)

★ ★ ☆ ☆ Expeller-pressed oil

★ ☆ ☆ ☆ Blended oil

☆ ☆ ☆ ☆ Refined oil

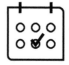

Purchase oil in **dark-colored glass** to protect the oil from exposure to sunlight. Non-reactive metal containers, such as **stainless steel** and **tin**, also help protect the oils from oxidizing. Avoid oils sold in plastic containers. Don't buy oils sold on the top shelf, where they're exposed to direct light.

57° **Store Oils Properly**
Be sure the oils are kept tightly sealed. The ideal temperature for storing oils is **57°F**, so a cool, dark pantry is best. Do NOT store oil next to the stove. Date when the oil was opened, and use it up within 6 months.

Know the Harvest Date
Extra virgin olive oil is best used within **18 months** from harvest. Some expiration dates are labeled with a 2- or 3-year expiration date, so it's important to know the harvest date.

HOW TO SELECT THE HEALTHIEST RICE
Since rice spends so much time growing in flooded areas, they absorb more arsenic than many other whole foods.

Tip #1: Know that organic does not mean arsenic-free. Organically grown rice takes up as much arsenic as conventionally grown rice since the metal is present in the soil and water. See "Cooking Tips to Reduce Arsenic in Rice" (pg. 257).

Tip #2: Check where the rice was grown. California rices contain significantly less arsenic than rice grown in Arkansas, Louisiana, and Texas. White rice from California has 38% less inorganic arsenic than white rices from other parts of the country. On average, brown rice has 80% more arsenic than white rice, but brown basmati from California,

India, or Pakistan has 33% less arsenic than other brown rices.[1] According to Lundberg®, their rice in the 1-lb, 2-lb, and 12-lb packages (except wild rice) comes from California.

Tip #3: Choose growers that are routinely testing for arsenic and are transparent about their growing practices. Lundberg tests their brown rice for arsenic and posts their results on their website.

Tip #4: Buy COLOR-ful rices and benefit from the various antioxidants. Look for brown, black, and red rice. They not only have different nutritional profiles, their flavors and textures vary too.

Tip #5: Rotate in other types of intact grains. By just switching up the grains, you can transform a single recipe into an entirely new dish. Different varieties of grains contain different amounts of arsenic:

- **Grains with negligible levels of arsenic:** amaranth, buckwheat, millet, polenta or grits, wild rice
- **Grains with very little arsenic:** barley, bulgur, and farro
- **Grains with average arsenic levels:** quinoa[1]

 TRY THESE REAL FOOD RECIPES!

Hibiscus Berry Tea pg. 244
Two-Minute Pizza Sauce pg. 283

PLAY 29 — REAL FOOD RECIPES FOR LONGEVITY JOCKS

Y ou don't cook – you have better things to do. Why sweat over a hot stove when you could be cooking up plans to play golf? Or master slicing on the tennis court? Or warming up the sofa with your favorite sports channel? Here's why. You feel sluggish, have high cholesterol, high blood pressure, or carry one spare tire too many. Or you just need a change from the same old burger and take-out. Honestly though, you crave a decent home-cooked meal.

Still not worth crying over onions and a sink full of dishes, you say? It *is* with the right tools, tips and recipes. *Athletes in Aprons* recipes will inspire you to fire up some homemade healthy fuel in record-breaking time. Whether you're a rookie cook or a veteran chowhound, these recipes are spoken in a language that great sports minds can comprehend.

Athletes in Aprons meals not only taste darn good, but will boost your energy, bolster your immune system, and help keep your ticker ticking. So get off the bench, suit up (that is, get on your apron), and hit the kitchen!

The Kickoff — Astounding Starters

Breakfasts Without Boxes — Fast Breaks

The 7th Inning Stretch — Snacks with Benefits

The End Zone — Fantastic Finishes

THE SIMPLEST WAY TO REMOVE PESTICIDE RESIDUES

Eating organic produce dramatically reduces your dietary exposure to pesticides, but does not eliminate it. Soak your fruits and vegetables for 12-15 minutes in a baking soda solution in these proportions:

• 1 teaspoon baking soda to 2 cups water

• 1 tablespoon baking soda to 6 cups water
(for larger batches).[1]

This is the most economical method compared to soaking in full-strength vinegar or a 10% salt solution — methods that have also been proven to be effective. Commercial produce washes tested to be no more effective than cleaning with plain tap water.

Don't forget to rub and scrub! The mechanical action of scrubbing with a vegetable brush under tap water helps remove pesticide residues. Also, rubbing dry with a clean dish towel or paper towel removes any remaining residues..

Coach Karen says

Wash produce just before you eat it (except berries). Any moisture left on them can harbor bacteria and speed spoilage. See "Keep the Fuzz Off Fresh Berries" on pg. 294.

CHOCOLATE HUMMUS
Makes 8 servings

Here's a chocolaty twist on traditional hummus. It's packed full of flavor, fiber, and BROWNs. Smear it on sliced apples, bananas, strawberries, celery sticks, and whole grain crackers for a high-protein satisfying snack.

The Line-Up

1 (15.5-oz) can chickpeas, drained

3 Fancy Medjool dates*

1/4 cup natural 100% unsweetened cocoa powder*

3 tablespoons organic date syrup*

1/3 cup, natural peanut butter*

1/2 teaspoon Hawaiian sea salt

Coach Karen says

Chill your chocolate hummus overnight, and enjoy it frosted on your favorite cupcake!

1/4 teaspoon vanilla*

1/4 cup water (up to 1/2 cup if needed)

*Coach Karen's First-Round Picks on pg. 206.

The Play-by-Play

1. Combine all ingredients in a food processor. Add 1/4 cup of water and blend. Increase the water to attain a smooth, creamy consistency.

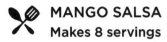 **MANGO SALSA**
Makes 8 servings

Mangos are filled with nutritious goodness, flavor, and ORANGEs. This succulent, aromatic fruit makes the A-list of anti-aging foods. Mango salsa is a refreshing topping for just about anything — from fish to home-baked chips. Combine it with your favorite guacamole, an amazingly healthy superfood that's rich in fiber, healthy fats, and GREENs, for a tropical 'creamy' salsa.

Coach Karen says

Look for honey mangos that have some 'wrinkling' on the outside. They may look like they're older, but that's when they are sweet, creamy in texture, and ripe!

The Line-Up

4 honey mangos (a.k.a. Manila or Ataulfo Mango)

1/4 of 1 small fresh pineapple

3/4 of 1 large red bell pepper

1/16 of 1 jalapeño (to taste)

1/2 cup cilantro

1/4 cup red onion

Juice from 1 lemon

Juice from 1 lime

The Play-by-Play

1. Dice all the ingredients and squeeze the fresh juice over them. Mix well to combine all the flavors. Chill.

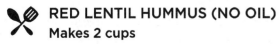 **RED LENTIL HUMMUS (NO OIL)**
Makes 2 cups

Red lentil hummus has everything you love about traditional chickpea hummus, but it's made with red lentils that are naturally sweet and nutty. Better yet, this take on a popular Middle Eastern dip and spread contains no added oil. When red lentils are cooked, they break down into a purée and make the perfect creamy base for dunking veggies, dipping crackers, spreading on sandwiches, or topping off a bowl of greenery. This recipe is simple to make and addictive with its bright, fresh flavor.

The Line-Up

1 cup red lentils (they're actually orange), uncooked

2 cups water

3 tablespoons tahini*

5 garlic cloves

2 tablespoons + 1 teaspoon lemon juice

1/2 tsp cumin

Cayenne (to taste)

Freshly ground pepper

Smoked paprika

Hawaiian sea salt (optional)

*Coach Karen's First-Round Picks on pg. 214.

The Play-by-Play

1. Sort out any discolored lentils. Rinse them in a strainer under cool running water. Place lentils and water in a saucepan, partially cover the pot, and bring to a boil. Reduce heat to low, and keep partially covered. Simmer for 20 minutes until lentils are tender and most of the water is absorbed. The lentils will "melt" into a purée. Let cool, or place in the refrigerator overnight.

2. Add garlic cloves and tahini to a small food processor. Add cooled lentils. Pulse until well blended. Add lemon juice, cumin, cayenne, black pepper, and sea salt. Adjust seasonings to taste. (Adding more lemon juice will brighten up the flavors.) Blend until smooth.

Pour hummus into a serving bowl, and dust with smoked paprika. Serve with COLOR-ful vegetables and Sprouted Grain 'Crackers' (pg. 293).

Coach Karen says

Eat lentils with foods high in vitamin C, such as bell peppers, to increase iron absorption. Lentils are an excellent source of iron.

SUMMER FRUIT BRUSCHETTA
Makes 8 servings

This sweet summery treat is the perfect pre-game snack — one you can whip up in minutes. It's a fresh tasting, super delicious blend of ORANGEs, REDs, and GREENs that'll keep you going back for more.

The Line-Up

10 organic strawberries, diced

3-1/2 ripe organic nectarines, diced

1 cup fresh basil leaves, chopped

2 tablespoon cherry balsamic vinegar*

1 (8-oz) tub of plain cream cheese alternative*

1 tablespoon + 1 teaspoon tart cherry butter*

1 box flax seed crackers* with sunflower seeds

*Coach Karen's First-Round Picks on pg. 206.

The Play-by-Play

1. Combine fruit and basil in a medium-sized bowl. Drizzle with cherry balsamic and combine well.

2. Stir the tart cherry butter into the cream cheese (optional). Smear the cream cheese on a cracker. Using a slotted spoon, place the fruit mixture on each cracker and enjoy!

Coach Karen says

If you can't wait until summer to eat this, use frozen organic strawberries and peaches while you wait.

BREAKFASTS WITHOUT BOXES — FAST BREAKS

 ## GRILLED OATMEAL WITH FRESH FRUIT 'N NUTS
Makes 9 servings

Take your oatmeal out of the bowl and into a form that's portable and finger lickin' good!

The Line-Up

1-1/2 cups steel-cut oats

2 cups soy milk*

2 cups water

Coach Karen says

For a quick fix, swap out the fresh fruit with organic 100% fruit spread or fruit butter.

Coach Karen says

Date sugar is just dehydrated dates ground into a sugar-like consistency. It's naturally sweet with a caramel-like flavor and looks like brown sugar.

1/4 cup organic date sugar*

Extra virgin avocado or olive oil*

Toppings: natural nut butter* or yogurt*, fresh fruit

*Coach Karen's First-Round Picks on pg. 206.

The Play-by-Play

1. Bring the oats, milk, water, oats, and date sugar to a boil in a large saucepan. Reduce heat to medium-low. Simmer for about 20 minutes. Stir often to prevent scorching and bubbling over.

2. Using a non-aerosol oil sprayer**, lightly mist an 8" x 8" pan with extra virgin oil. Pour oatmeal into the pan. Press down the oatmeal, and smooth it out into an even layer. Let cool in the fridge overnight — or cool quickly in the freezer. Just don't forget about it, and let it freeze! Slice the cooled oatmeal into 9 squares.

3. Heat a skillet over medium heat (300°F). Lightly mist it with oil using a non-aerosol oil sprayer** (1/4 teaspoon oil per trigger pull). Place a square of oatmeal into the heated pan. Gently press it down with a spatula. Cook until golden brown and heated through (about 5 minutes on each side).

Top with nut butter or yogurt and fresh fruit, like sliced or diced strawberries, raspberries, bananas, and nectarines.

**Coach Karen's Cool Tools on pg. 196.

PEPITAS VS PUMPKIN SEEDS

The term pepita is sometimes used interchangeably with pumpkin seed, but the two seeds are different. Pumpkin seeds are the thick white, oval-shaped seeds that you dig out of a pumpkin when making a jack-o-lantern. These whole seeds can be roasted and eaten with the white hull still on. Pepitas are the green seeds inside the hull, so they refer to the pumpkin seed with its hull removed. They actually come from specific types of pumpkins that contain these green ready-to-eat hulless seeds.

(continued on next page)

(continued from previous page)

Pepitas become more crisp and nuttier tasting when toasted. They add "crunch" to your foods and are a good source of protein, iron, and vitamin K. To toast them, place raw pepitas in a dry skillet over medium heat until they jump around a bit in the pan and puff up. It happens really fast (about 2 minutes), so keep both eyeballs on your pepitas — not on the sports channel. Remove the toasted seeds immediately from the heated skillet, so they don't get scorched. Set aside to cool.

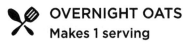 OVERNIGHT OATS
Makes 1 serving

Preparing oatmeal couldn't be easier! No cooking required. Oats make the perfect high-fiber, nutritious, and stick-to-your-ribs, grab 'n go meal. Instead of cooking your groats, just dump in some liquid and crunchy add-ins. Let them sit in the fridge overnight, and in the morning, toss in some flaxseeds and berries, and you're on your way to start your day!

The Line-Up

1/2 cup organic unsweetened soy milk*

1/3 cup old-fashioned rolled oats

1/4 cup of blueberries, fresh or frozen

1 tablespoon organic raisins

1 tablespoon dried or freeze-dried unsweetened organic cherries*

1 tablespoon pepitas, toasted

1 tablespoon organic ground golden flaxseed*

8-9 raw almonds, cut roughly into slivers

Optional: ground cinnamon*

*Coach Karen's First-Round Picks on pg. 206.

The Play-by-Play

1. Toast pepitas and cool.

2. Combine oats with raisins, cherries, almonds, and toasted pepitas in a bowl. Add milk, and stir thoroughly until all the ingredients are combined. Cover the bowl, and refrigerate overnight.

The next day, add the fresh or frozen blueberries and flaxseeds. Stir and serve. No cooking required...*really!*

Simple Substitutes

Chopped raw hazelnuts for almonds

Raw sunflower seeds for toasted pepitas

Organic natural dried blueberries for dried tart cherries

Chia seeds for the ground flaxseed

Fresh or frozen blackberries and/or raspberries for blueberries

Goji berries for unsweetened dried (tart) cherries

Chopped dates for the raisins

Chopped raw hazelnuts for raw almonds

One tablespoon almond butter for the raw almonds

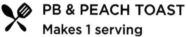 ### PB & PEACH TOAST
Makes 1 serving

Roasting fruit brings out their natural juices and sweetness. Enjoy them on your morning toast layered with your favorite nut butter and cinnamon for an easy-to-assemble breakfast or pre-game snack.

Coach Karen says

If fresh peaches are out of season, you can use defrosted frozen peaches instead.

The Line-Up

1 medium peach, pit removed and sliced in half

1 slice sprouted whole grain bread*, lightly toasted

1 tablespoon organic natural creamy peanut butter*

Organic date sugar* (optional)

8 to 9 raw almonds, chopped

Pinch ground cinnamon*

*Coach Karen's First-Round Picks on pg. 206.

The Play-by-Play

1. Preheat toaster oven to 325°F.

2. Place peach cut side up on a baking sheet. (Lining the pan with parchment paper will prevent sticking.) Bake peach for 5-10 minutes until softened, then slice.

3. Lightly spread toasted bread with peanut butter. Sprinkle toast lightly with date sugar (optional), then press chopped almonds into the peanut butter. Layer sliced peaches on top and dust with cinnamon.

 ### STEELY PROTEIN OATS
Makes 7 servings

Here's a way to beef up your morning oats — a textured blend of both steel-cut and rolled oats. Adding tofu, fruit, sunflower seeds, and flaxseed balance this bowl with high-fiber carbs, protein, and healthy fats that'll stick with you all morning.

The Line-Up

1 (14-oz) block of organic firm tofu*

3 cups water

1/2 cup steel-cut oats

1/2 cup of "old-fashioned" rolled oats

1/2 cup raisins

1/2 cup water or soy milk*

1-1/2 medium banana, sliced into small pieces

1/3 cup raw sunflower seeds, toasted

1-1/2 tablespoons ground flaxseed*

1 teaspoon ground cinnamon* (more if desired)

3/4 teaspoon vanilla* (more if desired)

*Coach Karen's First-Round Picks on pg. 206.

Coach Karen says

Refrigerate your cooked oats overnight. When oats are cooked and cooled, the carbohydrate resists digestion and won't raise glucose (a.k.a. resistant starch). Perfect for controlling blood sugar.[2]

The Play-by-Play

1. Let tofu stand on a plate to drain excess water. (No pressing is necessary.)

2. Bring 1-1/2 cups water to a boil in a saucepan. Add steel-cut oats. Reduce heat to medium-low. Cook for 10-15 minutes (longer for a creamier oatmeal), stirring often to prevent scorching.

3. Add 1-1/2 cups water to the partially cooked steel-cut oats, bring to a boil. Stir in rolled oats. Reduce heat to medium-low. Stir often for about 10-15 minutes (longer for a creamier oatmeal) to prevent scorching. Remove from heat.

4. Add the drained tofu to a bowl and mash. Add the vanilla and cinnamon, and blend together. Add tofu mixture and 1/2 cup water or soy milk to the cooked oatmeal. Stir constantly on medium-low for several minutes to warm up the tofu. Add chopped banana, raisins, sunflower seeds, flaxseed, and more cinnamon to taste. Mix well.

Serve hot or cold. Top with fresh berries.

HOW TO MAKE YOUR SMOOTHIES CREAMY

Thick, ice-cream like smoothies not only have more staying power, they're fun to make. Unlike a McD's milk shake (sugar, cream, corn syrup, and cream in a cup) that can leave you craving more food, here are a dozen anti-inflammatory ingredients that'll create a satisfying, frosty, rich smoothie.

- Avocado

- Chia seeds

- Flaxseeds

- Flour — almond, chickpea (garbanzo bean), oat, soy, walnut

- Frozen fruit

- Nut and seed butters

- Psyllium husk

- Quinoa

- Rolled oats (dry)

- Tofu

- Vegetable purées — e.g., cooked pumpkin, sweet potato, kabocha

- Yogurt

 ### CHOCOLATE RECOVERY MILK
Makes 1 serving

This version of chocolate milk is an excellent source of fluid, carbohydrate, protein, and essential vitamins and minerals, which makes it an effective post-exercise thirst quencher. Unlike commercial chocolate milk, it contains an ideal balance of macronutrients without refined sugars, oils, salt, phosphates, and growth hormones and without raising insulin-like growth factor-1, which is associated with several common cancers.

The Line-Up

1 cup organic unsweetened soy milk*

Coach Karen says

Drink Chocolate Recovery Milk 5 to 60 minutes after exercise, particularly following heavy strength training aimed to increase lean body mass and muscle growth.

1-1/2 tablespoons natural 100% unsweetened cocoa powder*

2 tablespoons Date Paste (pg. 280)

*Coach Karen's First-Round Picks on pg. 206.

The Play-by-Play

1. Combine all ingredients in a blender bottle (shaker cup with a stainless steel ball).

2. Shake well.

Serve immediately.

CAFFEINE BUZZ

Natural 100% cocoa powder contains high levels of BROWNs (flavonols) and some caffeine. Here's how it compares with other brews and bars:

- Natural 100% cocoa powder, 1 tablespoon = 12 mg caffeine
- Coffee, 8 oz = 100-175 mg caffeine
- Chocolate bar, 1.5 oz:
  - 90% cacao = 75 to 85 mg
  - 80% cacao = 68 mg
  - 70% cacao = 60 mg
- Green tea, 8 oz = 20 to 30 mg caffeine

CITRUS MANGO COOLER
Makes 3 servings

Chill out with a cool glass of blended COLORS! This slushy tropical drink is perfect for parties or post-exercise.

The Line-Up

2 cups frozen mango chunks/slices — or about 4 fresh Honey mangos (originally called Ataulfo mangos)

2 large juicy oranges

2 juicy limes

1 juicy lemons

6 fresh strawberries

1/2 cup of ice cubes/crushed ice

The Play-By-Play

1. Cut mango and put in blender. Remove stems on 3 strawberries and add to blender.

2. Freshly squeeze juice from fruits to make:

   - 3/4 cup orange juice

   - 1/4 cup lemon juice

   - 1/4 cup lime juice

3. Add fruit juices and ice to blender. Blend until smooth.

Divide among three frosted glasses garnished with a slice of lime and strawberry on the rim.

 ### COCOA ALMOND MILKSHAKE
Makes 2-3 servings

Here's a great way to enjoy the taste and benefits of chocolate without the added cocoa butter and sugar. This smoothie calls for 100% unsweetened cocoa powder, but the dates, bananas, and date syrup give it a whole food natural sweetness.

The Line-Up

1 serving of Five-Minute Almond Milk (pg. 244)

1/4 teaspoon vanilla*

2 small frozen bananas

3 tablespoons natural 100% unsweetened cocoa powder*

2 tablespoons organic almond butter*

1/4 teaspoon organic date syrup*

1-2 handfuls ice (optional)

*Coach Karen's First-Round Picks on pg. 206.

The Play-By-Play

1. Place all ingredients (except frozen bananas and ice) in a blender or food processor. Blend thoroughly. Add the frozen bananas, and blend *just until smooth*. Add ice to add more

Coach Karen says

The ice crystals in the frozen bananas give it the "creaminess". If you blend too long, the consistency will become more watery. If you'd like to eat it with a spoon (like an ultra thick milkshake), don't add any ice, and don't over-blend.

Coach Karen says

To freeze several bananas, slice them into 1" pieces, and set them on a parchment-lined baking sheet. Place in the freezer for at least 25 minutes. Then store in a freezer bag or glass container until you have a shake craving!

'slurriness' and volume. The ice will also chill it into a cold frosty shake.

Eat immediately or freeze in individual serving cups for a frozen snack/dessert.

 ### FIVE-MINUTE ALMOND MILK
Makes 1 serving

Making your own nut milk is a process — soaking nuts overnight, draining, rinsing, grinding, and straining. But you're out of milk *now*. Here's a quick solution for milking up your cereal, pancake batter, milkshakes, etc.

The Line-Up

1 cup purified water

1 dried organic Fancy Medjool date*, chopped

1/4 cup organic almond flour*

1/4 teaspoon vanilla*

*Coach Karen's First-Round Picks on pg. 206.

The Play-by-Play

1. Add chopped date and water in blender. Let stand for 5 minutes to soften. Add almond flour and vanilla. Blend thoroughly. Check to be sure the date is completely processed.

Chill and serve.

 ### HIBISCUS BERRY TEA
Makes 6 servings

Hibiscus tea is delicious and rich in powerful REDs and BLUEs, and the pomegranate juice and raspberries amp them up even more. Studies show hibiscus tea may be a safe and natural way to help lower blood pressure and significantly improve lipid profiles (decrease in total cholesterol, LDLs, and triglycerides and increase in HDL cholesterol).[3, 4] Include one cup of hibiscus tea as part of your daily beverages. Cheers!

The Line-Up

4 hibiscus tea bags*

3 cups purified water

1 cup organic 100% pomegranate juice*

12 half-round orange slices from an unpeeled organic orange

Garnish: 18 to 24 raspberries (about 1/2 cup), fresh or frozen

For a Single Serving

1 hibiscus tea bag*

3/4 cups purified water

1/4 cup organic 100% pomegranate juice*

2 half-round orange slices from an unpeeled organic orange

Garnish: 3 to 4 organic raspberries, fresh or frozen

*Coach Karen's First-Round Picks on pg. 206.

The Play-by-Play

1. Bring water to a boil in a medium saucepan. (For a single serving, you can microwave the water in a glass 2-cup measuring cup.) Add the juice, orange slices, and tea bags. Cover and steep for 6 minutes.

Drop one orange slice and 3 to 4 raspberries into each glass. Pour in the tea. Serve warm or chilled.

THE ANTI-AGING DENTAL DIET

Acidic foods, such as the following, soften precious tooth enamel:

- Alcoholic beverages (beer, liquor, mixed drinks, wine)
- Citrus fruits (including water or tea with lemon)
- Cranberry juice
- Grapes
- Hibiscus tea
- Pineapple
- Pomegranate juice
- Soda (Coca-Cola® is more acidic than vinegar.)

(continued on next page)

(continued from previous page)

- Sugar
- Tomatoes and tomato products
- Vinegar (including salad dressings, pickles, sauerkraut)

You may have been raised to "brush after every meal", but this is where you can relax that rule a bit. The abrasiveness of brushing when your enamel is 'soft' can further damage your enamel. Instead, rinse with tap water to wash away some of the acid, then wait at least 30-60 minutes before brushing. Saliva helps to restore the pH balance.

Pair vegetables, nuts, and whole grains with acids. These fibrous foods act like little toothbrushes, increase saliva production, and increase chewing, which help to keep your teeth and gums healthy. Add intact grains, crunchy veggies (like bell peppers, broccoli, carrots, cauliflower, celery, and radishes), and nuts to your salads dressed with vinaigrette.

MANGO BERRY FREEZE
Makes 3 servings

Chill out with a glass of ORANGEs, BLUEs, and a healthy dose of vitamin C (an antioxidant). An analysis of over 13,000 older men and women (aged 42 to 82 years old) found that those with adequate blood levels of vitamin C had an average of 1.6% to 3.4% more muscle mass, respectively, than those with lower levels of the vitamin.[6]

The Line-Up

2 cups frozen mango chunks

1/2 cup frozen wild blueberries

2 medium oranges, fresh squeezed juice

1/2 lemon, fresh squeezed juice

2 tablespoons chia seeds*

1/2 cup seltzer water

1/2 cup ice

The Play-by-Play

1. Blend all ingredients in a blender until combined and thick.

Serve immediately.

 ## WATERMELON ICE
Makes 6 servings

This 'snow cone in a cup' is *soooo* refreshing, while being full of REDs (particularly lycopene) and ORANGEs. Not an ounce of sugar is added — contains just the natural sweetness of the fruit, the cool effect of the mint, and zesty lime.

The Line-Up

9 heaping cups watermelon, cut in chunks

1 Honey mango (originally called Ataulfo mango)

2-3 sprigs fresh mint leaves

1/2 cup fresh squeezed juice (about 2 to 3 limes)

Lime zest from 1 lime

The Play-by-Play

1. Combine all the ingredients in a blender, and mix well. Divide into individual cups. Freeze until slushy.

Serve immediately.

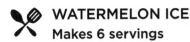 **GREAT GREENS — SALADS AND SALAD DRESSINGS**

LEMON DILL POTATO SALAD
Makes 8 servings

Potato salad is synonymous with gobs of mayo, but this version is full of flavor and bound without fat.

The Line-Up

2 pounds baby red potatoes, unpeeled, diced into bite-sized pieces

1 Fuji apple, unpeeled, diced

2 tablespoons freshly squeezed lemon juice

Coach Karen says

Refrigerate cooked potatoes or potato salad overnight. When potatoes are cooked and cooled, the carbohydrate resists digestion and won't raise glucose (a.k.a. resistant starch). Perfect for controlling blood sugar.[10]

1/2 cup small red bell pepper, diced

1/2 cup small red onion, diced

2-3 stalks green onions, sliced

Smoked or sweet paprika

Creamy Lemon Dill Vinaigrette (pg. 248)

The Play-by-Play

1. Fill a large pot with about 2 inches of water. Place a steamer basket inside the pot, add potatoes. Cover and bring water to a boil. Turn heat down, and simmer on low until potatoes are soft and tender, and a fork pierces easily though them, about 25-30 minutes. Cool. Place cooked potatoes in the fridge for faster cooling.

2. Add diced apple, bell pepper, red onion, and green onions to large mixing bowl, and mix together. (Save some green onions for garnish.) Stir in cooled potatoes.

3. Pour vinaigrette over the potato mixture. Mix gently until completed coated. (If you have extra dressing, save it for steamed veggies and salads.)

Garnish with sprinkling of paprika and green onions, then serve.

Coach Karen says

Add potato salad to a bowl of leafy greens, steamed veggies (such as broccolini, asparagus), avocado, and grilled tofu. Drizzle with extra dressing. Top with a dollop of tofu mayo.

 ## 'CREAMY' LEMON DILL VINAIGRETTE
Makes 1 cup

The Line-Up

1/2 cup Tofu Mayonnaise (pg. 281)

3 tablespoons organic rice vinegar* (Not to be confused with "seasoned" rice vinegar that contains sugar and salt.)

3 tablespoons balsamic vinegar

2 tablespoons freshly squeezed lemon juice

1 tablespoon Dijon mustard

2 tablespoons freeze-dried dill* (or 2 tablespoons fresh, chopped)

1 large shallot, minced

2-3 cloves garlic, minced

*Coach Karen's First-Round Picks on pg. 206.

Coach Karen says

Try Eden® "brown" rice vinegar. It's sweet, smooth, and mellow in contrast to the sharpness associated with vinegar.

The Play-by-Play

Whisk ingredients in a small bowl and serve.

MAPLE MUSTARD VINAIGRETTE
Makes ~1/2 cup

This is an absolutely delicious dressing — a team favorite. The savory fig balsamic vinegar is a *must-have*. This vinaigrette pairs well with any leafy green, but it's a grand slam when drizzled on baby kale and arugula.

The Line-Up

3 tablespoons extra virgin olive oil*

3 tablespoons savory fig balsamic vinegar*

3 teaspoons organic amber maple syrup

1-1/2 teaspoons organic stoneground mustard*

3/4 teaspoon sea salt

3/8 teaspoon freshly ground black pepper

*Coach Karen's First-Round Picks on pg. 206.

The Play-by-Play

Whisk ingredients in a small bowl, or shake them in a jar and serve.

MELLOW MISO LIME DRESSING
Makes 6 servings

This to-die-for dressing combines the umami of miso ("MEE-soh"), a gut-healthy probiotic, with the brightness of fresh limes and spiciness of fresh ginger. Perfect for your bowls (pg. 160).

The Line-Up

1/2 cup organic rice vinegar*

1/2 cup mirin*

1/4 cup freshly squeezed lime juice (2-3 limes)

2 tablespoons organic white miso*

2 teaspoons fresh ginger, grated

1 teaspoon lime zest

Freshly ground pepper and Hawaiian sea salt (optional)

*Coach Karen's First-Round Picks on pg. 206.

The Play-by-Play

Whisk ingredients in a small bowl, or shake them in a jar and serve.

BERRIES

The Natural Starch Blockers

Berries are rich in REDs and BLUEs. They've been shown to act as 'starch blockers' making them especially healthy for your brain, gut, and blood sugar. In vitro studies suggest berries may reduce the digestion and absorption of starch, leaving more to feed your good gut bacteria.[7] Raspberries, for example, completely block the enzyme that breaks down starches into sugar. The result? Berries can suppress blood sugar spikes and support your immune system. If you have diabetes, make berries your best friend — fresh, frozen, or freeze-dried. Pair them with starchy foods like cereals, toast, and pancakes!

 ## POMEGRANATE BALSAMIC VINAIGRETTE
Makes 8 servings

This light and refreshing vinaigrette is packed with REDs and BLUEs and can be made in minutes. Making your own dressing is a condiment that far exceeds the taste and nutrition of store-bought dressings. You know exactly what's in them too — fresh ingredients that you can pronounce!

The Line-Up

1/3 cup white balsamic vinegar

1/4 cup organic 100% pomegranate juice*

3 tablespoons extra virgin olive oil*

1 tablespoon Dijon mustard

1 teaspoon organic date syrup*

Coach Karen says

Fresh pomegranate arils come ready-to-eat (September through December) and are also available frozen.

1 teaspoon garlic powder

1/4 cup pomegranate seeds

Black pepper, freshly ground (to taste)

Sea salt (to taste)

*Coach Karen's First-Round Picks on pg. 206.

Pomegranate Pairings

(Fruit) apples, berries, citrus, mango, pear, pineapple
(Veggies) arugula, cucumber, ginger, kale, spinach, Swiss chard, squash

The Play-by-Play

Whisk ingredients in a small bowl, or shake them in a jar and serve.

RASPBERRY PECAN SALAD WITH RASPBERRY CHAMPAGNE VINAIGRETTE
Makes 4 servings

The Line-Up

2 cups fresh raspberries

5 oz (about 6 cups) fresh baby spinach leaves

1/3 cup pecans, raw, coarsely chopped

1/4 cup red onions, slivered

2 tablespoons ground flaxseed*

Raspberry Champagne Vinaigrette (pg. 252)

The Play-by-Play

1. In a large bowl, combine spinach, onion, flaxseed, and vinaigrette. Toss gently to coat. Add raspberries and walnuts, and gently toss again.

Serve immediately.

RASPBERRY CHAMPAGNE VINAIGRETTE
Makes 1-1/4 cups

Pair this crushed raspberry vinaigrette with a bed of leafy greens and toasted chopped walnuts. One cup of raspberries contains a whopping eight grams of fiber in their tiny seeds. Don't be tempted to press the raspberry mixture through a sieve and discard these amazing seeds — embrace the 'seedy' texture!

The Line-Up

2 cups fresh raspberries

3 tablespoons champagne vinegar

1 tablespoon organic date syrup*

1 teaspoon Dijon mustard

1/2 teaspoon lemon zest

1/8 teaspoon sea salt

1/8 teaspoon freshly ground black pepper

*Coach Karen's First-Round Picks on pg. 206.

The Play-by-Play

1. In a small saucepan, combine the raspberries, vinegar, date syrup, and mustard. Bring to a boil, then reduce heat. Simmer uncovered 8 to 10 minutes or until berries have broken down, and mixture is slightly thick. Cool slightly.

2. Whisk in the lemon zest, salt, and pepper. Thin with a little water if desired.

Cool completely and serve.

Coach Karen says

Champagne vinegar is more delicate in flavor and acidity than other types of vinegar. Since it's less pungent, you can use more vinegar and less oil on your salad.

 TROPICAL BERRY QUINOA SALAD WITH ZESTY CITRUS DRESSING
Makes 4 servings

This salad is rich in vitamin C, which is needed for the growth, development, and repair of all body tissues. When playing your sport or working out, you need more of this vitamin. If you're deficient or even marginally deficient in vitamin C, your muscle mass and physical performance may decline.[6] Vitamin C is a potent antioxidant that also aids in your skin's ability to regenerate — that is, to heal wounds and battle crinkles. Your skin renews itself roughly every 27 days, but that process slows down with age, so feed your face and body well with a healthy bowl of vitamin C!

The Line-Up

1 large mango, fresh or frozen, diced into bite-size pieces

2 Gold Nugget or Sumo mandarin oranges, diced (Can be substituted with one 15-oz can mandarin oranges in it's own juice.)

2 kiwis, diced

1 pint (6 oz) container raspberries, fresh or frozen

1 heaping cup blueberries, fresh or frozen

1 lime

1/3 cup almonds, slivered or sliced

1 cup uncooked sprouted quinoa blend*

1-1/2 cups water

Zesty Citrus Dressing (pg. 253)

Freshly ground black pepper

*Coach Karen's First-Round Picks on pg. 211.

The Play-by-Play

1. Bring 1-1/2 cups of water to a boil. Add the sprouted quinoa, and simmer on low heat for 15 minutes.
2. Put the quinoa in another bowl and cool. You can fan the quinoa or put the bowl in an ice bath to chill quickly.
3. Combine the fruit, almonds, and cooled quinoa in a large bowl.
4. Add the Zesty Citrus Dressing, and mix well.
5. Season with freshly ground black pepper.

Serve with a lime wedge, and squeeze lime juice over the salad.

 ### ZESTY CITRUS DRESSING
Makes 1/2 cup

The Line-Up

1/4 cup extra virgin avocado or olive oil*

Coach Karen says

Adjust the amount of date paste or date syrup to your taste since the sweetness or tartness of the citrus fruits will vary.

2 tablespoons orange juice + 1 teaspoon zest from an orange

1 tablespoon lemon juice + 1/4 teaspoon zest from a lemon

1-1/4 tablespoon homemade Date Paste (pg. 280) —
For a quick fix, sub with organic date syrup*.

1 teaspoon Dijon mustard

*Coach Karen's First-Round Picks on pg. 206.

The Play-By-Play

Whisk ingredients in a small bowl, or shake them in a jar and serve.

SUPER BOWLS — SOUPS TO SUPPERS

BASIL TOMATO CORN SOUP
Makes 4 servings

This recipe is the high-speed version of this soup. Throw down a homemade RED-rich soup *fast!*

The Line-Up

1 yellow onion, quartered

4 cloves garlic, whole

2 Enoya peppers or red bell peppers, quartered

1 jalapeño pepper, halved

1 (24-oz) glass bottle of strained tomatoes*

2 teaspoons dried basil to taste

1/4 teaspoon dried thyme

2 cups dark leafy greens (e.g., spinach, arugula, Swiss chard or a combination of all)

5-oz frozen organic sweet corn (white or yellow)

8-oz firm tofu*, cubed

1-1/2 cups low-sodium vegetable broth*

1/8-1/4 teaspoon red pepper flakes

Freshly ground black pepper and salt (optional)

Coach Karen says

The more herbs you use to flavor your food, the more antioxidants you'll consume.

Extra virgin avocado or olive oil*

*Coach Karen's First-Round Picks on pg. 206.

The Play-by-Play

1. Heat a large pot over medium heat (300°F). Lightly mist it with oil using a non-aerosol oil sprayer** (1/4 teaspoon oil per trigger pull). Sauté onions until soft. Add garlic and peppers, then sauté for 1 minute. Cook until veggies are soft and tender.

2. Add cooked veggies and some vegetable broth to a blender**, and purée to desired texture (very smooth to slightly chunky), then pour into the pot.

3. Stir in strained tomatoes, basil, and thyme. Cover and continue cooking for another 5-8 minutes, stirring occasionally. Add the greens, corn, tofu, and more broth (adjust to your preferred consistency). Cook until the corn is soft and no longer tastes 'raw', about 5 minutes. Season to taste with red pepper flakes, black pepper, and dash of salt (optional).

Serve immediately.

**Coach Karen's Cool Tools on pg. 196.

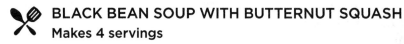 **BLACK BEAN SOUP WITH BUTTERNUT SQUASH**
Makes 4 servings

Here's a hearty high-protein, high-fiber soup that packs some heat! Full of flavor in a wholesome base of REDs, ORANGEs, GREENs, and BLUEs.

The Line-Up

1-1/2 to 1-3/4 cups onions, chopped

1-1/2 cups red and green sweet peppers, chopped

1 jalapeño, chopped

2 teaspoons cumin seeds

2 teaspoons dried oregano, crushed

1/4 teaspoon ground allspice

1/4 teaspoon crushed red pepper

4 cloves garlic, minced

1-1/2 cups organic butternut squash or kabocha*, fresh or frozen

3 (15-oz) cans salt-free black beans, rinsed and drained

2-1/2 to 3 cups low-sodium vegetable broth*

2 tablespoons tomato paste

2 tablespoons lime juice

1 tablespoon balsamic vinegar

1 teaspoon date syrup*

1 bay leaf

Freshly ground black pepper and sea salt (optional)

Snipped fresh cilantro or chopped avocado (optional)

Lime wedges

Extra virgin avocado or olive oil*

*Coach Karen's First-Round Picks on pg. 206.

The Play-by-Play

Coach Karen says

Exposing spices to direct heat releases the oils, and their flavors become more vibrant.

1. Heat a large pot over medium heat (300°F). Lightly mist it with oil using a non-aerosol oil sprayer** (1/4 teaspoon oil per trigger pull). Add the first seven ingredients, and sauté until soft, stirring occasionally for about 6-8 minutes. Add garlic and butternut squash, and cook for another 2 minutes, stirring frequently.

2. Add 2 cans of beans, 2-1/2 cups vegetable broth, tomato paste, lime juice, vinegar, and date syrup. Bring to a boil, reduce heat to simmer for 15-20 minutes. Purée the contents with an immersion blender or in small batches in your blender** or food processor until fully smooth.

3. Return the purée to the pot. Add bay leaf and remaining can of beans. Add more broth for a thinner consistency. Simmer for about 10 minutes, stirring occasionally. Season with black pepper and sea salt (optional).

Garnish with cilantro or chopped avocado, and serve immediately with lime wedges.

**Coach Karen's Cool Tools on pg. 196.

COOKING TIPS TO REDUCE ARSENIC IN RICE

First, don't fret. Arsenic is a heavy metal and carcinogen that occurs naturally in our Earth and is present in our environment from industrial pollution. It's in our soil, air, and water. Since rice spends so much time growing in flooded areas, they absorb more arsenic than many other whole foods.

Regular exposure to small amounts of arsenic can increase the risk of heart disease, type 2 diabetes, and some cancers (bladder, lung, and skin cancer), but you can still enjoy rice. First, pick your rice carefully (pg. 226). Second, cook it in lots of water (just like pasta) since arsenic is soluble in water, and moderate your weekly servings. Instead of eating rice every day, change it up, and rotate in some other intact grains, such as amaranth, buckwheat, barley, bulgur, oats, farro, millet, and quinoa.

The Method

1. **Select water-to-rice ratio (three options), and cook over medium-high heat.**

   - **6-to-1 Ratio** — Cook the rice in 6 parts boiling water per 1 part rice (the traditional method of cooking rice in Asia).[8] This ratio drastically reduces arsenic levels by 40%

   - **10-to-1 Ratio** — Cook the rice in 10 parts boiling water per 1 part rice. *For example, for 1 cup rice, use 10 cups water; for 1-1/2 cups of rice, use 15 cups water (about 4 quarts).* This ratio reduces arsenic levels by 60%.

   - **5-to-1 Ratio (Overnight Method)** — Soak the rice overnight, then cook in 5 parts boiling water per 1 part. Drain the water, and rinse thoroughly with clean fresh water again. Soaking rice opens up the grain's structure, and allows arsenic to permeate into the water. This process reduces arsenic levels by 82%.

2. **Cook the rice until tender, about 20 to 25 minutes.** Drain rice through a strainer. Optional: Rinse one more time with hot water.

3. **Dry out the rice.** Spread the rice on a baking sheet to dry. For smaller amounts, you can just stir the rice around in a warm pot to dry out.

(continued on next page)

(continued from previous page)

Should you rinse the rice first? Research shows rinse washing rice (5 to 6 rinses with agitation) removed 28% of arsenic compared to raw rice.[9]

Don't let the rice absorb the water. Arsenic escapes into the cooking water and is removed when water is drained, but if all the water evaporates, the arsenic is reabsorbed back into the rice. Don't let the rice boil dry, such as when you cook rice in an electric rice cooker (the modern technique of cooking rice).

Arsenic vs Anthocyanins (BLUEs)

Watching all those BLUEs from your black rice wash down the drain can be unsettling when you're making the effort to upgrade your consumption of rice. You will be reducing the BLUE concentration by cooking rice like pasta, but you will also be reducing arsenic concentration considerably too. Coin toss? On the bright side, cooking rice this way may actually promote the partial migration of BLUEs from the outer bran layer into the inner bran layer of rice (the endosperm), so all is *not* lost.

 ### BLACK RICE SALMON BENTO BOWL WITH MELLOW MISO LIME DRESSING
Makes 4 servings

Black rice is the new brown! It's full of BLUEs, more protein, more fiber, and fewer carbs. Miso is a probiotic — it's good for your healthy gut bacteria and supports your immune system. This Japanese-style rice bowl with the miso lime dressing is a winning combination of texture, taste, and nutrition.

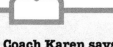

Coach Karen says

To save time, prepare dressing the night before and refrigerate.

The Line-Up

4 (4- to 6-oz) wild-caught salmon fillets, 1" thick, skin on

1-1/2 cups organic black rice*, uncooked

8 radishes, trimmed, halved, sliced thin

2 avocados, halved, pitted, sliced thin

2 cucumbers, halved lengthwise, sliced thin

4 scallions, sliced thin

Black sesame seeds*

Yuzu furikake*

Mellow Miso Lime Dressing (pg. 249)

*Coach Karen's First-Round Picks on pg. 206.

The Play-by-Play

1. Using the 10-to-1 ratio, follow the rice cooking directions in "Cooking Tips to Reduce Arsenic in Rice" (pg. 256).

2. Drizzle 3/8 cup dressing over cooked rice. Set aside the remaining dressing. Let rice cool completely, about 20 minutes, tossing occasionally.

3. Follow cooking directions in "How to Cook Incredibly Moist Salmon" (pg. 271). Seasoning: Mellow Miso Lime Dressing.

4. Portion rice into 4 bowls, and sprinkle with furikake. Flake salmon into large 3-inch pieces. Top rice with salmon, radishes, avocado, and cucumber. Sprinkle with scallions and black sesame seeds. Drizzle with 3/8 cup dressing.

Serve and pass around the furikake. Refrigerate extra dressing.

Coach Karen says

In Japan, "bento" (a convenient Japanese home-packed meal) is an integral part of the food culture. A traditional bento box (lunch box) is visually appealing and holds a main dish and several side dishes.

HOW TO PRESS TOFU WITHOUT A TOFU PRESS

Place tofu between layers of paper towels in a rimmed plate or baking sheet. Weigh down the tofu with a heavy object, such as a heavy cast iron skillet filled with something heavy, like a bag of flour, cans of beans, etc. Let sit until the paper towels stop absorbing moisture, a minimum of 10 minutes. Change paper towels as needed. For a firmer, drier tofu, press for 30 to 60 minutes. Unwrap tofu and slice.

KOREAN-STYLE TOFU BOWL
Makes 2 servings

Spice up your rice bowl with an explosion of flavor with some Korean-style marinated tofu and your favorite COLOR-ful toppings. If you ever thought tofu was tasteless, here's where bland meets bold.

Coach Karen says

Make a batch of Korean-style tofu in advance to have on hand in the fridge. Cut it into cubes, and toss it into grains, salads, and stir-fries.

The Line-Up

1 (14-oz) block organic firm tofu*, pressed

2 scallions, thinly sliced (separate the sliced dark green tops from the white/pale green parts)

Extra virgin olive oil*

Black sesame seeds* (garnish)

Cooked rice

For the Sauce

3 tablespoons low-sodium soy sauce*

3 tablespoons mirin* (Japanese rice cooking wine)

2 cloves garlic, minced or 1 teaspoon freeze-dried garlic*

1 teaspoon fresh ginger root, peeled, finely chopped or 1 teaspoon freeze-dried ginger*

1 teaspoon dry mustard*

1 teaspoon onion powder

1 teaspoon garlic powder

1 teaspoon toasted sesame oil

3/4 teaspoon gochugaru* (Korean-style red pepper) or red pepper flakes

3 tablespoons water

White/pale green parts of the scallion

*Coach Karen's First-Round Picks on pg. 206.

The Play-by-Play

1. Press the tofu in a tofu press** for 20 minutes. Then slice the pressed tofu vertically into eight rectangular segments, about 3/8-inch thick. Pat dry with paper towels.

2. Whisk the sauce ingredients in a small bowl. Set aside.

3. Heat a large skillet over medium heat (300°F). Lightly mist it with oil using a non-aerosol oil sprayer** (1/4 teaspoon oil per trigger pull). When the oil is heated, add the tofu. Brown lightly on both sides. Pour in the sauce, and reduce heat to medium-low. Simmer the tofu until the sauce is reduced by

half, about 4 minutes. Turn the tofu over to simmer on both sides.

Serve tofu over a bowl of hot rice with some Wilted Power Greens (pg. 286), shredded carrots, mushrooms, or favorite seasonal vegetable. Sprinkle with sesame seeds and the dark green scallion tops.

**Coach Karen's Cool Tools on pg. 191.

RASPBERRY LIME GAZPACHO
Makes 6 servings

Gazpacho is cold soup made of raw, blended vegetables. Here's a version made with a refreshing and COLOR-ful purée of brain-boosting berries.

The Line-Up

1-1/2 pints fresh raspberries (about 3-1/2 cups)

20 oz frozen unsweetened raspberries, defrosted

5 kiwi fruits, peeled

2-3 tablespoons freshly squeezed lime juice

6 fresh mint leaves, cut into thin strips

16 oz seltzer water, plain

Garnish

1 cup blueberries, fresh or frozen

1 cup pineapple, diced, fresh or frozen

1-1/2 teaspoons organic date sugar*

The Play-by-Play

1. Process the fresh and frozen raspberries in a food processor until they are smooth. Transfer to a big bowl. Add the seltzer water, mint, and stir.

2. Process the kiwis and the lime juice in the food processor until smooth. Pour equal amounts of the raspberry purée into 6 small chilled soup bowls. Pour equal amounts of the kiwi-lime juice purée in each of the bowls.

Sprinkle equal amounts of blueberries and diced pineapple on each. Add a dash of date sugar on top, and serve immediately.

Coach Karen says

Seltzer water is simply plain water with added carbon dioxide for bubbles. Club soda contains added sodium bicarbonate, disodium phosphate, and other minerals. Sparkling mineral water contains naturally occurring carbonation and minerals, e.g., sodium.

ROASTED KABOCHA AND APPLE SOUP
Makes 4-5 servings

This soup is rich in ORANGEs and will have you going back for more. You can make this soup all year round with organic kabocha that's conveniently diced and frozen. Kabocha (Japanese pumpkin) is sweet with a very tender, 'fluffy' texture that boosts sweetness in any dish without adding extra sugar.

The Line-Up

2-1/2 packages (2-1/2 pounds) of frozen organic kabocha*

4 cups (2 medium) yellow onion, peeled and quartered

3-4 cloves garlic

2-1/4 firm organic Honey Crisp apples, peeled, cored, and quartered

4-5 cups low-sodium vegetable stock*

1/2 to 1 teaspoon New Mexico ground chile (not "chili powder")

Red pepper flakes or cayenne pepper, to taste

Freshly ground black pepper and kosher salt (optional)

Extra virgin avocado or olive oil*

Walnut Cilantro Pesto (pg. 285)

Garnish: toasted pepitas (pg. 236)

*Coach Karen's First-Round Picks on pg. 206.

The Play-By-Play

1. Preheat oven to 350°F. Arrange produce on a parchment-lined rimmed baking sheet. Lightly mist with oil using a non-aerosol oil sprayer** (1/4 teaspoon oil per trigger pull). Season with salt and pepper. Roast for about 25-30 minutes.

2. Transfer roasted vegetables to a blender** or food processor. Add 2 cups vegetable stock, and purée until smooth. Repeat with remaining vegetables and stock. Transfer purée to a large pot. Add more stock if the soup is too thick. Add seasonings, and bring to a simmer. Cover, and allow flavors to commingle.

Garnish with pepitas and a dollop of pesto. Serve immediately.

**Coach Karen's Cool Tools on pg. 191.

Coach Karen says

This soup is also delicious made with sugar pie pumpkin and butternut squash.

Coach Karen says

When roasting veggies, arrange the rack in the top third of the oven. Cut veggies to the same size, and don't overcrowd them on the baking sheet. You want plenty of hot air all around them.

BAMBURGERS™ WITH CHIPOTLE MAYO
Makes 4 servings

Black Beans, Black rice, Almond butter, and Mushrooms are the BAM in these burgers. They're made with black soy beans, known as the 'Crown Prince' of beans in Japan. They're not only rich in BLUEs, a 1/2-cup serving contains 6 gm of dietary fiber, nearly half the carbs (11 gm) of regular black beans and twice the protein (11 gm). Keep your kitchen locker stocked with the following basics, and you can throw down a muscle-building meal real fast.

The Line-Up

1 (15-oz) can black soybeans*, drained and rinsed

2 tablespoons organic raw creamy almond butter*

1/4 cup + 2 tablespoons oat flour*

1 flax egg (pg. 97)

4-oz can chunky portobello mushrooms, drained (reserve liquid)

1/4 cup liquid from mushrooms

1/4 cup hot diced green chiles, undrained (half of a 4-oz can)

1/2 cup cooked black rice*

Extra virgin avocado or olive oil*

Chipotle Mayo (pg. 277)

Sprouted whole grain burger buns*

Topping ideas: arugula, smashed avocado, beefsteak tomatoes, lettuce, microgreens, red onions

Seasoning

3/4 teaspoon ground cumin

3/4 teaspoon dried minced onions

1/2 teaspoon ground chipotle chile powder

1/4 teaspoon garlic powder

1/4 teaspoon oregano

Coach Karen says

If you don't have black soy beans, you can sub with traditional black beans. But put black soy beans on your grocery list for next time, and give them a try!

Coach Karen says

To make a flax egg, mix 3 TBSP of water with 1 TBSP of ground flaxseeds (3-to-1 ratio) in a small bowl. Stir and let the mixture stand for 5 minutes to thicken.

1/4 teaspoon kosher salt

1/8 teaspoon smoked paprika

Freshly ground black pepper

*Coach Karen's First-Round Picks on pg. 206.

The Play-by-Play

Prepping the Burgers

1. Preheat oven to 300°F. Line a rimmed baking sheet with foil or parchment paper. Spread the beans onto the baking sheet. Bake for 10-12 minutes, or until beans are dry to the touch and begin to split. Once dried, place the beans in a small bowl, and mash with a potato masher.

2. Add almond butter, oat flour, flax egg, and seasoning. Mix well. Add mushrooms, mushroom liquid, green chiles, and black rice. Stir to incorporate.

3. Let the black bean mixture rest in the fridge for 20 minutes before shaping into patties. **Do not skip this step.**

Cooking the Burgers

1. Heat a large cast iron or heavy skillet over medium heat (300°F). Lightly mist it with oil using a non-aerosol oil sprayer** (1/4 teaspoon oil per trigger pull).

2. Drop 1/4 of the mixture directly into the heated skillet. Shape the patties right in the hot pan by molding gently into a 4-1/4" round patty using the tip of a dinner knife. Repeat until all patties are made.

3. Cook the burgers until firm and a dark crust forms on the bottom of the burgers, about 9 minutes on the first side, then flip over, and cook 5 minutes on the other side.

Serve on lightly toasted sprouted grain bread. Slather on Chipotle Mayo, then pile on the toppings.

**Coach Karen's Cool Tools on pg. 196.

Coach Karen says

Letting the burgers rest helps the dry ingredients incorporate with the wet ingredients, which creates a more homogenized burger that'll hold together.

Coach Karen says

Tomatoes add crunch and REDs, but remove the seeds. The seeds tend to make your burger a little slippery and shoot out of your bun. Pick a large beefsteak tomato to cover your patty.

BLT (BARBECUE-SEASONED TOFU, LETTUCE, AND TOMATO)
Makes 2 servings

When you're craving barbecue, pull together these grilled spicy and smoky tofu slabs with grilled onions.

The Line-Up

1 (16-oz) block organic firm tofu*, pressed

Extra virgin avocado or olive oil*

For the Marinade

2 tablespoons low-sodium soy sauce*

1 tablespoon maple syrup

1 tablespoon Chipotle Sauce (pg. 277)

1/2 teaspoon smoked paprika

Freshly ground black pepper

For the BLT

4 slices sprouted whole grain bread*

1 teaspoon organic stoneground mustard*

Lettuce leaves

1 large tomato, sliced

1 large yellow onion, sliced

*Coach Karen's First-Round Picks on pg. 206.

The Play-by-Play

1. Press the tofu using a tofu press** for 20 minutes. Meanwhile, thoroughly whisk all marinade ingredients in a small bowl.

2. Transfer pressed tofu to a baking dish. Coat with the marinade, and let the tofu marinate for 10 minutes per side (longer is better).

3. While the tofu is marinating, heat a large cast iron or heavy skillet over medium heat (300°F). Lightly mist it with oil using a non-aerosol oil sprayer** (1/4 teaspoon oil per trigger pull). Add the onions, and cook until softened and golden (about 20

Coach Karen says

Azumaya makes a 16-oz "square" block of tofu, which makes four 4-oz squares of tofu that fit perfectly on a slice of bread. Other tofu brands are 14-oz and more rectangular in shape.

Coach Karen says

If you don't have a tofu press, see "How to Press Tofu Without a Tofu Press" on pg. 195.

minutes). Season with pepper. Transfer onions to a plate and reserve skillet (no need to wipe out).

4. Keep heat on medium, and add the marinated tofu. Pour the marinade over the tofu, and cook for about 5 minutes per side until the tofu is golden brown.

Serve on lightly toasted sprouted grain bread with mustard and a layer of lettuce, tomato, and grilled onions.

**Coach Karen's Cool Tools on pg. 191.

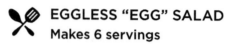 EGGLESS "EGG" SALAD
Makes 6 servings

This eggless egg salad is much easier to make than the traditional egg salad. It's fuss-free — no boiling, cooling, and peeling eggs! Whip this up in 10 minutes for a super easy protein-rich, cholesterol-free lunchtime classic.

Coach Karen says

Serve eggless salad on a sprouted grain English muffin or wrapped in a crunchy Romaine heart or tender butter leaf. Dust with paprika.

The Line-Up

For the Salad

1 (14-oz) package organic medium firm tofu*, pressed

1/4 cup organic celery, chopped (about 1 stalk)

2 tablespoons green onions, chopped (about 1 stalk)

1 tablespoon fresh parsley, chopped

1 tablespoon freeze-dried dill* (or 1 tablespoon fresh, chopped)

For the Dressing

1/4 cup Tofu Mayonnaise (pg. 281)

2 tablespoons nutritional yeast*

1 tablespoon yellow mustard

1 tablespoon apple cider vinegar

1 teaspoon garlic powder

1 teaspoon hot dry mustard powder*

1/4 teaspoon smoked paprika

1/4 teaspoon turmeric

1/4 teaspoon kala namak* (Indian black salt)

1/2 teaspoon freshly ground black pepper

Dash of cayenne

*Coach Karen's First-Round Picks on pg. 206.

The Play-by-Play

1. Press the tofu in a tofu press** for 20 minutes. Meanwhile, place all the dressing ingredients in a large bowl, and whisk together.

2. Place the pressed tofu in a small bowl, and mash with a potato masher or large dinner fork. Add the rest of the salad ingredients to the tofu. Mix thoroughly.

3. Add the salad mixture to the dressing. Mix well. Cover and chill in the fridge for at least 30 minutes (longer is better) to allow the flavors to meld together. Refrigerate in a glass container for up to 5 days.

Refrigerate in a glass container for up to 5 days.

**Coach Karen's Cool Tools on pg. 191.

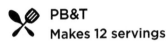 ### PB&T
Makes 12 servings

Peanut butter is a great source of healthy fat, but it's also pretty dense in calories. Lighten it up with some WHITEs and complete plant protein. PB&T (peanut butter and tofu) is a fluffier spread for your crackers and sandwiches and makes a flavorful veggie dip for post-game snacking. Give it a try!

The Line-Up

8 oz. organic soft tofu*, drained

1/2 cup organic natural nutty peanut butter*

1/4 cup organic raisins or other dried fruit

2 tablespoons organic raw sunflower seeds, toasted

1/4 teaspoon sesame seeds, toasted

Optional add-in: 1 tablespoon of organic fruit spread or fruit butter*

*Coach Karen's First-Round Picks on pg. 206.

The Play-By-Play

1. Drain the tofu by letting it sit on a plate for about 5-10 minutes. No need to press it.
2. Lightly toast the sunflower seeds in a sauté pan on medium-low heat.
3. Add the drained tofu and remaining ingredients to a medium bowl, then mix well to blend together.

Store in the fridge in a tightly covered container.

CENTER COURT — EXCITING ENTRÉES

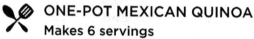

ONE-POT MEXICAN QUINOA
Makes 6 servings

This dish is extremely versatile. Enjoy it also as a dip, side dish, on your salad, in a sprouted grain tortilla, or fresh butter leaf.

The Line-Up

1 small red onion, chopped

3 cloves of garlic, minced

2 bell peppers (one orange, one yellow or red), chopped

2 green onions, chopped

1 cup fresh parsley or cilantro, chopped

1 avocado, cut into cubes

2 cups frozen corn

1 to 2 limes

1 cup sprouted quinoa*

1-1/2 cup low-sodium vegetable broth*

1 (15-oz) can black beans, no salt added*

2 (14.5-oz) cans diced tomatoes

Extra virgin avocado or olive oil*

Seasonings

1 tablespoon smoked paprika

1/2 tablespoon cumin

2 teaspoon New Mexico ground chili

Freshly ground black pepper

Red pepper flakes (to your taste)

Serving Options

Sprouted grain tortillas or sprouted grain corn tortillas*

Live butter lettuce*

Hot sauce (your favorite)

*Coach Karen's First-Round Picks on pg. 206.

The Play-by-Play

1. Heat a large skillet over medium heat (300°F). Lightly mist it with oil using a non-aerosol oil sprayer** (1/4 teaspoon oil per trigger pull). Sauté onions for 2-3 minutes until they're translucent. Add garlic and bell pepper. Cook for another 2 minutes. Add in sprouted quinoa, broth, beans, tomatoes, and corn. Stir in seasonings.

2. Cover and bring to a boil. Simmer on low heat for 20 minutes. Stir occasionally to keep ingredients from sticking. Squeeze lime over ingredients (to taste). Stir in parsley just before serving, or add as a garnish when served.

Serve with fresh lime slice. Top with avocado and your favorite hot sauce.

**Coach Karen's Cool Tools on pg. 196.

Coach Karen says

Instead of sautéing veggies in oil, you can cook them in some low-sodium vegetable broth.

 PLANT-POWERED PIZZA
Makes 3-4 servings

Move over ooey-gooey pizzas that clog your pipes. What makes this pizza unique: a sprouted grain flatbread pizza crust and a healthy mix of COLORS. For max flavor and texture, the key is to *cook* the toppings before adding them to your pizza. Makes a nutritious, satisfying starter, snack, or main attraction.

The Line-Up

1 sprouted reduced-sodium flatbread pizza crust*

1/2 yellow onion, chopped

Coach Karen says

Root vegetables, like butternut squash or sweet potato, also make great pizza toppings.

2 cloves garlic, minced

1 red bell pepper, chopped

6 oz. fresh Organic Girl® SuperGreens (a combo of baby red/green Swiss chard, tatsoi, arugula, spinach)

7 oz firm organic tofu*

One 7-oz. can of sliced mushrooms, drained

One 4.25-oz can of chopped black olives

About 1+ tablespoon date sugar*

Low-sodium vegetable broth* or extra virgin avocado or olive oil* (about 1 tablespoon)

Two-Minute Pizza Sauce (pg. 283)

Vegan 'Parmesan' (pg. 285)

Seasonings

1/4 teaspoon garlic powder

1/4 teaspoon freshly ground black pepper

1/8 teaspoon paprika

Dried Italian parsley

Dried oregano

*Coach Karen's First-Round Picks on pg. 206.

The Play-by-Play

1. Preheat oven to 350°F.

2. Place tofu on a plate, and allow the liquid to drain. No need to "press". Cut into small bite-sized cubes.

3. Heat vegetable broth or oil in a large pot or wok over medium heat (300°F). Add onion and garlic. Cook until onions are transparent and soft. Add bell pepper and mushrooms. Cook for 2-3 minutes. Add leafy greens, and cook until wilted. Add the drained tofu, garlic powder, black pepper, and paprika. When the ingredients are combined and heated through, remove from heat.

4. Place Flatzza on a pizza pan or parchment-lined baking sheet, and cover generously with pizza sauce (about 1 cup). Sprinkle sauce generously with date sugar and Vegan Parmesan. Add

Coach Karen says

Mushrooms are 92% water and release a lot of it when cooked. To avoid diluting your topping mixture, use canned mushrooms, which are cooked before canning.

Coach Karen says

By sprinkling the pizza with date sugar, it ensures every bite gets a bit of sweetness, which offsets the acidity of the tomatoes.

the topping evenly, then spread 1/2 can of chopped olives evenly over the topping. Add more pizza sauce (about 1/2 cup). Sprinkle with parsley and more Vegan Parmesan.

5. Place pizza pan in the oven. If using a parchment-lined baking sheet, slide the paper directly onto the oven rack. (The baking sheet is only used to carry the pizza and help slide it onto the rack.) Bake for 20-30 minutes until pizza is crisp and warm.

Slice and serve with red pepper flakes, oregano, and Vegan Parmesan.

HOW TO COOK INCREDIBLY MOIST SALMON

Baking salmon in a low-temperature oven (275°F) is gentler on the salmon, which slowly melts the fat between the flesh. The fillets are flaky on the outside and the middle is incredibly melt-in-your-mouth moist and buttery soft. When salmon is cooked 'aggressively' at high heat, more of that weird white stuff will get squeezed out of the fish. This white substance is protein called albumin. You want as much of the protein to stay in the flesh, so cook slowly at a lower temperature.

The tough and durable skin acts as a protective barrier between the fish and the hot pan, and helps to hold the fish together while cooking. So even if you plan to remove the skin before eating the fish, keep the skin on.

The Method

1. **Line a baking sheet with parchment paper.**

2. **Remove fillets 15 to 20 minutes before cooking,** so it's closer to room temperature. For even cooking, don't put a cold fillet straight from the fridge into a hot pan.

3. **Preheat oven to 275°F.**

4. **Pat fillets dry** — or they'll be more likely to stick to the pan.

5. **Sprinkle with salt and pepper on both sides** (optional).

6. **Place fillets (skin side down) on the prepared pan.**

(continued on next page)

Coach Karen says

For a flavorful, easy Lemon-Herb Salmon: Season fillets with fresh-squeezed lemon juice, garlic powder, thyme, rosemary, and parsley flakes, then cover with rows of lemon slices. Bake slowly.

Coach Karen says

It's best to use an instant-read thermometer to ensure the salmon isn't undercooked or well-done.

(continued from previous page)

7. **Add preferred seasoning** — e.g., herbs, spices, fresh squeezed lemon juice, or glaze

8. **Bake slowly to 145°F.**

Test for Doneness

The USDA suggests cooking salmon until the center reaches an internal temperature of 145°F (medium). Remove immediately. Above 145°F, and you'll end up with a dry, sad piece of fish.

At this point, you can push on the top of the salmon with a fork at its thickest part, and the layers of flesh separate easily into moist sections. If it resists being flaked with a fork, it's not done yet. This may take about 15 to 20 minutes, but cooking times will vary depending on the size and thickness of the fish and your oven.

 SLOW-BAKED MISO-MAPLE SALMON
Makes 2 servings

Once you try slow cooking salmon, you won't want it any other way.

The Line-Up

4 skin-on wild salmon fillets

3 tablespoons maple syrup

2 tablespoons organic mellow white miso*

1 tablespoon toasted sesame oil

Sesame seeds, white or black*

*Coach Karen's First-Round Picks on pg. 206.

The Play-by-Play

1. In a small bowl, whisk together the maple syrup, miso paste, and sesame oil.

2. Follow cooking directions in "How to Cook Incredibly Moist Salmon" (pg. 271). Seasoning: Miso-Maple Glaze.

Sprinkle with sesame seeds, and serve immediately.

TOFU LETTUCE WRAPS
Makes 8 servings

These versatile wraps are filled with lots of COLORS — from crumbled tofu (plant-based protein), a variety of veggies, and dark leafy greens. You can use whatever vegetables you have on hand. They make a perfect side dish, appetizer, or can be a meal all by itself. Asian-inspired dishes can contain high amounts of sodium from the sauces, but this recipe contains lower sodium components that make these wraps much more acceptable in the sodium category.

The Line-Up

For the Sauce

3 tablespoons hoisin sauce*

3 tablespoons low-sodium soy sauce*

2 tablespoons organic rice vinegar*

1 teaspoon sesame oil

For the Filling

1 (14-oz) block organic firm or extra firm tofu*, pressed

8 oz baby bella cremini mushrooms, diced

1 can water chestnuts, drained, finely chopped

1 medium carrot, cut into 1" matchsticks (or grated)

4 green onions, thinly sliced (divided in half)

3 cloves garlic, minced

2 teaspoons fresh ginger, grated or 2 teaspoons freeze-dried ginger*

1/4 teaspoon red pepper flakes

1/8 teaspoon gochugaru*

Extra virgin olive oil*

The Wrap

1/2 head of butter lettuce

The Toppings

Toasted sesame seeds

Chopped peanuts

Cilantro (optional)

*Coach Karen's First-Round Picks on pg. 206.

The Play-by-Play

Coach Karen says

If you don't have a tofu press, see "How to Press Tofu Without a Tofu Press" on pg. 258.

1. Press the tofu in a tofu press** for 20 minutes. Crumble pressed tofu in a bowl using a potato masher or fork.

2. In a small bowl, mix all the sauce ingredients together.

3. Heat a large skillet over medium heat (300°F). Lightly mist it with oil using a non-aerosol oil sprayer** (1/4 teaspoon oil per trigger pull). Add crumbled tofu, and cook for 5 minutes. Add diced mushrooms and carrots. Cook until soft, about 3 more minutes. Add water chestnuts, garlic, ginger, red pepper flakes, gochugaru, and half of the green onions. Cook briefly, about 30 seconds.

4. Pour sauce over the tofu mixture, and mix to coat throughout. Cook until sauce is heated through, about 30 to 60 seconds.

Spoon tofu mixture into individual lettuce leaves. Sprinkle with sesame seeds, chopped peanuts, cilantro, and remaining green onions.

**Coach Karen's Cool Tools on pg. 191.

WILD SALMON OR TOFU TACOS WITH CITRUS SALSA
Makes 8 tacos

The Line-Up

1 pound skin-on wild salmon

1 (14-oz) block organic firm tofu*, pressed

2 cups baby arugula

1/4 cup almond flour*

1 tablespoon New Mexico ground chile (not "chili powder")

1 teaspoon Cajun Spice (pg. 276)

Sea salt and freshly ground black pepper

8 sprouted corn tortillas*

Citrus Salsa (pg. 279)

Extra virgin avocado or olive oil*

*Coach Karen's First-Round Picks on pg. 206.

The Play-by-Play

For the Tofu

1. Press the tofu in a tofu press** for 20 minutes. Slice the pressed tofu vertically into eight rectangular segments, about 3/8-inch thick. Pat dry with paper towels.

2. In a small bowl, combine the flour, ground chile, and Cajun Spice. Dust the pressed tofu with the flour mixture.

3. Heat a large skillet over medium heat (300°F). Lightly mist it with oil using a non-aerosol oil sprayer** (1/4 teaspoon oil per trigger pull). When the oil is heated, add the tofu. Brown lightly on both sides.

For the Salmon

1. Follow cooking directions in "How to Cook Incredibly Moist Salmon" (pg. 271). Seasoning: ground chile and Cajun Spice.

Divide the cooked tofu and/or salmon evenly among the tortillas, and top with the Citrus Salsa and arugula.

**Coach Karen's Cool Tools on pg. 191.

ON THE SIDELINES — SIDES, SAUCES, AND SEASONINGS

BARLEY WITH FRESH FIGS, ARUGULA, AND MAPLE MUSTARD VINAIGRETTE
Makes 2 servings

This side dish is a definite "go to" when fresh figs are in season. It's super easy to toss together, and the flavors of the sweet figs compliment the peppery arugula and toasted nuts. Toss in your leftover grains for a well-rounded, satisfying meal or side dish.

The Line-Up

1-1/2 cup organic hulless barley or purple barley*, cooked (1/2 cup dry)

2 to 3 cups organic baby arugula, chopped

4 fresh figs, quartered or sliced in half

Coach Karen says

Hulless barley contains 34 carbs, a whopping 8 gm fiber, and 6 gm protein per serving, while 'pearled' barley has been stripped of its bran layer and is no longer an "intact" grain.

Coach Karen says

Fig season is short. If you missed it, use dried figs. To rehydrate them, place the figs in a small bowl, and pour boiling hot water over them. Let them steep for 10 to 15 minutes to plump up, then strain.

1/8 to 1/4 cup red onion, thinly sliced

1/8 cup raw walnuts, toasted (or hazelnuts, pecans, pistachios)

1 tablespoon hemp seeds*

Freshly ground black pepper

Maple Mustard Vinaigrette (pg. 249)

Optional add-ins: chopped organic apples, pears, peaches, or raspberries

*Coach Karen's First-Round Picks on pg. 206.

The Play-by-Play

1. Cook barley according to "How to Cook No-Fail Farro" (pg. 278).

2. Toast nuts in a dry skillet over low to medium heat, stirring occasionally until lightly toasted (about 5 to 6 minutes).

3. Place barley, arugula, nuts, and onions in a large bowl. Drizzle with some Maple Mustard Vinaigrette, and toss until all the ingredients are lightly coated with dressing. Add the figs, toasted nuts, and hemp seeds, then toss lightly to incorporate.

Serve immediately.

Coach Karen says

Spice up whole grains, soups, stews, pasta, roasted chickpeas, and roasted soybeans (a.k.a. soy nuts), fish, grilled tofu, veggies, dressings, and popcorn with a bit o' Cajun! No worries about the salt. Try it on anything!

CAJUN SPICE (NO SALT)
Makes 7 tablespoons (a little less than 1/2 cup)

Cajun seasoning contains loads of super antioxidants and flavor components, such as paprika, garlic powder, onion powder, oregano, and thyme. For heat, cajun seasoning contains cayenne pepper, black pepper, white pepper, and red chili flakes. Here's how to get the kick without a whole day's worth of sodium.

The Line-Up

2 tablespoon paprika

1 tablespoon garlic powder

1 tablespoon onion powder

2 teaspoons black pepper

2 teaspoons cayenne pepper

2 teaspoons dried thyme

Coach Karen says

Label ground spices with the date you prepared it or purchased it. Ground spices lose their fresh-ness the quickest since more of their surface area is exposed to air, light, and moisture.

2 teaspoons dried oregano

1/2 to 1 teaspoon red pepper flakes

The Play-by-Play

1. Combine all the ingredients in a small bowl. Stir well to fully mix all the spices.

Use immediately and store the remainder in an airtight glass spice jar.

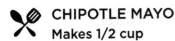 ## CHIPOTLE MAYO
Makes 1/2 cup

For a smoky, spicy, zesty taste, smear this no-oil mayo liberally on your BLTs, tacos, and BAMburgers.

The Line-Up

1/2 cup Tofu Mayonnaise (pg. 281)

4 teaspoons Chipotle Sauce (pg. 277)

The Play-by-Play

1. Whisk ingredients in a small bowl. Adjust the amount of sauce to your taste, and serve.

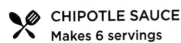 ## CHIPOTLE SAUCE
Makes 6 servings

This sauce is a *must-have* for your hot 'n spicy BLT (barbecue-seasoned tofu, lettuce, and tomato sandwich on pg. 265).

The Line-Up

1 tablespoon ketchup*

1 tablespoon organic apple cider vinegar

1 teaspoon chipotle chili powder

1/2 teaspoon cumin

1/8 teaspoon cayenne

Pinch of oregano and garlic powder, to taste

*Coach Karen's First-Round Picks on pg. 218.

Coach Karen says

A "pinch" is the tiny bit you pick up between the tip of your index finger and thumb — about 1/16 of a teaspoon.

The Play-by-Play

1. Whisk ingredients in a small bowl and serve.

HOW TO COOK NO-FAIL FARRO

Farro, pronounced "fah-roh" (rhymes with "sorrow"), is an heirloom variety of wheat, meaning it has not been genetically modified and continues to be grown as nature intended. Farro varies in cooking times because every farro is different, and depending on how you cook it, you could end up with something *very, very* chewy. So here's a no-fail way to cook farro — cook it like pasta.

The Method

1. **Bring a large pot of water to a full, roaring boil.** If you like, add aromatics to the water (e.g., onion, garlic, fresh herbs, etc).

2. **Sort through the farro.** Discard any debris. Rinse the grain to remove any not-so-savory residue. Don't skip this step.

3. **Add the rinsed farro to the boiling water.** Stir, and bring back to a full boil. Turn down the heat, and simmer for about 30 to 40 minutes. Don't let the water evaporate — add more water if necessary or cover. It's done when you taste it, and you like the texture. Whole farro tastes slightly sweet and nutty because its bran layer is still intact.

4. **Drain the cooked farro through a sieve.** Discard the aromatics.

5. **Dry out farro.** Spread farro on a baking sheet to dry out. Pop it into the oven at 250°F to speed up the drying and to stay warm. For smaller amounts, stir the cooked farro around in a warm nonstick skillet to dry out.

CILANTRO LIME FARRO
Makes 4 servings

Here's an easy, fresh-tasting side dish that goes with just about anything! Plate it with roasted veggies, salmon, and salads for a filling protein and fiber boost. Farro and barley can be used interchangeably.

The Line-Up

1 cup organic whole farro* (not pearled), uncooked or 2 cups cooked

3/4 cup (4 oz) avocado

1/3 cup fresh cilantro, finely chopped

Zest and juice from 1 lime (about 2 tablespoons juice)

1 scallion, diced

Pinch of garlic powder

Freshly ground black pepper and sea salt (optional)

Optional (but highly recommended) add-in: fresh or frozen diced mango

*Coach Karen's First-Round Picks on pg. 210.

Coach Karen says

There are three types of farro, a so-called "ancient grain". The varieties include einkorn, emmer, and spelt. The one sold most often in the U.S. is emmer.

The Play-by-Play

1. Follow cooking directions in "How to Cook No-Fail Farro" (pg. 277). Allow cooked farro to cool. Transfer cooled farro to a mixing bowl. Add avocado, and smash it with a fork.

2. Add lime juice, lime zest, scallion, garlic powder, fresh cilantro (save some for garnishing), black pepper, and sea salt. Mix well to combine all the flavors.

Garnish with fresh cilantro and serve.

CITRUS SALSA
Makes 2 cups

This salsa makes a scrumptious topping for fish and fish tacos.

The Line-Up

1 Hass avocado, chopped

3 large Roma tomatoes, diced (don't remove the seeds)

1/2 cup red onion, finely chopped (about 1/4 onion)

1 orange, peeled, cut into segments, then chopped into bite-size pieces

1 large lime, peeled, cut into segments, then chopped into bite-sized pieces

3 green onions, sliced

1 jalapeño, finely chopped (keep the seeds if you like it hot)

1/4 cup fresh cilantro leaves, chopped

1/2 teaspoon Hawaiian sea salt, to taste

1/4 teaspoon freshly ground black pepper

The Play-by-Play

1. Mix all the ingredients together in a glass bowl. Cover and refrigerate for an hour.

Mix again and serve.

Coach Karen says

Substitute date paste for dry sweeteners using a 1-to-1 ratio.

Coach Karen says

Make small batches, so your date paste is 'fresh'. If you prefer making a larger batch, freeze what you won't be using right away in silicone bottom ice cube trays.

 ## DATE PASTE
Makes 6 servings

Date paste is the best way to naturally sweeten almost ANY recipe. Dates are an excellent source of BROWNs, soluble fiber, and essential minerals, like potassium and magnesium. Use date paste in place of refined sugar, brown sugar, agave syrup, maple syrup, honey, and coconut sugar, which contain twice as much sugar per serving. Whisk date paste into salad dressings, spread it on toast, and swirl it into yogurt, smoothies, or oatmeal.

The Line-Up

6 Fancy Medjool dates*, pitted

1 cup water, boiled

*Coach Karen's First-Round Picks on pg. 209.

The Play-by-Play

1. Place pitted dates in boiling hot water for 10 minutes to soften.
2. Add the dates and 1/4 cup of the soaking water into food processor. Process until smooth, scraping down the side of the bowl to be sure all of the dates are incorporated. Use more or less water to make paste thinner (less sweet) or thicker.

Pour into a clean, air-tight glass container or Mason jar, and store in the fridge for up to one week.

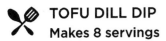

TOFU DILL DIP
Makes 8 servings

Finally, a creamy protein-based dip made with lots of GREENs but without the cream. You won't find a trace of emulsified fat (mayo) or sour cream here. Dunk your favorite fresh veggies and chips in this oh-so delicious dip, but don't stop there. This dill-infused sauce pairs well with salmon, baked potatoes, and roasted spuds too. Be prepared to make a double batch!

The Line-Up

1 (12.3-oz) carton of organic silken tofu*

1/4 cup fresh parsley, minced

1 stalk green onion

1 tablespoon fresh squeezed lemon juice

1 tablespoon organic apple cider vinegar

1-1/8 teaspoon dried dill or 1-3/8 tablespoons fresh or freeze-dried dill*

1/2 teaspoon onion powder

1/4 teaspoon Dijon mustard

1/4 teaspoon sea salt

*Coach Karen's First-Round Picks on pg. 206.

The Play-by-Play

1. Pat the tofu dry before processing (if needed). Place all the ingredients in a food processor, and blend until smooth.

Refrigerate in a glass jar for up to 5 days.

TOFU MAYONNAISE (NO OIL)
Makes 16 servings (2 cups)

This mayo recipe is made with **Mori-Nu Silken 'Firm' Tofu**, which is packaged in a 4" x 3" blue aseptic carton without water and needs no refrigeration until opened. This particular tofu has a smooth creamy texture and is perfect for making this vegan mayonnaise.

Coach Karen says

This dill dip is made with **Mori-Nu Silken 'Nigari' Tofu**. It's packaged in a 4" x 3" aqua (greenish-blue) aseptic carton without water and needs no refrigeration until opened. This particular brand and type of tofu is silky smooth and creamy.

Coach Karen says

Use Mori-Nu Silken 'Firm' tofu to achieve the creaminess of mayonnaise. Making tofu mayo with a tofu that's packed in water will have a different texture and consistency.

Coach Karen says

Keep a batch of Tofu Mayo on hand to flavor veggies, salads, and sandwiches and to make a quick dressing or sauce.

The Line-Up

1 (12.3-oz) package of organic silken tofu*

2 tablespoons fresh lemon juice

1 tablespoon Dijon mustard

2 small cloves garlic

1/4 teaspoon kala namak* (a.k.a. Indian black salt)

1/8 tsp white pepper

*Coach Karen's First-Round Picks on pg. 206.

The Play-by-Play

1. Pat the tofu dry before processing (if needed). Place all the ingredients in a food processor, and blend until smooth.

Refrigerate in a glass jar for up to 5 days.

Coach Karen says

Umami literally means "pleasant, savory taste" in Japanese.

Coach Karen says

The recommended daily amount of B12 for adults is 2.4 mcg. B12 is essential for brain health and is naturally present in foods of animal origin.

GET ON THE "NOOCH" BANDWAGON

Nutritional yeast, a savory food seasoning (nicknamed "nooch" for short) became popular in health food stores in the 1960s and '70s and has long been a staple in the vegan culture. Because of its flavor and healthy profile, nooch (rhymes with 'pooch') has since made its way into non-vegan pantries. When you want a hit of 'umami' (one of the five basic tastes), and your dish doesn't need salt, add some nooch.

These mustard-yellow flakes taste like a nutty, aged cheese, but contains little sodium and no fat. One tablespoon contains 5 gm protein, 2 gm fiber, and 11.16 mcg vitamin B12.

Sprinkle nooch on anything in lieu of cheese: salads, soups, veggies, dips, potatoes, popcorn, pizza, pasta, rice, kale chips, crackers, and mixed nuts. Use it as a base for making 'cheesy' sauces, vegan 'ricotta', and 'Parmesan' cheese. Nutritional yeast is a dried deactivated (dead) yeast and not a live yeast like baker's or brewer's yeast. Don't buy nutritional yeast that's stored in an open bin or exposed to direct sunlight. UV light destroys vitamin B2 (riboflavin).

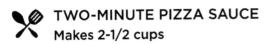 **TOFU 'RICOTTA'**
Makes 6 servings

Dollop this easy, cheesy 'ricotta' on pizza, in lasagna, savory crepes; stuff it in manicotti, ravioli, and rolled eggplant; or slather it on toast with pesto. The fresh basil leaves are a must!

The Line-Up

1/2 cup chopped (1-oz) fresh basil leaves

1 (12-oz) block organic extra-firm tofu*, pressed

Juice of 2 lemons (about 1/3 cup juice)

3 tablespoons nutritional yeast*

1 tablespoon dried oregano

1/2 teaspoon freshly ground black pepper

2 tablespoons extra virgin olive oil*

Vegan 'Parmesan' (pg. 285)

*Coach Karen's First-Round Picks on pg. 206.

The Play-by-Play

1. Press the tofu in a tofu press** for 20 minutes.

2. Add basil leaves to the food processor, and chop into small bits. Add pressed tofu, lemon juice, nutritional yeast, oregano, black pepper, and Vegan Parmesan. Purée, but only until the tofu mixture is blended, and you can still see bits of basil leaves. Blend in about 2 tablespoons oil to create a smooth, creamy, less dry purée.

3. Adjust seasoning (more nutritional yeast for cheesiness, more lemon for brightness).

Serve immediately, or refrigerate until ready to use.

**Coach Karen's Cool Tools on pg. 195.

TWO-MINUTE PIZZA SAUCE
Makes 2-1/2 cups

If you love homemade pizza, this RED-rich sauce is a refrigerator staple. Hey, hockey fans...you can literally whip this up during a TV timeout. Always have some ready for your next pizza creation — or just eat it by the spoonful as part of your daily RED requirement.

The Line-Up

15 oz. organic salt-free tomato sauce

6 oz. organic salt-free tomato paste

2 tablespoons oregano leaves, dried

2 tablespoons Italian seasoning

1/2 teaspoon garlic powder

1/2 teaspoon onion powder

1/4 teaspoon freshly ground black pepper

The Play-by-Play

1. Mix tomato paste and sauce together in a medium-sized bowl until smooth and thoroughly combined.
2. Add seasonings and mix well.

Refrigerate in an airtight glass container for up to one week or freeze for up to two months.

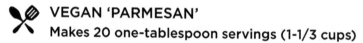

VEGAN 'PARMESAN'
Makes 20 one-tablespoon servings (1-1/3 cups)

Sprinkle this savory crumb-style topping on pasta, pizza, popcorn, veggies, avocado toast — anything that you'd usually top with Parmesan cheese. It's made from a base of cashews and nutritional yeast, so it doesn't melt, but adds the "cheesy" flavor. If you're out of or sensitive to cashews, you can sub with blanched almonds.

The Line-Up

1 cup (150 gm) raw, unsalted cashews

1/4 cup (20 gm) nutritional yeast*

1/2 teaspoon garlic powder

1/4 teaspoon onion powder

1 teaspoon Hawaiian sea salt

*Coach Karen's First-Round Picks on pg. 217.

The Play-by-Play

1. Pulse, don't blend, all ingredients in a small food processor until fine. Do not overprocess, or you could end up with 'cashew butter'. It should mimic grated Parmesan in texture and consistency.

Refrigerate and store in an airtight shaker jar for up to two months.

 ### VEGAN HEMP 'PARMESAN'
Makes 12 one-tablespoon servings (3/4 cup)

If you love hemp seeds or you're sensitive to nuts, this "cheesy" version is nut-free.

Coach Karen says

Don't use a Vitamix for making this as it will start to "cream" the cashews —and you can end up with cashew butter.

The Line-Up

1/2 cup (68 gm) hemp seeds*

1/4 cup (20 gm) nutritional yeast*

1/2 teaspoon garlic powder

1/2 teaspoon onion powder

1/2 teaspoon Hawaiian sea salt

*Coach Karen's First-Round Picks on pg. 209.

The Play-by-Play

1. Pulse all ingredients in a small food processor until the hemp seeds are a slightly powdery texture and have combined well with the nutritional yeast.

Store in an airtight shaker jar, and keep in the fridge or freezer for up to 3 months.

 ### WALNUT CILANTRO PESTO (NO OIL)
Makes 16 servings

This spin on classic pesto is super-concentrated in bright GREENs and nitrates. It's made from a base of omega-3 fat, protein, and fiber (walnuts), and unlike the traditional green sauce, it contains no added oil or cheese. The jalapeño pepper and cayenne give it a little kick! Spread it on pizza, pasta, crackers, and toast.

The Line-Up

1 cup walnut pieces

4 cloves garlic

2 cups cilantro leaves, stems removed

1/4 cup purified water (approximate)

1 jalapeño pepper, seeded and chopped

2-3 tablespoons fresh squeezed lemon juice

1 tablespoon organic apple cider vinegar, unfiltered

1/2 teaspoon paprika

1/8 teaspoon cayenne

Coarsely ground black pepper

1/2 teaspoon Hawaiian sea salt, to taste

1/2 teaspoon cumin, optional (Cumin gives the pesto a more 'earthy' flavor.)

The Play-by-Play

1. Put the walnuts and garlic in a food processor, and grind them until they are fine.
2. Add cilantro, 2-3 tablespoons water, and the remaining ingredients and blend. Add more water as needed until the pesto is more of a thick sauce. Taste it and add more seasonings to your liking.

Store in the fridge in a tightly covered container.

 WILTED POWER GREENS
Makes 4 servings

Eating a boatload of dark leafy greens couldn't be easier! Choose from sturdier greens, such as spinach, arugula, red and green Swiss chard, kale, bok choy, Napa cabbage, and tatsoi. Tatsoi (pronounced "taht-SOY") is an Asian green that's also known as "spoon mustard" with its small, dark green spoon-shaped leaves and mild mustard flavor. Tatsoi, one of the best kept secrets in the nutrition space, is packed with a slew of nutrients, like vitamin A, vitamin C, calcium, and potassium.

Coach Karen says
Use as a dip, spread, and condiment to soups. Add a dollop of pesto to tomato soup and roasted winter squash soup when serving.

Coach Karen says
When adding pesto to pasta, keep the pasta warm. Do not heat the pesto. It will change the color, taste, and texture of the fresh cilantro.

The Line-Up

5 oz (about 4 cups) dark leafy greens

Extra virgin avocado or olive oil*

Sea salt and freshly ground black pepper

*Coach Karen's First-Round Picks on pg. 223.

The Play-by-Play

1. Heat a large skillet over medium heat (300°F). Lightly mist it with oil using a non-aerosol oil sprayer** (1/4 teaspoon oil per trigger pull). Add crumbled tofu, and cook for 5 minutes.

2. Add leafy greens. Cook, stirring occasionally until wilted (about 2-3 minutes). Season to taste.

Serve immediately as a side dish, over hot rice, or in ramen (Japanese noodle soup).

**Coach Karen's Cool Tools on pg. 196.

Coach Karen says

Stir up some other quick-cooking COLORS like shredded or match-style carrots, thinly sliced cabbage, bean sprouts, scallions, or sliced mushrooms.

Coach Karen says

"Baby" versions of greens like kale and Swiss chard are sweeter and perfect for salads and smoothies.

THE 7TH INNING STRETCH — SNACKS WITH BENEFITS

 ### BAKED KALE CHIPS
Makes 3 servings

Baked kale chips are a great way to get in your daily GREENs. When baked properly, they're a healthy alternative to potato chips — betcha can't eat just one!

The Line-Up

1 bunch kale

1 tablespoon extra virgin avocado or olive oil*

Nutritional yeast seasoning*

Cajun Spice (pg. 276)

Sea salt, optional

*Coach Karen's First-Round Picks on pg. 206.

The Play-by-Play

1. Preheat oven to 275°F. Line a large rimmed baking sheet with parchment paper.

2. Wash kale and pat dry. Remove the leaves from the thick stems (ribs). Use knife, kitchen shears, or a Kale and Herb Stripper. Cut or roughly tear kale into 1-1/2" pieces, which are bigger than bite-size pieces because they'll shrink when cooked. Add them to the salad spinner. Spin the leaves until thoroughly dry.

3. Place dried leaves in a large bowl. Using a non-aerosol oil sprayer**, lightly mist kale with extra virgin olive oil (no more than 1 tablespoon). Don't use too much oil, or you'll end up with soggy chips. Sprinkle with Cajun Spice. Mix to distribute the oil, then spread out the leaves in a single layer on the prepared baking sheet.

4. Bake until crispy (about 20-25 min), turning leaves halfway through. Do not let the leaves burn. The chips should be crispy and definitely not burnt or soggy.

Sprinkle generously with nutritional yeast for a cheesy finish and a pinch of sea salt (optional), then serve immediately. Store any leftovers in an airtight container.

**Coach Karen's Cool Tools on pg. 191.

Coach Karen says

Remember, the goal is to "crisp" the kale, not scorch it. Low-heat baking for a longer period of time is the key to perfect chips.

 ### CAJUN SOY NUTS
Makes 12 servings

Organic soy nuts are a portable, protein-rich powerhouse. Add them to salads, trail mix, yogurt, stir-fries, and pasta dishes for some crunch. By making your own soy nuts, you control the amount of salt and oil. They're the perfect snack when you crave something 'crunchy'. A one-ounce serving (about 1/4 cup) of homemade soy nuts contains about 170 calories, 15 gm of soy protein, 14 gm of carbohydrate, and 10 gm of fiber. Black soybeans are a delicacy in Japan and contain substantial amounts of WHITEs and BLUEs and contain more vitamin C and nearly twice the iron as the more familiar yellow soybeans.

Coach Karen says

Let the soybeans "dry out" in the fridge for a day. If the beans are too moist inside, they won't get crunchy.

The Line-Up

1-1/2 cups dry organic black (or yellow) soybeans*

6 cups water

Extra virgin avocado or olive oil*

Cajun Spice (pg. 276)

Sea salt (optional)

*Coach Karen's First-Round Picks on pg. 206.

The Play-by-Play

1. Pick out any broken or discolored beans. Rinse well. Soak the beans for 15 hours in 6 cups of water. (Since the beans are absorbing the water, change the water periodically, so the water is fresh.) Rinse the beans in fresh water. Drain them thoroughly.

2. Roll the soybeans around on a clean kitchen towel to remove excess moisture, or pat the beans dry. Place beans in a bowl, cover lightly, and place in the refrigerator for a day to "dry out".

3. Preheat oven to 300°F. Line a rimmed baking sheet with parchment paper. Spread the beans out evenly. Using a non-aerosol oil sprayer**, lightly mist beans with oil. Roast for about an hour, stirring every 15 minutes, until the beans are lightly browned and crunchy. While the beans are still hot, dust them with Cajun Spice. (Sea salt is optional.)

Store in an airtight container.

**Coach Karen's Cool Tools on pg. 196.

Coach Karen says

Most soybeans grown in the U.S. (94%) are GMO soy. The use of genetic engineering or genetically modified organisms (GMOs) is prohibited in organic products.

CHOCOLATE 101

Cacao ("kuh-KOW") and cocoa have historically been used interchangeably, but the two are different ingredients. Cacao, cocoa, Dutch cocoa, and chocolate...what's the difference? Here's how it all breaks down along with the kinds to eat and which to avoid.

Cacao

Cacao refers to the tree and the raw, unrefined bean (or seed). Raw cacao is touted as a "superfood" because it's either not roasted at all, or if roasted, it's roasted below 118°F. Processing conditions during roasting of the raw cacao bean affect the

(continued on next page)

(continued from previous page)

levels of BROWNs, but roasted cacao beans are still a good source of these antioxidants.[12]

Warning! Raw cacao beans are handled by many hands and may contain toxic molds and undesirable pathogens since they haven't been treated with high heat. Many of the farmers in West Africa and Central and South America, primary producers of cacao, live in extreme poverty and lack proper sanitary conditions.

From Cacao to Cocoa

When raw cacao is processed at high temperatures, it's called cocoa. Cocoa powder is what remains after cacao beans have been fermented, dried, roasted, then ground into a fine powder.

This is the powder that's used to bake brownies, chocolate cakes, cookies, and puddings. There are two types of cocoa: Dutch-processed and natural.

100% Dutch-Processed Cocoa Powder — Cacao is naturally acidic. Dutch-processed cocoa powder has been treated with alkali to neutralize the acids, so it has a smoother, more mellow flavor than natural cocoa and imparts a cocoa powder that has a darker hue. However, a significant amount of BROWNs are lost when processed with alkali.

Researchers found that a heavily alkalized cocoa powder contained about 2.0 mg per gram of total BROWNs compared to a natural cocoa powder with 40 mg per gram.[13] In baking, Dutched cocoa powder is paired with baking powder (acid) to make up for the acid that was removed from the cocoa. Acid is needed for leavening (making it rise)

100% Natural Cocoa Powder — Natural cocoa powder retains its acidity and BROWNs since it hasn't been processed with alkali, which gives this powder a sharp finish. It's usually lighter brown in color. If you bake with it, pair it with baking soda (alkali) since it hasn't lost any of its acidity.

(continued on next page)

(continued from previous page)

Chocolate — Cocoa is the key ingredient in chocolate, which is many steps away from the original cacao pod. The greater percentage of cocoa solids and additives (e.g., milk fat, sugar, and butter fat) used to make the chocolate will result in varying degrees of bitterness and BROWNs. Finished dark chocolate, which contains no milk, has two to three times more BROWNs than milk chocolate, so choose 70% dark chocolate or higher to obtain the most antioxidants. Find ways to consume cocoa in forms other than chocolate bars and chips due to the processing that neutralizes the benefits of the BROWNs in chocolate. Consider adding 100% natural cocoa powder to a creamy frozen banana smoothie for an antioxidant-rich snack. Try the Cocoa Almond Milkshake (pg. 243).

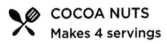
COCOA NUTS
Makes 4 servings

The dusting of pure cocoa, hint of ginger, and dates add some healthy BROWNs and a twist of flavor to your naked nuts.

The Line-Up

1 cup whole raw walnuts (or a mix of walnuts, almonds, and pecans)

4 teaspoons (1 tablespoon + 1 teaspoon) organic date sugar*

1 tablespoon organic date syrup*

1/2 teaspoon Hawaiian sea salt

1/4 teaspoon powdered ginger

1 tablespoon natural 100% unsweetened cocoa powder*

*Coach Karen's First-Round Picks on pg. 206.

The Play-by-Play

1. Preheat oven to 300°F.

2. Mix date sugar, date syrup, salt, and ginger in a small bowl. Mix well. Add nuts and combine. Spread nuts on a parchment-lined baking sheet. Bake for 10 min.

3. While still hot, dust the nuts with the cocoa powder and toss together.

Serve immediately. Store in an airtight container and refrigerate.

 FUDGY OATMEAL BARS
Makes 16 servings

These chocolate bars make nutritious pre- and post-game snacks that are naturally sweet, full of fiber, free of added oil, and a treat to eat.

The Line-Up

Dry Ingredients

1 cup rolled oats

1/2 cup organic almond flour*

1/4 cup natural 100% unsweetened cocoa powder*

6 tablespoons (1/4 cup + 2 tablespoons) organic date sugar*

1/2 tsp baking soda

1/2 tsp baking powder

Flax Eggs (2)

2 tablespoons organic ground golden flaxseed*

6 tablespoons water (1/4 cup + 2 tablespoons)

Add-Ins

1/4 cup Fancy Medjool dates (about 3 dates), chopped

1/4 cup walnuts, roughly chopped

3 tablespoons avocado

*Coach Karen's First-Round Picks on pg. 206.

The Play-by-Play

1. Preheat oven to 350°F. Make 2 flax eggs. Set aside.
2. Add all dry ingredients to a large bowl and mix. Add chopped dates and nuts, then mix. Add flax eggs and avocado. Combine well, but do not over-mix.

How to Make a Flax Egg

Mix 3 TBSP water with 1 TBSP ground flaxseed (3-to-1 ratio). To make 2 flax eggs, mix 6 TBSP (1/4 cup + 2 TBSP) water with 2 TBSP flaxseed. Combine well, and set aside for 5 minutes to thicken.

Coach Karen says

Chopped dates can be sticky and clump together. Roll chopped dates in a little almond or oat flour to separate them.

3. Using a non-aerosol oil sprayer**, lightly mist an 8" x 8" pan with extra virgin oil. Press mixture into the pan. (It will be a thick and dry dough, not a 'pourable' batter.)

4. Bake 10 to 11 minutes until the top/edges begin to set. (Bars will be soft, but will set when cooled.) Let the pan cool for 10 minutes on a cooling rack.

When completely cooled, cut into bars. Store in an airtight container, and refrigerate for up to a week.

**Coach Karen's Cool Tools on pg. 196.

SPROUTED GRAIN 'CRACKERS'
Makes 1 serving

If you're in need of a healthy platform for your favorite hummus or guac, here's an ultra-simple solution that bumps up your whole grain, fiber, and protein intake. Ditch the 'flour-y' pita chips. Store-bought crackers or pita chips made with high-quality ingredients, no added oil or sugar, and acceptable sodium levels are hard to find.

The Line-Up

1 large sprouted grain tortilla*

*Coach Karen's First-Round Picks on pg. 211.

The Play-by-Play

1. Preheat oven to 300°F.

2. Lay 1 tortilla on a baking sheet for about 5 to 6 minutes, then flip over and repeat. Your "cracker" is done when the edges start to curl up and the center is hard. At that point, they'll be 'crisp' enough to break into pieces.

Break the cooled tortilla into large pieces, and dunk into your favorite dip!

Coach Karen says

Make a batch of crackers (6 tortillas) or make them single-serve style to control portions.

HOW TO KEEP THE FUZZ OFF FRESH BERRIES

Bathe your berries in diluted vinegar as soon as you bring them home. Yes, vinegar. Rinsing produce with a 10% vinegar solution reduces viruses by 95% and bacteria on strawberries, like E. coli and salmonella, by 90%.[14] Vinegar also kills the mold spores that are on the surface of the berries. They'll stay mold-free, plump, and firm for a week or more (that is, if you don't eat them all). You won't taste the vinegar because it's so diluted, plus you can give them a final clear rinse as well.

Prepare a mixture of one part white distilled or apple cider vinegar with 10 parts warm water (72° to 109°F). Rinse the berries first in fresh water, then gently agitate the berries by swirling them around in this solution for two minutes:

- **For a small basket:** 2 tablespoons vinegar + 1-1/4 cups water
- **For a large basket:** 1/4 cup vinegar + 2-1/2 cups water

Don't oversoak, or you'll lose valuable water-soluble vitamins. After the vinegar wash, you can rinse your berries in a colander under clear running water. Pat the berries dry. Gently place them in a towel-lined berry colander or bowl, and store them in your produce drawer. No more gray fuzzy berries!

 FRUIT PLATE WITH DARK CHOCOLATE CURLS
Makes 4 servings

Dark chocolate + sweet fruit = healthy harmony. For an elegant end to a nice meal (and no fuss), garnish a plate of COLOR-ful, naturally sweet fruit with dark, nearly unsweetened chocolate. Sprinkle some coarsely chopped almonds on the plate for some bits of crunch. Dark chocolate is the most 'bitter' of the chocolate bunch, especially as you venture into the higher percentages of cocoa, so balance it with fruits that are extra sweet. (That's why strawberries dipped in dark chocolate make a delicious pair.) Raspberries are both sweet and tart, but pair well too. Their bit of tartness adds a nice 'brightness' to the rich, deep dark chocolate.

The Line-Up

4-oz dark chocolate bar, 70% to 90% cocoa

4 oz raw organic almonds, roughly chopped

Assortment of fresh fruits, such as, apricots, grapes, honeydew, kiwi, mango, orange, passion fruit, plums, and strawberries. Top pairing picks: bananas, cherries, pears, and raspberries.

The Play-by-Play

For Chocolate Curls

1. Let the chocolate bar stand in a warm place (80° to 85°F) until thoroughly warm, but not melted — or microwave briefly on medium (50%) power.

2. Using a vegetable peeler, scrape the blade along the thin, flat side of the bar (lengthwise). Refrigerate the curls on a plate until ready to use.

Arrange fruits on each plate, then sprinkle with chopped almonds. Garnish each plate with the chocolate curls. Serve immediately.

PEAR AND BLUEBERRY CRUMBLE
Makes 4 servings

Cooked pears are great alongside grilled salmon or grains, but they're also scrumptious when served with Greek yogurt, oatmeal, frozen yogurt, or vanilla bean 'Nice Cream' (pg. 298).

The Line-Up

2 pears, unpeeled, sliced (not *too* thin or they may fall apart)

1 cup blueberries, frozen or fresh

1 cup unsweetened 100% organic pomegranate juice*

2 teaspoons freshly squeezed lemon juice

1 teaspoon ground cinnamon (1/2 teaspoon for pears + 1/2 teaspoon for crumble)

3/4 teaspoon powdered ginger

1/2 teaspoon nutmeg

1/2 cup rolled oats

1/2 cup raw almonds

Coach Karen says

Some of the best pears for sautéing and grilling are Bosc, Concorde, and D'Anjou. They keep their shape when heated and have a nice taste and texture. Ripe Bartlett pears tend to turn to mush under the slightest bit of heat.

1/4 cup organic date sugar*

1/4 cup (56 gm) Earth Balance® vegan buttery spread

2 tablespoons almond flour*

2 tablespoons ground flaxseeds*

Extra virgin avocado or olive oil*

*Coach Karen's First-Round Picks on pg. 206.

The Play-by-Play

1. Preheat oven to 300°F.

2. Toast nuts in a dry skillet over low to medium heat, stirring occasionally until lightly toasted (about 5 to 6 minutes).

3. Combine date sugar and 1/2 teaspoon cinnamon in a small bowl. Add vegan butter and smash with a fork to mix. Add oats, almonds, almond flour, and flaxseeds, then combine well. Set aside.

For the Pears

1. Heat a large skillet over medium heat (300°F). Lightly mist it with oil using a non-aerosol oil sprayer** (1/4 teaspoon oil per trigger pull). Add sliced pears, stirring occasionally until pears are light gold (about 4 to 5 minutes). Add pomegranate juice, lemon juice, 1/2 teaspoon cinnamon, ginger, and nutmeg to the pears. Stir, then mix in the blueberries. Cook until all liquid is absorbed and pears are just tender (about 3-5 minutes).

2. Place the pears in an 8" pie pan. Sprinkle with the crumble topping. Bake for 15-20 minutes to toast the crumble topping. Remove from oven.

Serve immediately. Refrigerate leftovers.

**Coach Karen's Cool Tools on pg. 196.

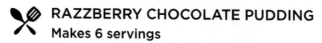

RAZZBERRY CHOCOLATE PUDDING
Makes 6 servings

This rich and dreamy pudding is luscious and decadent, but contains no cream, egg yolks, or refined sugar. Serve also as a lightened-up chocolate topping or dip for fresh strawberries.

The Line-Up

16 Fancy Medjool dates*, pitted, coarsely chopped

32 frozen raspberries

12 oz. avocado

1 cup + 1 tablespoon organic unsweetened soy milk*

1 cup natural 100% unsweetened cocoa powder*

1/4 cup organic date syrup*

2 teaspoons vanilla*

Pinch of Hawaiian sea salt

Garnish: fresh raspberry and mint leaf

*Coach Karen's First-Round Picks on pg. 206.

The Play-by-Play

1. Soak dates in boiling hot water until soft (about 5 to 10 minutes). Drain. Add the dates and milk to a food processor. Process until smooth.

2. Add the remaining ingredients, and blend until creamy. Divide into individual dessert cups (if desired). Refrigerate until cold (about 3 hours).

Garnish with a fresh raspberry and mint leaf, and serve immediately.

 ## SPICED APPLES WITH CINNAMON CRUNCH
Makes 4 servings

These cinnamon-spiced apples are naturally delicious. Enjoy their calming and homey aroma while they simmer on the stove.

The Line-Up

2 organic Honey Crisp apples, unpeeled, cored, trimmed, halved

3/4 cup unsweetened organic apple juice

1 teaspoon freshly squeezed lemon juice

1/2 cup walnuts, roughly chopped

1/3 cup Ezekiel 4:9 Sprouted Crunchy Cereal, Golden Flax*

1/4 cup almond flour*

1/4 cup organic date sugar*

3 tablespoons (42 gm) Earth Balance® vegan buttery spread, melted

3/4 teaspoon ground cinnamon* (1/2 teaspoon for the apples and 1/4 teaspoon for the topping)

1/8 teaspoon ground nutmeg

Extra virgin avocado or olive oil*

*Coach Karen's First-Round Picks on pg. 206.

The Play-by-Play

For the Crunch

1. Preheat oven to 300°F.
2. Combine date sugar and 1/4 teaspoon cinnamon in a small bowl. Pour in melted vegan butter and mix. Add almond flour, cereal, walnuts, and combine well.
3. Press mixture into an ungreased 8" x 8" baking pan. Bake for 35 minutes.

For the Apples

1. While the topping is baking, cut each apple half, so you have five slices per half.
2. Heat a large skillet over medium heat (300°F). Lightly mist it with oil using a non-aerosol oil sprayer** (1/4 teaspoon oil per trigger pull). Add apples, stirring occasionally until apples are light gold (about 4 to 5 minutes). Add apple juice, lemon juice, 1/2 teaspoon cinnamon, and nutmeg to the apples. Cook until all liquid is absorbed and apples are just tender (about 3-5 minutes).

Serve the apples with the crunchies on top. Sprinkle with date sugar (if desired).

**Coach Karen's Cool Tools on pg. 196.

 VANILLA BEAN 'NICE CREAM'
Makes 2 servings

Banana ice cream (a.k.a. Nice Cream) is a super simple, whole food, plant-based take on soft-serve ice cream that's made with a base of just one ingredient...the good ol' banana! No need to break out the

Coach Karen says

These spiced apples are delicious with or without the topping. Make a batch and refrigerate. Add them to oatmeal, yogurt, and toast, or enjoy over vanilla bean 'Nice Cream' for a treat!

Coach Karen says

For a different flavor Nice Cream, mix in 1/2 to 3/4 cup frozen organic strawberries; 1 to 2 tablespoons natural unsweetened 100% cocoa powder*; or 1 to 2 tablespoons nut/seed butter; 1 to 2 teaspoons matcha*.

ice cream maker. There's no dairy, no sweeteners, no eggs, and no saturated fat. How easy can healthy get? Give it a try!

The Line-Up

The Base

2 medium-large 8" ripe (but not overripe) bananas, frozen, 1/2" slices

1 vanilla bean

Optional: a few chopped almonds and/or dark chocolate chunks

The Play-by-Play

1. Split the vanilla bean lengthwise, and scrape the seeds from the vanilla bean. Spread the vanilla seeds over the frozen bananas.

2. Add the frozen sliced bananas and vanilla to a powerful blender** or small food processor. Blend until creamy like soft serve.

Eat immediately and enjoy!

**Coach Karen's Cool Tools on pg. 196.

Coach Karen says

To freeze several ripe bananas, slice them into 1/2-inch pieces, and set them on a parchment-lined baking sheet in a single layer. Place in the freezer for at least 25 minutes. Then transfer to a freezer bag or glass container for at least 2 hours (ideally overnight), and you'll always be prepared for a Nice Cream craving!

*I know once people get connected to real food,
they never change back.*

ALICE WATERS

POST-GAME WRAP

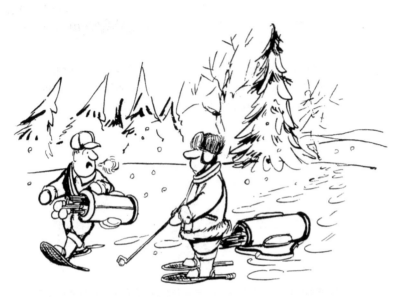

"This might be our last round of the year."

You've finally reached the end of your nutrition playbook, and like all great competitions in both life and sport, here's the takeaway. Care about your food — and by its own nature, you will upgrade your lifestyle. When you care about what you're eating and why it's good for you, your food choices become much clearer and easier to make. You naturally clear the field of all the clutter — everything that's refined, over-processed, over-salted, over-sweetened, and artificially colored. Get real food — the most wholesome, nutritious, and colorful you can find. Remember, what you eat becomes a part of you.

As you start to change the way you fuel your body, gauge your progress — but not by how much you weigh, but by how you *feel*. Do you feel good? Do your jeans fit better? How do you feel when you climb several flights of stairs? Can you scale them without a fire blazing in your thighs or without gasping for an inhaler?

Eat a variety of colors, enjoy your food, and move your body, which is the essence of this playbook's anti-aging message. Aim for progress, not perfection. With the right plan, you can undermine the aging process. You aren't doomed to have shrunken biceps, belly fat, brittle bones, brain farts, balance problems, and bifocals. Nor are you doomed to be sidelined with age-related game-changing diseases.

You can't extinguish old habits, but you can create new ones. One of the essential ingredients of transforming your life is belief. Researchers say what can make the difference between achieving your goals (or not) is *believing* you can do something different. Belief is the most powerful component of change.

Finally, you can control how well you feel and how fast you age. You can break 100. Shake off previous win-loss records. You're starting a new season. You know the plays. Now it's all up to YOU.

Knowing is not enough; we must apply.
Willing is not enough; we must do.

JOHANN WOLFGANG VON GOETHE

APPENDIX

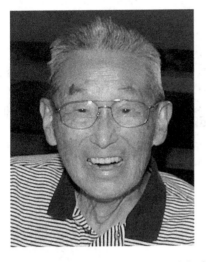

My dear dad is the inspiration behind writing this book, and I wrote the following on his 96th birthday. I learned many valuable life lessons from my father over the years, and I thought I'd share what I've observed to be "My Dad's Seven Keys to Longevity". I hope you'll find them helpful in your quest for health and wellness.

My Dad's Seven Keys to Longevity

1 Get a good night's sleep.	Don't let things bother you if there's nothing you can do about it. Just "worrying" doesn't do anything to make the situation better. My mom claimed that my dad fell asleep as soon as his head hit the pillow. The only thing that kept him awake at night was comforting me after a nightmare or when I had one of my many stomachaches.
2 Stay physically active.	Dad hardly ever sat down. He always found things to do and was always moving. His family and friends would encourage him to "sit down and relax", but I think his vitality emerged when he found ways to help others.

3 Respect life, nature, & the environment.	Grow, nurture, recycle, renew, and don't be wasteful. My dad practiced this long before it was "fashionable" to be green. He is a man of infinite patience and has a caring hand. Dad can bring the most neglected house plants back to life and would never think to throw them away.
4 Eat simply & "cleanly".	Dad loves to eat and isn't fussy. He could make any cook feel appreciated. But his favorite meal was just good ol' homegrown vegetables, tofu, fresh-picked fruit, and fish. Looking back, he ate "clean" way back when clean actually meant 'not dirty'.
5 Drink green tea & black coffee, not alcohol & soda.	All those healthy antioxidants have served him well. As my dad has aged though, it's harder to get him to drink enough fluids as water can be pretty boring — especially when he's not thirsty. Offer him a hot cup of tea or coffee though, and he won't refuse.
6 Learn new things & meet new people.	One of the things my dad told me once when I complained about a seminar as having been a "waste of time", he said, "If you learned just one new thing or met just one new person, then it was worth it." I live by those wise words to this day.
7 Live life & look ahead.	Dad always told me, "Things happen for a reason." That is, there is good buried under what may seem sad, tragic, or painful at the time. It was my dad's way to survive (and teach me to survive) hardship and grief, to stay positive, and be optimistic.

GAME NOTES

Notes from the Coach

1. Arias, Elizabeth, and Xu, Jiaquan. "United States Life Tables, 2017." *National Vital Statistics Reports.* 24 Jun 2019. https://www.cdc.gov/nchs/data/nvsr/nvsr68/nvsr68_07-508.pdf

2. National Institutes of Health/National Institute of Aging. *"Aging Under the Microscope – A Biological Quest."* 2002.

3. Coresh J, Selvin E, Stevens LA, Manzi J, Kusek JW, Eggers P, Van Lente F, Levey AS. Prevalence of chronic kidney disease in the United States. JAMA. 2007 Nov 7;298(17):2038-47. doi: 10.1001/jama.298.17.2038. PMID: 17986697.

4. Centers for Disease Control and Prevention. "Chronic Kidney Disease in the United States, 2021." *Chronic Kidney Disease Initiative.* March 04, 2021.

5. Odermatt A. The Western-style diet: a major risk factor for impaired kidney function and chronic kidney disease. Am J Physiol Renal Physiol. 2011 Nov;301(5):F919-31. doi: 10.1152/ajprenal.00068.2011. Epub 2011 Aug 31. PMID: 21880837.

Play 2: Free Agents — Understanding Free Radicals and Why You Age

1. Zolkipli-Cunningham, Zarazuela, and Marni J Falk. "Clinical effects of chemical exposures on mitochondrial function." *Toxicology* vol. 391 (2017): 90-99. doi:10.1016/j.tox.2017.07.009

2. Jia, Guanghong et al. "Mitochondrial functional impairment in response to environmental toxins in the cardiorenal metabolic syndrome." *Archives of toxicology* vol. 89,2 (2015): 147-53. doi:10.1007/s00204-014-1431-3

3. Neustadt, John, and Pieczenik, Steve R. "Medication-induced mitochondrial damage and disease." *Molecular Nutrition and Food Research.* 2008 Jul;52(7):780-8. doi: 10.1002/mnfr.200700075.

4. Pieczenik SR, Neustadt J. Mitochondrial dysfunction and molecular pathways of disease. Exp Mol Pathol. 2007 Aug;83(1):84-92. doi: 10.1016/j.yexmp.2006.09.008. Epub 2007 Jan 18. PMID: 17239370.

Play 3: The Benchwarmers — Foods to Ditch

1. Strong JP, Malcom GT, McMahan CA, et al. Prevalence and Extent of Atherosclerosis in Adolescents and Young Adults: Implications for Prevention From the Pathobiological Determinants of Atherosclerosis in Youth Study. *JAMA.* 1999;281(8):727–735. doi:10.1001/jama.281.8.727

2. de la Monte, Suzanne M, and Jack R Wands. "Alzheimer's disease is type 3 diabetes-evidence reviewed." *Journal of diabetes science and technology* vol. 2,6 (2008): 1101-13. doi:10.1177/193229680800200619

3. Monro JA, Leon R, Puri BK. The risk of lead contamination in bone broth diets. Med Hypotheses. 2013 Apr;80(4):389-90. doi: 10.1016/j.mehy.2012.12.026. Epub 2013 Jan 31. PMID: 23375414.

4. Hsu, Der-Jen et al. "Essential and toxic metals in animal bone broths." *Food & nutrition research* vol. 61,1 1347478. 18 Jul. 2017, doi:10.1080/16546628.2017.1347478

5. Farquhar, William B et al. "Dietary sodium and health: more than just blood pressure." *Journal of the American College of Cardiology* vol. 65,10 (2015): 1042-50. doi:10.1016/j.jacc.2014.12.039

6. Dickinson KM, Clifton PM, Keogh JB. Endothelial function is impaired after a high-salt meal in healthy subjects. Am J Clin Nutr. 2011 Mar;93(3):500-5. doi: 10.3945/ajcn.110.006155. Epub 2011 Jan 12. PMID: 21228265.

7. Uribarri, Jaime et al. "Advanced glycation end products in foods and a practical guide to their reduction in the diet." *Journal of the American Dietetic Association* vol. 110,6 (2010): 911-16.e12. doi:10.1016/j.jada.2010.03.018

8. Anderson GH, Liu Y, Smith CE, Liu TT, Nunez MF, Mollard RC, Luhovyy BL. The acute effect of commercially available pulse powders on postprandial glycaemic response in healthy young men. Br J Nutr. 2014 Dec 28;112(12):1966-73. doi: 10.1017/S0007114514003031. Epub 2014 Oct 20. PMID: 25327223.

9. Zafar TA, Al-Hassawi F, Al-Khulaifi F, Al-Rayyes G, Waslien C, Huffman FG. Organoleptic and glycemic properties of chickpea-wheat composite breads. J Food Sci Technol. 2015 Apr;52(4):2256-63. doi: 10.1007/s13197-013-1192-7. Epub 2013 Oct 20. PMID: 25829607; PMCID: PMC4375205.

10. Almekinder, Elisabeth, "20 Healthy Flours form Lowest to Highest Carbohydrates." TheDiabetesCouncil.com *2020 May*. https://www.thediabetescouncil.com/20-healthy-flours/

11. Törrönen R, Kolehmainen M, Sarkkinen E, Poutanen K, Mykkänen H, Niskanen L. Berries reduce postprandial insulin responses to wheat and rye breads in healthy women. J Nutr. 2013 Apr;143(4):430-6. doi: 10.3945/jn.112.169771. Epub 2013 Jan 30. PMID: 23365108.

12. Ferris, Heather and Kahn, Ronald. "Unraveling the Paradox of Selective Insulin Resistance in the Liver: the Brain–Liver Connection." *Diabetes* 2016 Jun; 65(6): 1481-1483. https://doi.org/10.2337/dbi16-0010

13. Zhou Y, Rui L. Leptin signaling and leptin resistance. *Front Med.* 2013;7(2):207–222. doi:10.1007/s11684-013-0263-5

14. Vighi, G et al. "Allergy and the gastrointestinal system." *Clinical and experimental immunology* vol. 153 Suppl 1,Suppl 1 (2008): 3-6. doi:10.1111/j.1365-2249.2008.03713.x

15. Yacoub, Rabi et al. "Advanced glycation end products dietary restriction effects on bacterial gut microbiota in peritoneal dialysis patients; a randomized open label controlled trial." *PloS one* vol. 12,9 e0184789. 20 Sep. 2017, doi:10.1371/journal.pone.0184789

16. Claesson MJ, Jeffery IB, Conde S, Power SE, O'Connor EM, Cusack S, Harris HM, Coakley M, Lakshminarayanan B, O'Sullivan O, Fitzgerald GF, Deane J, O'Connor M, Harnedy N, O'Connor K, O'Mahony D, van Sinderen D, Wallace M, Brennan L, Stanton C, Marchesi JR, Fitzgerald AP, Shanahan F, Hill C, Ross RP, O'Toole PW. Gut microbiota composition correlates with diet and health in the elderly. Nature. 2012 Aug 9;488(7410):178-84. doi: 10.1038/nature11319. PMID: 22797518.

17. Heiman ML, Greenway FL. A healthy gastrointestinal microbiome is dependent on dietary diversity. Mol Metab. 2016 Mar 5;5(5):317-320. doi: 10.1016/j.molmet.2016.02.005. PMID: 27110483; PMCID: PMC4837298.

18. Langdon, Amy et al. "The effects of antibiotics on the microbiome throughout development and alternative approaches for therapeutic modulation." *Genome medicine* vol. 8,1 39. 13 Apr. 2016, doi:10.1186/s13073-016-0294-z

19. Bressa C, Bailén-Andrino M, Pérez-Santiago J, González-Soltero R, Pérez M, et al. (2017) Differences in gut microbiota profile between women with active lifestyle and sedentary women. PLOS ONE 12(2): e0171352. https://doi.org/10.1371/journal.pone.0171352

20. Biedermann, Luc et al. "Smoking cessation induces profound changes in the composition of the intestinal microbiota in humans." *PloS one* vol. 8,3 (2013): e59260. doi:10.1371/journal.pone.0059260

21. Benedict, Christian et al. "Gut microbiota and glucometabolic alterations in response to recurrent partial sleep deprivation in normal-weight young individuals." *Molecular metabolism* vol. 5,12 1175-1186. 24 Oct. 2016, doi:10.1016/j.molmet.2016.10.003

22. Galley JD, Nelson MC, Yu Z, Dowd SE, Walter J, Kumar PS, Lyte M, Bailey MT. Exposure to a social stressor disrupts the community structure of the colonic mucosa-associated microbiota. BMC Microbiol. 2014 Jul 15;14:189. doi: 10.1186/1471-2180-14-189. PMID: 25028050; PMCID: PMC4105248.

23. Francescone, Ralph et al. "Microbiome, inflammation, and cancer." *Cancer journal (Sudbury, Mass.)* vol. 20,3 (2014): 181-9. doi:10.1097/PPO.0000000000000048

Play 4: Fired Up Means Aging Up — Chronic Inflammation

1. Musunuru, K., Kral, B., Blumenthal, R. et al. The use of high-sensitivity assays for C-reactive protein in clinical practice. *Nat Rev Cardiol* 5, 621–635 (2008). https://doi.org/10.1038/ncpcardio1322

2. Ridker, Paul M et al. "C-Reactive Protein and Other Markers of Inflammation in the Prediction of Cardiovascular Disease in Women." New England Journal of Medicine 2000 Mar; 342:836-843. doi: 10.1056/NEJM200003233421202.

3. Calder PC, Ahluwalia N, Brouns F, Buetler T, Clement K, Cunningham K, Esposito K, Jönsson LS, Kolb H, Lansink M, Marcos A, Margioris A, Matusheski N, Nordmann H, O'Brien J, Pugliese G, Rizkalla S, Schalkwijk C, Tuomilehto J, Wärnberg J, Watzl B, Winklhofer-Roob BM. Dietary factors and low-grade inflammation in relation to overweight and obesity. Br J Nutr. 2011 Dec;106 Suppl 3:S5-78. doi: 10.1017/S0007114511005460. PMID: 22133051.

4. Pahwa R, Singh A, Jialal I. Chronic Inflammation. [Updated 2019 Dec 13]. In: StatPearls [Internet]. Treasure Island (FL): StatPearls Publishing; 2020 Jan. https://www.ncbi.nlm.nih.gov/books/NBK493173/

5. Simpson, Norah and Dinges, David. "Sleep and Inflammation". *International Life Sciences Institute* 2007 Dec; S244-S252. doi: 10.1301/nr.2007.dec.S244–S252.

6. Drewnowski A, Rehm CD. Consumption of added sugars among US children and adults by food purchase location and food source. Am J Clin Nutr. 2014;100(3):901–907. https://www.ncbi.nlm.nih.gov/pmc/articles/PMC4135498/

7. Ohnishi, Mutsuko, Razzaque, Shawkat. "Dietary and genetic evidence for phosphate toxicity accelerating mammalian aging." *FASEB Journal* 23 Apr 2010.

8. Yamada S, Tokumoto M, Tatsumoto N, Taniguchi M, Noguchi H, Nakano T, Masutani K, Ooboshi H, Tsuruya K, Kitazono T. Phosphate overload directly induces systemic inflammation and malnutrition as well as vascular calcification in uremia. *Am J Physiol Renal Physiol*. 2014 Jun 15;306(12):F1418-28. doi: 10.1152/ajprenal.00633.2013. Epub 2014 May 7. PMID: 24808541.

9. Sacks, Frank M. Dietary Fats and Cardiovascular Disease: A Presidential Advisory from the American Heart Association. *Circulation*. 15 Jun 2017;136:e1–e23. doi.org/10.1161/CIR.0000000000000510

10. Sacks, Frank M. Coconut Oil and Heart Health, Fact or Fiction? *Circulation*. 10 Mar 2020;141:815-817. doi.org/10.1161/CIRCULATIONAHA.119.044687

11. Nicholls SJ, Lundman P, Harmer JA, Cutri B, Griffiths KA, Rye KA, Barter PJ, Celermajer DS. Consumption of saturated fat impairs the anti-inflammatory properties of high-density lipoproteins and endothelial

function. J Am Coll Cardiol. 2006 Aug 15;48(4):715-20. doi: 10.1016/j.
jacc.2006.04.080. Epub 2006 Jul 24. PMID: 16904539.

12. Tang, W.H. Wilson et al. "Intestinal Microbial Metabolism of
Phosphatidylcholine and Cardiovascular Risk." *N Engl J Med* 2013;
368:1575-1584. 25 Apr 2013. doi: 10.1056/NEJMoa1109400

13. Heianza, York et al. "Gut Microbiota Metabolites and Risk of Major
Adverse Cardiovascular Disease Events and Death: A Systematic
Review and Meta-Analysis of Prospective Studies." *Journal of the
American Heart Association* 2017. 29 Jun 2017. https://doi.org/10.1161/
JAHA.116.004947

14. Zeneng Wang, Nathalie Bergeron, Bruce S Levison, Xinmin S Li, Sally
Chiu, Xun Jia, Robert A Koeth, Lin Li, Yuping Wu, W H Wilson Tang,
Ronald M Krauss, Stanley L Hazen, Impact of chronic dietary red meat,
white meat, or non-meat protein on trimethylamine N-oxide metabolism
and renal excretion in healthy men and women, *European Heart
Journal*, Volume 40, Issue 7, 14 February 2019, Pages 583–594, https://
doi.org/10.1093/eurheartj/ehy799

15. Zhu, Weifei et al. "Gut Microbe-Generated Trimethylamine N-Oxide
From Dietary Choline Is Prothrombotic in Subjects." *Circulation* vol.
135,17 (2017): 1671-1673. doi:10.1161/CIRCULATIONAHA.116.025338

16. Genoni, Angela et al. "Long-term Paelolithic diet is associated with
lower resistant starch intake, different gut microbiota composition and
increased serum TMAO concentrations." *European Journal of Nutrition*
2019, 59:1845–1858. 5 July 2019.

17. Carolyn A Miller, Karen D Corbin, Kerry-Ann da Costa, Shucha Zhang,
Xueqing Zhao, Joseph A Galanko, Tondra Blevins, Brian J Bennett,
Annalouise O'Connor, Steven H Zeisel, Effect of egg ingestion on
trimethylamine-N-oxide production in humans: a randomized, controlled,
dose-response study, *The American Journal of Clinical Nutrition*,
Volume 100, Issue 3, September 2014, Pages 778–786, https://doi.
org/10.3945/ajcn.114.087692

18. American Heart Association. "Heavy Meals May Trigger Heart Attacks."
ScienceDaily. ScienceDaily, 21 November 2000. <www.sciencedaily.com/
releases/2000/11/001120072759.htm>.

19. de Pablo P, Cooper MS, Buckley CD. Association between bone mineral
density and C-reactive protein in a large population-based sample.
Arthritis Rheum. 2012 Aug;64(8):2624-31. doi: 10.1002/art.34474. PMID:
22487938.

20. Li, Dang et al. "Trimethylamine-N-oxide promotes brain aging and
cognitive impairment in mice." *Aging cell* vol. 17,4 (2018): e12768.
doi:10.1111/acel.12768

Play 5: Your Defensive Line — How Colorful Is Your Food?

1. Thiede, Ashley and Sheri Zidenberg-Cherr, "Nutrition and Health Info Sheet: Phytochemicals for Health Professionals." *UC Davis Department of Nutrition* 2016. Jun 2016. https://nutrition.ucdavis.edu/sites/g/files/dgvnsk426/files/content/infosheets/factsheets/fact-pro-phytochemical.pdf

2. Roher, Alex E et al. "Cerebral blood flow in Alzheimer's disease." *Vascular health and risk management* vol. 8 (2012): 599-611. doi:10.2147/VHRM.S34874

3. Presley, Tennille D et al. "Acute effect of a high nitrate diet on brain perfusion in older adults." *Nitric oxide : biology and chemistry* vol. 24,1 (2011): 34-42. doi:10.1016/j.niox.2010.10.002

4. Borlinghaus, Jan et al. "Allicin: chemistry and biological properties." *Molecules (Basel, Switzerland)* vol. 19,8 12591-618. 19 Aug. 2014, doi:10.3390/molecules190812591

5. Vinson JA, Zubik L, Bose P, Samman N, Proch J. Dried fruits: excellent in vitro and in vivo antioxidants. J Am Coll Nutr. 2005 Feb;24(1):44-50. doi: 10.1080/07315724.2005.10719442. PMID: 15670984.

6. Claudine Manach, Augustin Scalbert, Christine Morand, Christian Rémésy, Liliana Jiménez, Polyphenols: food sources and bioavailability, *The American Journal of Clinical Nutrition,* Volume 79, Issue 5, May 2004, Pages 727–747, https://doi.org/10.1093/ajcn/79.5.727

7. American Institute for Cancer Research. "Freeze-Dried Fruits Are a Good Health Choice." 2006. *Ever Green, Ever Healthy.* May 2006 Edition. http://aicr.org

8. Shofian, Norshahida Mohamad et al. "Effect of freeze-drying on the antioxidant compounds and antioxidant activity of selected tropical fruits." *International journal of molecular sciences* vol. 12,7 (2011): 4678-92. doi:10.3390/ijms12074678

9. Orak HH, Aktas T, Yagar H, Isbilir SS, Ekinci N, Sahin FH. Effects of hot air and freeze drying methods on antioxidant activity, colour and some nutritional characteristics of strawberry tree (Arbutus unedo L) fruit. Food Sci Technol Int. 2012 Aug;18(4):391-402. doi: 10.1177/1082013211428213. Epub 2012 Apr 20. PMID: 22522307.

Play 6: Raw vs Cooked — Which is the Winner?

1. Giovannucci E, Rimm EB, Liu Y, Stampfer MJ, Willett WC. A prospective study of tomato products, lycopene, and prostate cancer risk. J Natl Cancer Inst. 2002 Mar 6;94(5):391-8. doi: 10.1093/jnci/94.5.391. PMID: 11880478

2. Karppi J, Laukkanen JA, Sivenius J, Ronkainen K, Kurl S. Serum lycopene decreases the risk of stroke in men: a population-based follow-up study. Neurology. 2012 Oct 9;79(15):1540-7. doi: 10.1212/WNL.0b013e31826e26a6. PMID: 23045517

3. Cornell University. "Cooking Tomatoes Boosts Disease-Fighting Power." ScienceDaily. *ScienceDaily,* 23 April 2002. www.sciencedaily.com/releases/2002/04/020422073341.htm

4. United States Department of Agriculture. "Lycopene." *USDA National Nutrient Database* 2018. https://www.nal.usda.gov/sites/www.nal.usda.gov/files/lycopene.pdf

5. Fielding JM, Rowley KG, Cooper P, O' Dea K. Increases in plasma lycopene concentration after consumption of tomatoes cooked with olive oil. Asia Pac J Clin Nutr. 2005;14(2):131-6. PMID: 15927929

6. Pellegrini N, Chiavaro E, Gardana C, Mazzeo T, Contino D, Gallo M, Riso P, Fogliano V, Porrini M. Effect of different cooking methods on color, phytochemical concentration, and antioxidant capacity of raw and frozen brassica vegetables. J Agric Food Chem. 2010 Apr 14;58(7):4310-21. doi: 10.1021/jf904306r. PMID: 20218674

7. Palermo M, Pellegrini N, Fogliano V. The effect of cooking on the phytochemical content of vegetables. J Sci Food Agric. 2014 Apr;94(6):1057-70. doi: 10.1002/jsfa.6478. Epub 2013 Dec 13. PMID: 24227349

8. Memnune Şengül, Hilal Yildiz & Arzu Kavaz (2014) The Effect of Cooking on Total Polyphenolic Content and Antioxidant Activity of Selected Vegetables, International Journal of Food Properties, 17:3, 481-490, DOI: 10.1080/10942912.2011.619292

9. Sun, Yang et al. "Association of fried food consumption with all cause, cardiovascular, and cancer mortality: prospective cohort study." *British Medical Journal* 2019;364:k5420. doi: https://doi.org/10.1136/bmj.k5420

10. Uribarri, Jaime et al. "Advanced glycation end products in foods and a practical guide to their reduction in the diet." *Journal of the American Dietetic Association* vol. 110,6 (2010): 911-16.e12. doi:10.1016/j.jada.2010.03.018

11. Mojska H, Gielecińska I. Studies of acrylamide level in coffee and coffee substitutes: influence of raw material and manufacturing conditions. Rocz Panstw Zakl Hig. 2013;64(3):173-81. PMID: 24325083

12. Mojska H, Gielecińska I, Cendrowski A. Acrylamide content in cigarette mainstream smoke and estimation of exposure to acrylamide from tobacco smoke in Poland. Ann Agric Environ Med. 2016 Sep;23(3):456-61. doi: 10.5604/12321966.1219187. PMID: 27660868

Play 7: Starting Lineup — The Fab 15 Recruits

1. Carlsen et al.: The total antioxidant content of more than 3100 foods, beverages, spices, herbs and supplements used worldwide. *Nutrition Journal* 2010 9:3.

2. American Chemical Society. "Eating berries may activate the brain's natural housekeeper for healthy aging." ScienceDaily. ScienceDaily, 24

August 2010. www.sciencedaily.com/releases/2010/08/100823142927. htm.

3. Zhou, Hui et al. "Proteomic analysis of the effects of aged garlic extract and its FruArg component on lipopolysaccharide-induced neuroinflammatory response in microglial cells." *PloS* one vol. 9,11 e113531. 24 Nov. 2014, doi:10.1371/journal.pone.0113531

4. Song, Hailong et al. "Bioactive components from garlic on brain resiliency against neuroinflammation and neurodegeneration." *Experimental and therapeutic medicine* vol. 19,2 (2020): 1554-1559. doi:10.3892/etm.2019.8389

5. Miller KB, Hurst WJ, Payne MJ, Stuart DA, Apgar J, Sweigart DS, Ou B. Impact of alkalization on the antioxidant and flavanol content of commercial cocoa powders. J Agric Food Chem. 2008 Sep 24;56(18):8527-33. doi: 10.1021/jf801670p. Epub 2008 Aug 19. PMID: 18710243.

6. Fan, Frank S. "Iron deficiency anemia due to excessive green tea drinking." *Clinical case reports* vol. 4,11 1053-1056. 5 Oct. 2016, doi:10.1002/ccr3.707

7. Gerry Schwalfenberg, Stephen J. Genuis, Ilia Rodushkin, "The Benefits and Risks of Consuming Brewed Tea: Beware of Toxic Element Contamination", *Journal of Toxicology*, vol. 2013, Article ID 370460, 8 pages, 2013. https://doi.org/10.1155/2013/370460

8. Ka He, Yiqing Song et al, "Fish Consumption and Incidence of Stroke," *American Heart Association Journal Stroke*. 2004;35:1538–1542. https://doi.org/10.1161/01.STR.0000130856.31468.47

9. Lin PY, Chiu CC, Huang SY, Su KP. A meta-analytic review of polyunsaturated fatty acid compositions in dementia. J Clin Psychiatry. 2012 Sep;73(9):1245-54. doi: 10.4088/JCP.11r07546. Epub 2012 Aug 7. PMID: 22938939.

10. "Omega-3 Fatty Acids." *National Institutes of Health / Office of Dietary Supplements*. 1 Oct 2020. https://ods.od.nih.gov/factsheets/Omega3FattyAcids-HealthProfessional/

11. Vardavas CI, Linardakis MK, Hatzis CM, Saris WH, Kafatos AG. Prevalence of obesity and physical inactivity among farmers from Crete (Greece), four decades after the Seven Countries Study. Nutr Metab Cardiovasc Dis. 2009 Mar;19(3):156-62. doi: 10.1016/j.numecd.2008.10.008. Epub 2009 Jan 26. PMID: 19176283.

12. Constantine I Vardavas, Manolis K Linardakis, Christos M Hatzis, Wim H M Saris, Anthony G Kafatos, Cardiovascular disease risk factors and dietary habits of farmers from Crete 45 years after the first description of the Mediterranean diet, *European journal of cardiovascular prevention and rehabilitation*, Volume 17, Issue 4, 1 August 2010, Pages 440–446, https://doi.org/10.1097/HJR.0b013e32833692ea

13. Kafatos A, Diacatou A, Voukiklaris G, Nikolakakis N, Vlachonikolis J, Kounali D, Mamalakis G, Dontas AS. Heart disease risk-factor status

and dietary changes in the Cretan population over the past 30 y: the Seven Countries Study. Am J Clin Nutr. 1997 Jun;65(6):1882-6. doi: 10.1093/ajcn/65.6.1882. PMID: 9174487.

14. Vrentzos GE, Papadakis JA, Malliaraki N, Zacharis EA, Mazokopakis E, Margioris A, Ganotakis ES, Kafatos A. Diet, serum homocysteine levels and ischaemic heart disease in a Mediterranean population. Br J Nutr. 2004 Jun;91(6):1013-9. doi: 10.1079/BJN20041145. PMID: 15182405.

Play 8: One-on-One Drills — Salt Assaults

1. Farquhar WB, Edwards DG, Jurkovitz CT, Weintraub WS. Dietary sodium and health: more than just blood pressure. J Am Coll Cardiol. 2015 Mar 17;65(10):1042-50. doi: 10.1016/j.jacc.2014.12.039. PMID: 25766952; PMCID: PMC5098396.

2. Roher, Alex E et al. "Cerebral blood flow in Alzheimer's disease." *Vascular health and risk management* vol. 8 (2012): 599-611. doi:10.2147/VHRM.S34874

3. Kwong, Jeffrey et al. "Acute Myocardial Infarction After Laboratory-Confirmed Influenza Infection." *New England Journal of Medicine.* 2018; 378:345-353. DOI: 10.1056/NEJMoa1702090

4. American Society of Nephrology. "Low Potassium Linked To High Blood Pressure." ScienceDaily. ScienceDaily, 12 November 2008. <www.sciencedaily.com/releases/2008/11/081109074611.htm

5. De Clerck I, Boussery K, Pannier JL, Van De Voorde J. Potassium potently relaxes small rat skeletal muscle arteries. Med Sci Sports Exerc. 2003 Dec;35(12):2005-12. doi: 10.1249/01.MSS.0000099101.39139.FA. PMID: 14652495.

6. Haddy FJ, Vanhoutte PM, Feletou M. Role of potassium in regulating blood flow and blood pressure. Am J Physiol Regul Integr Comp Physiol. 2006 Mar;290(3):R546-52. doi: 10.1152/ajpregu.00491.2005. PMID: 16467502.

7. Chatterjee, Ranee et al. "Serum potassium and the racial disparity in diabetes risk: the Atherosclerosis Risk in Communities (ARIC) Study." *The American journal of clinical nutrition* vol. 93,5 (2011): 1087-91. doi:10.3945/ajcn.110.007286

8. U.S Department of Agriculture, Agricultural Research Service, Nutrient Data Laboratory. 2014. USDA National Nutrient Database for Standard Reference, Release 27. http://www.ars.usda.gov/nutrientdata

9. Weaver, Connie M. "Potassium and health." *Advances in nutrition (Bethesda, Md.)* vol. 4,3 368S-77S. 1 May. 2013, doi:10.3945/an.112.003533

Play 9: The Fundamentals — How to Play the Eating Game

1. Shishehbor F, Mansoori A, Shirani F. Vinegar consumption can attenuate postprandial glucose and insulin responses; a systematic

review and meta-analysis of clinical trials. Diabetes Res Clin Pract. 2017 May;127:1-9. doi: 10.1016/j.diabres.2017.01.021. Epub 2017 Mar 2. PMID: 28292654.

2. Carolyn A Miller, Karen D Corbin, Kerry-Ann da Costa, Shucha Zhang, Xueqing Zhao, Joseph A Galanko, Tondra Blevins, Brian J Bennett, Annalouise O'Connor, Steven H Zeisel, Effect of egg ingestion on trimethylamine-N-oxide production in humans: a randomized, controlled, dose-response study, *The American Journal of Clinical Nutrition*, Volume 100, Issue 3, September 2014, Pages 778–786, https://doi.org/10.3945/ajcn.114.087692

3. Zeng ST, Guo L, Liu SK, et al. Egg consumption is associated with increased risk of ovarian cancer: Evidence from a meta-analysis of observational studies. Clinical nutrition (Edinburgh, Scotland) 2015;34:635-41.

4. Si R, Qu K, Jiang Z, Yang X, Gao P. Egg consumption and breast cancer risk: a meta-analysis. Breast cancer (Tokyo, Japan) 2014;21:251-61.

5. Alicja Wolk, Christos S. Mantzoros, Swen-Olof Andersson, Reinhold Bergström, Lisa B. Signorello, Pagona Lagiou, Hams-Olov Adami, Dimitrios Trichopoulos, Insulin-Like Growth Factor 1 and Prostate Cancer Risk: A Population-Based, Case-Control Study, *JNCI: Journal of the National Cancer Institute*, Volume 90, Issue 12, 17 June 1998, Pages 911–915, https://doi.org/10.1093/jnci/90.12.911

6. Murphy, N et al. "Insulin-like growth factor-1, insulin-like growth factor-binding protein-3, and breast cancer risk: observational and Mendelian randomization analyses with ~430 000 women." *Annals of oncology : official journal of the European Society for Medical Oncology* vol. 31,5 (2020): 641-649. doi:10.1016/j.annonc.2020.01.066

7. Xi P and Liu RH. Whole food approach for type 2 diabetes prevention. Mol Nutr Food Res. 2016 May 9. doi: 10.1002/mnfr.201500963.

Play 10: Your Best Offense — Eat More Beans!

1. Lin, Long-Ze et al. "The polyphenolic profiles of common bean *(Phaseolus vulgaris L.)." Food chemistry* vol. 107,1 (2008): 399-410. doi:10.1016/j.foodchem.2007.08.038

2. Dolan, Laurie C et al. "Naturally occurring food toxins." *Toxins* vol. 2,9 (2010): 2289-332. doi:10.3390/toxins2092289

3. Peumans, Willy J. and Van Damme, Els J. M. "Lectins as Plant Defense Proteins." *Plant Physiology*. 109: 347-352 (1995).

4. Allen, Karen and Proctor, Debra. "Killer Kidney Beans?" *Utah State University Extension*. Oct 2014.

5. Thompson, Lilian et al. "Effect of Heat Processing on Hemagglutinin Activity in Red Kidney Beans." *Journal of Food Science*. Volume 48, Issue 1, January 1983. doi.org/10.1111/j.1365-2621.1983.tb14831.x

Play 11: Fixing the Chronic Slice — Slurp Up Some Souper Stuff

1. Penn State. "Eating Soup Will Help Cut Calories At Meals." ScienceDaily. ScienceDaily, 2 May 2007. <www.sciencedaily.com/releases/2007/05/070501142326.htm>.

2. Conrad Z, Niles MT, Neher DA, Roy ED, Tichenor NE, Jahns L (2018) Relationship between food waste, diet quality, and environmental sustainability. PLoS ONE 13(4): e0195405. https://doi.org/10.1371/journal.pone.0195405

Play 12: No. 1 Seed — Eat This Food Every Day

1. Francis, Andrew et al. "Effects of dietary flaxseed on atherosclerotic plaque regression." *American Journal of Physiology - Heart and Circulatory Physiology*. 15 Jun 2013. doi.org/10.1152/ajpheart.00606.2012

2. Patade A, Devareddy L, Lucas EA, Korlagunta K, Daggy BP, Arjmandi BH. Flaxseed reduces total and LDL cholesterol concentrations in Native American postmenopausal women. J Womens Health (Larchmt). 2008 Apr;17(3):355-66. doi: 10.1089/jwh.2007.0359. PMID: 18328014.

3. Hidden, Jane and Barbar Delage. "Essential Fatty Acids." *Linus Pauling Institute, Oregon State University* 2003. https://lpi.oregonstate.edu/mic/other-nutrients/essential-fatty-acids

4. National Institutes of Health. "Omega-3 Fatty Acids — Fact Sheet for Health Professionals." https://ods.od.nih.gov/factsheets/Omega3FattyAcids-HealthProfessional/

5. Rodriguez-Leyva, Delfin, and Grant N Pierce. "The cardiac and haemostatic effects of dietary hempseed." *Nutrition & metabolism* vol. 7 32. 21 Apr. 2010, doi:10.1186/1743-7075-7-32

6. Zhang W, Wang X, Liu Y, Tian H, Flickinger B, Empie MW, Sun SZ. Dietary flaxseed lignan extract lowers plasma cholesterol and glucose concentrations in hypercholesterolaemic subjects. Br J Nutr. 2008 Jun;99(6):1301-9. doi: 10.1017/S0007114507871649. Epub 2007 Dec 6. PMID: 18053310.

7. Milder IE, Arts IC, van de Putte B, Venema DP, Hollman PC. Lignan contents of Dutch plant foods: a database including lariciresinol, pinoresinol, secoisolariciresinol and matairesinol. Br J Nutr. 2005 Mar;93(3):393-402. doi: 10.1079/bjn20051371. PMID: 15877880.

8. Nieman DC, Gillitt N, Jin F, Henson DA, Kennerly K, Shanely RA, Ore B, Su M, Schwartz S. Chia seed supplementation and disease risk factors in overweight women: a metabolomics investigation. J Altern Complement Med. 2012 Jul;18(7):700-8. doi: 10.1089/acm.2011.0443. PMID: 22830971.

9. U.S. Food & Drug Administration, "What You Should Know About Using Cannabis, Including CBD, When Pregnant or Breastfeeding," October 2019.

Play 13: Whole Grain Analysis — The 5-to-1 Fiber Rule

1. Anderson GH, Liu Y, Smith CE, Liu TT, Nunez MF, Mollard RC, Luhovyy BL. The acute effect of commercially available pulse powders on postprandial glycaemic response in healthy young men. Br J Nutr. 2014 Dec 28;112(12):1966-73. doi: 10.1017/S0007114514003031. Epub 2014 Oct 20. PMID: 25327223.

2. Zafar TA, Al-Hassawi F, Al-Khulaifi F, Al-Rayyes G, Waslien C, Huffman FG. Organoleptic and glycemic properties of chickpea-wheat composite breads. J Food Sci Technol. 2015 Apr;52(4):2256-63. doi: 10.1007/s13197-013-1192-7. Epub 2013 Oct 20. PMID: 25829607; PMCID: PMC4375205.

3. Genoni A, Christophersen CT, Lo J, Coghlan M, Boyce MC, Bird AR, Lyons-Wall P, Devine A. Long-term Paleolithic diet is associated with lower resistant starch intake, different gut microbiota composition and increased serum TMAO concentrations. Eur J Nutr. 2020 Aug;59(5):1845-1858. doi: 10.1007/s00394-019-02036-y. Epub 2019 Jul 5. PMID: 31273523; PMCID: PMC7351840.

4. Whole Grains Council. "Fiber in Whole Grains". https://wholegrainscouncil.org/whole-grains-101/identifying-whole-grain-products/fiber-whole-grains

5. Gupta, Raj Kishor et al. "Reduction of phytic acid and enhancement of bioavailable micronutrients in food grains." *Journal of food science and technology* vol. 52,2 (2015): 676-84. doi:10.1007/s13197-013-0978-y

6. Lee YR, Kim CE, Kang MY, Nam SH. Cholesterol-lowering and antioxidant status-improving efficacy of germinated giant embryonic rice (Oryza sativa L.) in high cholesterol-fed rats. Ann Nutr Metab. 2007;51(6):519-26. doi: 10.1159/000112733. Epub 2007 Dec 20. PMID: 18097137.

Play 14: Breakfast of Champions — Picking a Winning Cereal

1. Irina Uzhova, Valentín Fuster, Antonio Fernández-Ortiz, José M. Ordovás, Javier Sanz, Leticia Fernández-Friera, Beatriz López-Melgar, José M. Mendiguren, Borja Ibáñez, Héctor Bueno, José L. Peñalvo. The Importance of Breakfast in Atherosclerosis Disease. *Journal of the American College of Cardiology*, 2017; 70 (15): 1833 DOI: 10.1016/j.jacc.2017.08.027

2. Shuang Rong MD, PhD et al. "Association of Skipping Breakfast With Cardiovascular and All-Cause Mortality." *Journal of the American College of Cardiology* 73(16): 2025-2032: DOI: 10.1016/j.jacc.2019.01.065

3. El Khoury, D et al. "Beta glucan: health benefits in obesity and metabolic syndrome." *Journal of nutrition and metabolism* vol. 2012 (2012): 851362. doi:10.1155/2012/851362

4. Ho HV, Sievenpiper JL, Zurbau A, Blanco Mejia S, Jovanovski E, Au-Yeung F, Jenkins AL, Vuksan V. A systematic review and meta-

analysis of randomized controlled trials of the effect of barley β-glucan on LDL-C, non-HDL-C and apoB for cardiovascular disease risk reductioni-iv. Eur J Clin Nutr. 2016

5. Loreto Gesualdo et al. The role of whole-grain barley on human fecal microbiota and metabolome. *Applied and Environmental Microbiology*, September 2015 DOI: 10.1128/AEM.02507-15

Play 15: Game Day Roster — Who's on First?

1. Jenkins, David J. A. et al. "Cumulative Meta-Analysis of the Soy Effect Over Time." *Journal of the American Heart Association* online 27 Jun 2019. https://doi.org/10.1161/JAHA.119.012458

2. Lanou, Amy J. "Soy foods: are they useful for optimal bone health?." *Therapeutic advances in musculoskeletal disease* vol. 3,6 (2011): 293-300. doi:10.1177/1759720X11417749

3. Levis, Silvina, and Marcio L Griebeler. "The role of soy foods in the treatment of menopausal symptoms." *The Journal of nutrition* vol. 140,12 (2010): 2318S-2321S. doi:10.3945/jn.110.124388

4. Nechuta SJ, Caan BJ, Chen WY, Lu W, Chen Z, Kwan ML, Flatt SW, Zheng Y, Zheng W, Pierce JP, Shu XO. Soy food intake after diagnosis of breast cancer and survival: an in-depth analysis of combined evidence from cohort studies of US and Chinese women. Am J Clin Nutr. 2012 Jul;96(1):123-32. doi: 10.3945/ajcn.112.035972. Epub 2012 May 30. PMID: 22648714; PMCID: PMC3374736.

5. Ziaei, Samira, and Reginald Halaby. "Dietary Isoflavones and Breast Cancer Risk." *Medicines (Basel, Switzerland)* vol. 4,2 18. 7 Apr. 2017, doi:10.3390/medicines4020018

6. Messina M. Soybean isoflavone exposure does not have feminizing effects on men: a critical examination of the clinical evidence. Fertil Steril. 2010 May 1;93(7):2095-104. doi: 10.1016/j.fertnstert.2010.03.002. Epub 2010 Apr 8. PMID: 20378106.

7. Jane Higdon, Ph.D. "Soy Isoflavones." *Oregon State University, Linus Pauling Institute website.* 2004. https://lpi.oregonstate.edu/mic/dietary-factors/phytochemicals/soy-isoflavones

8. Marina Touillaud, Amandine Gelot, Sylvie Mesrine, Catherine Bennetau-Pelissero, Françoise Clavel-Chapelon, Patrick Arveux, Fabrice Bonnet, Marc Gunter, Marie-Christine Boutron-Ruault, Agnès Fournier, Use of dietary supplements containing soy isoflavones and breast cancer risk among women aged >50 y: a prospective study, *The American Journal of Clinical Nutrition*, Volume 109, Issue 3, March 2019, Pages 597–605, https://doi.org/10.1093/ajcn/nqy313

Play 16: Sports Nuts — What's Your Nut Knowledge?

1. Hayes, Joy, and Gretchen Benson. "What the Latest Evidence Tells Us About Fat and Cardiovascular Health." *Diabetes spectrum : a publication*

of the American Diabetes Association vol. 29,3 (2016): 171-5. doi:10.2337/diaspect.29.3.171

Play 18: The Five-Pound Payoff

1. Whelton PK, Carey RM, Aronow WS, et al. 2017 ACC/AHA/AAPA/ABC/ACPM/AGS/APhA/ASH/ASPC/NMA/PCNA Guideline for the prevention, detection, evaluation, and management of high blood pressure in adults: A report of the American College of Cardiology/American Heart Association Task Force on Clinical Practice Guidelines. Journal of the American College of Cardiology. 2018;71:e127.

2. Modest weight loss through a 12-week weight management program with behavioral modification seems to attenuate inflammatory responses in young obese Koreans. Nutr Res. 2015 Apr;35(4):301-8. doi: 10.1016/j.nutres.2015.02.004. Epub 2015 Feb 24. PMID: 25753918.

3. Calder, Philip & Ahluwalia, Namanjeet & Brouns, Fred & Buetler, Timo & Clément, Karine & Cunningham, Karen & Esposito, Katherine & Jönsson, Lena & Kolb, Hubert & Lansink, Mirian & Marcos, Ascensión & Margioris, Andrew & Matusheski, Nathan & Nordmann, Herve & O'Brien, John & Pugliese, Giuseppe & Rizkalla, Salwa & Schalkwijk, Casper & Tuomilehto, Jaakko & Winklhofer-Roob, Brigitte. (2011). Dietary factors and low-grade inflammation in relation to overweight and obesity. The British journal of nutrition. 106 Suppl 3. S5-78. 10.1017/S0007114511005460.

4. Gorina, Y., Schappert, S., Bercovitz, A., Elgaddal, N., & Kramarow, E. (2014). Prevalence of incontinence among older Americans. Vital & Health Statistics. Series 3, Analytical And Epidemiological Studies, (36), 1-33

5. Subak LL, Wing R, West DS, Franklin F, Vittinghoff E, Creasman JM, Richter HE, Myers D, Burgio KL, Gorin AA, Macer J, Kusek JW, Grady D; PRIDE Investigators. Weight loss to treat urinary incontinence in overweight and obese women. N Engl J Med. 2009 Jan 29;360(5):481-90. doi:10.1056/NEJMoa0806375. PMID: 19179316; PMCID: PMC2877497.

6. Messier SP, Gutekunst DJ, Davis C, DeVita P. Weight loss reduces knee-joint loads in overweight and obese older adults with knee osteoarthritis. Arthritis Rheum. 2005 Jul;52(7):2026-32. doi: 10.1002/art.21139. PMID: 15986358.

Play 19: Fumbles and Fixes — Why You're Not Losing Weight

1. Patel, Alpa V et al. "Leisure time spent sitting in relation to total mortality in a prospective cohort of US adults." *American journal of epidemiology* vol. 172,4 (2010): 419-29. doi:10.1093/aje/kwq155

2. Owen, Neville et al. "Too much sitting: the population health science of sedentary behavior." *Exercise and sport sciences reviews* vol. 38,3 (2010): 105-13. doi:10.1097/JES.0b013e3181e373a2

3. Genevieve N. Healy, Charles E. Matthews, David W. Dunstan, Elisabeth A.H. Winkler, Neville Owen, Sedentary time and cardio-metabolic biomarkers in US adults: NHANES 2003–06, *European Heart Journal*, Volume 32, Issue 5, March 2011, Pages 590–597, https://doi.org/10.1093/eurheartj/ehq451

4. Melanson, Kathleen et al. Research on BMI and gender influence on amounts of food consumed and eating speed. Presented at *The Obesity Society*, Orlando, FL, October 2011.

5. Epel EE, Moyer AE, Martin CD, Macary S, Cummings N, Rodin J, Rebuffe-Scrive M. Stress-induced cortisol, mood, and fat distribution in men. Obes Res. 1999 Jan;7(1):9-15. doi: 10.1002/j.1550-8528.1999.tb00385.x. PMID: 10023725.

6. Epel ES, McEwen B, Seeman T, Matthews K, Castellazzo G, Brownell KD, Bell J, Ickovics JR. Stress and body shape: stress-induced cortisol secretion is consistently greater among women with central fat. Psychosom Med. 2000 Sep-Oct;62(5):623-32. doi: 10.1097/00006842-200009000-00005.

7. Chao, Ariana et al. "Food cravings mediate the relationship between chronic stress and body mass index." *Journal of health psychology* vol. 20,6 (2015): 721-9. doi:10.1177/1359105315573448

8. Schmid SM, Hallschmid M, Jauch-Chara K, Born J, Schultes B. A single night of sleep deprivation increases ghrelin levels and feelings of hunger in normal-weight healthy men. J Sleep Res. 2008 Sep;17(3):331-4. doi: 10.1111/j.1365-2869.2008.00662.x. Epub 2008 Jun 28. PMID: 18564298.

9. Calvin, Andrew D et al. "Effects of experimental sleep restriction on caloric intake and activity energy expenditure." *Chest* vol. 144,1 (2013): 79-86. doi:10.1378/chest.12-2829

10. Kripke DF, Garfinkel L, Wingard DL, Klauber MR, Marler MR. Mortality associated with sleep duration and insomnia. Arch Gen Psychiatry. 2002 Feb;59(2):131-6. doi: 10.1001/archpsyc.59.2.131. PMID: 11825133.

Play 20: Building Your Body After 50 — How to Reverse Muscle Loss

1. U.S. Census Bureau, Population Projections.

2. Bhasin, Shalender et al. "Design of a randomized trial to determine the optimum protein intake to preserve lean body mass and to optimize response to a promyogenic anabolic agent in older men with physical functional limitation." *Contemporary clinical trials* vol. 58 (2017): 86-93. doi:10.1016/j.cct.2017.05.004

3. Douglas Paddon-Jones, Wayne W Campbell, Paul F Jacques, Stephen B Kritchevsky, Lynn L Moore, Nancy R Rodriguez, Luc JC van Loon, Protein and healthy aging, *The American Journal of Clinical Nutrition*, Volume 101, Issue 6, June 2015, Pages 1339S–1345S, https://doi.org/10.3945/ajcn.114.084061

4. Adela Hruby, PhD, MPH, Shivani Sahni, PhD, Douglas Bolster, PhD, Paul F Jacques, DSc, Protein Intake and Functional Integrity in Aging: The Framingham Heart Study Offspring, *The Journals of Gerontology: Series A*, Volume 75, Issue 1, January 2020, Pages 123–130, https://doi.org/10.1093/gerona/gly201

5. Velissaris, Dimitrios et al. "C-Reactive Protein and Frailty in the Elderly: A Literature Review." *Journal of clinical medicine research* vol. 9,6 (2017): 461-465. doi:10.14740/jocmr2959w

6. Nutrition and Athletic Performance, Medicine & Science in Sports & Exercise: March 2009 - Volume 41 - Issue 3 - p 709-731 doi: 10.1249/MSS.0b013e31890eb86

7. Deutz, Nicolaas E P et al. "Protein intake and exercise for optimal muscle function with aging: recommendations from the ESPEN Expert Group." *Clinical nutrition* (Edinburgh, Scotland) vol. 33,6 (2014): 929-36. doi:10.1016/j.clnu.2014.04.007

8. Antonio, J., Peacock, C.A., Ellerbroek, A. et al. The effects of consuming a high protein diet (4.4 g/kg/d) on body composition in resistance-trained individuals. *J Int Soc Sports Nutr* 11, 19 (2014). https://doi.org/10.1186/1550-2783-11-19

9. Kripke DF, Garfinkel L, Wingard DL, Klauber MR, Marler MR. Mortality Associated With Sleep Duration and Insomnia. *Arch Gen Psychiatry*. 2002;59(2):131–136. doi:10.1001/archpsyc.59.2.131

10. Picca, Anna et al. "Gut Dysbiosis and Muscle Aging: Searching for Novel Targets against Sarcopenia." *Mediators of inflammation* vol. 2018 7026198. 30 Jan. 2018, doi:10.1155/2018/7026198

11. Ding, Kai et al. "Gut Microbiome and Osteoporosis." *Aging and disease* vol. 11,2 438-447. 9 Mar. 2020, doi:10.14336/AD.2019.0523

Play 21: Extra Innings — Pre- and Post-Game Snacks

1. Nutrition and Athletic Performance, Medicine & Science in Sports & Exercise: March 2009 - Volume 41 - Issue 3 - p 709-731 doi: 10.1249/MSS.0b013e31890eb86

2. Herbert Yu, Thomas Rohan, Role of the Insulin-Like Growth Factor Family in Cancer Development and Progression, *JNCI: Journal of the National Cancer Institute*, Volume 92, Issue 18, 20 September 2000, Pages 1472–1489, https://doi.org/10.1093/jnci/92.18.1472

3. Douglas Paddon-Jones, Wayne W Campbell, Paul F Jacques, Stephen B Kritchevsky, Lynn L Moore, Nancy R Rodriguez, Luc JC van Loon, Protein and healthy aging, *The American Journal of Clinical Nutrition*, Volume 101, Issue 6, June 2015, Pages 1339S–1345S, https://doi.org/10.3945/ajcn.114.084061

Play 22: Basic Training — Bowl Like a Pro

1. Zduńczyk Z, Flis M, Zieliński H, Wróblewska M, Antoszkiewicz Z, Juśkiewicz J. In vitro antioxidant activities of barley, husked oat, naked oat, triticale, and buckwheat wastes and their influence on the growth and biomarkers of antioxidant status in rats. J Agric Food Chem. 2006 Jun 14;54(12):4168-75. doi: 10.1021/jf060224m. PMID: 16756343.

2. Zieliński H, Kozłowska H. Antioxidant activity and total phenolics in selected cereal grains and their different morphological fractions. J Agric Food Chem. 2000 Jun;48(6):2008-16. doi: 10.1021/jf990619o. PMID: 10888490.

Play 26: Team Meeting — What You and Your Doctor Should Discuss

1. Adrienne L. Jones, B.S.; Lauren Harris-Kojetin, Ph.D.; and Roberto Valverde, M.P.H., Division of Health Care Statistics. "Characteristics and Use of Home Health Care by Men and Women Aged 65 and Over". *National Health Statistics Reports,* Number 52, April 18, 2012, https://www.cdc.gov/nchs/data/nhsr/nhsr052.pdf

2. Yamamoto K, Kawano H, Gando Y, Iemitsu M, Murakami H, Sanada K, Tanimoto M, Ohmori Y, Higuchi M, Tabata I, Miyachi M. Poor trunk flexibility is associated with arterial stiffening. *Am J Physiol Heart Circ Physiol.* 2009 Oct;297(4):H1314-8. doi: 10.1152/ajpheart.00061.2009. Epub 2009 Aug 7. PMID: 19666849.

3. Elflein, John. Home Care in the U.S. — Statistics & Facts. *Statistica. com,* July 28, 2020. https://www.statista.com/topics/4049/home-care-in-the-us/

4. Stamps, Jennifer J et al. "A brief olfactory test for Alzheimer's disease." *Journal of the neurological sciences* vol. 333,1-2 (2013): 19-24. doi:10.1016/j.jns.2013.06.033

5. Eveline Nüesch, Paul Dieppe, Stephan Reichenbach, Susan Williams, Samuel Iff, Peter Jüni. "All cause and disease specific mortality in patients with knee or hip osteoarthritis: population based cohort study." *BMJ* 2011;342:d1165. https://doi.org/10.1136/bmj.d1165

6. Leritz, Elizabeth C et al. "Cardiovascular Disease Risk Factors and Cognition in the Elderly." *Current cardiovascular risk reports* vol. 5,5 (2011): 407-412. doi:10.1007/s12170-011-0189-x

7. Reed B, Villeneuve S, Mack W, DeCarli C, Chui HC, Jagust W. Associations between serum cholesterol levels and cerebral amyloidosis. *JAMA Neurol.* 2014 Feb;71(2):195-200. doi: 10.1001/jamaneurol.2013.5390. PMID: 24378418; PMCID: PMC4083819.

8. Thibodeau, Jennifer T.; Turer, Aslan T.; Gualano, Sarah K.; Ayers, Colby R.; Velez-Martinez, Mariella; Mishkin, Joseph D.; Patel, Parag C.; Mammen, Pradeep P.A.; Markham, David W.; Levine, Benjamin D.; Drazner, Mark H. (2014). "Characterization of a Novel Symptom of

Advanced Heart Failure: Bendopnea". *JACC: Heart Failure*. 2 (1): 24–31. doi:10.1016/j.jchf.2013.07.009. ISSN 2213-1779. PMID 24622115.

9. Spector, June T et al. "Migraine headache and ischemic stroke risk: an updated meta-analysis." *The American journal of medicine* vol. 123,7 (2010): 612-24. doi:10.1016/j.amjmed.2009.12.021

10. Weinberg, Ido et al. "The systolic blood pressure difference between arms and cardiovascular disease in the Framingham Heart Study." *The American journal of medicine* vol. 127,3 (2014): 209-15. doi:10.1016/j.amjmed.2013.10.027

11. Yasuharu Tabara, Yoko Okada, Maya Ohara, Eri Uetani, Tomoko Kido, Namiko Ochi, Tokihisa Nagai, Michiya Igase, Tetsuro Miki, Fumihiko Matsuda, and Katsuhiko Kohara. Association of Postural Instability With Asymptomatic Cerebrovascular Damage and Cognitive Decline: The Japan Shimanami Health Promoting Program Study. *Stroke*, December 2014 DOI: 10.1161/STROKEAHA.114.006704

12. Mirmiran, Parvin et al. "Relationship between Diet and Non-alcoholic Fatty Liver Disease: A Review Article." *Iranian journal of public health* vol. 46,8 (2017): 1007-1017.

13. American Heart Association. "Liver, belly fat may identify high risks of heart disease in obese people." ScienceDaily. ScienceDaily, 22 July 2011. www.sciencedaily.com/releases/2011/07/110721163021.htm.

14. Oliver J. Rider , Rajarshi Banerjee , Jennifer J. Rayner , Ravi Shah , Venkatesh L. Murthy , Matthew D. Robson , and Stefan Neubauer. "Investigating a Liver Fat: Arterial Stiffening Pathway in Adult and Childhood Obesity." *Arteriosclerosis, Thrombosis, and Vascular Biology. 2016;36:198–203.* 12. doi.org/10.1161/ATVBAHA.115.306561

15. Sutton-Tyrrell K, Najjar SS, Boudreau RM, Venkitachalam L, Kupelian V, Simonsick EM, Havlik R, Lakatta EG, Spurgeon H, Kritchevsky S, Pahor M, Bauer D, Newman A; Health ABC Study. Elevated aortic pulse wave velocity, a marker of arterial stiffness, predicts cardiovascular events in well-functioning older adults. Circulation. 2005 Jun 28;111(25):3384-90. doi: 10.1161/CIRCULATIONAHA.104.483628. Epub 2005 Jun 20. PMID: 15967850.

16. Vilar-Gomez E, Martinez-Perez Y, Calzadilla-Bertot L, Torres-Gonzalez A, Gra-Oramas B, Gonzalez-Fabian L, Friedman SL, Diago M, Romero-Gomez M. Weight Loss Through Lifestyle Modification Significantly Reduces Features of Nonalcoholic Steatohepatitis. Gastroenterology. 2015 Aug;149(2):367-78.e5; quiz e14-5. doi: 10.1053/j.gastro.2015.04.005. Epub 2015 Apr 10. PMID: 25865049.

17. Chalasani N, Younossi Z, Lavine JE, Charlton M, Cusi K, Rinella M, Harrison SA, Brunt EM, Sanyal AJ. The diagnosis and management of nonalcoholic fatty liver disease: Practice guidance from the American Association for the Study of Liver Diseases. Hepatology. 2018 Jan;67(1):328-357. doi: 10.1002/hep.29367. Epub 2017 Sep 29. PMID: 28714183.

Play 27: The Equipment Room — Tools to Fire Up Fast Food

1. Fatemeh Hajiaghaalipour, Junedah Sanusi, M. S. Kanthimathi. "Temperature and Time of Steeping Affect the Antioxidant Properties of White, Green, and Black Tea Infusions." *Journal of Food Science*, 2015; DOI: 10.1111/1750-3841.13149

Play 28: Stock Your Locker — The Go-To Pantry (Your Reserves)

1. "How Much Arsenic Is in Your Rice?" *Consumer Reports magazine*, January 2015. https://www.consumerreports.org/cro/magazine/2015/01/how-much-arsenic-is-in-your-rice/index.htm

2. U.S. Food & Drug Administration, "Agricultural Biotechnology — Feed Your Mind," September 2020. https://www.fda.gov/food/consumers/agricultural-biotechnology

3. American Cancer Society, "Known and Probable Human Carcinogens." August 14, 2019. https://www.cancer.org/cancer/cancer-causes/general-info/known-and-probable-human-carcinogens.html

4. Han WY, Zhao FJ, Shi YZ, Ma LF, Ruan JY. Scale and causes of lead contamination in Chinese tea. Environ Pollut. 2006 Jan;139(1):125-32. doi: 10.1016/j.envpol.2005.04.025. Epub 2005 Jul 5. PMID: 15998560.

5. Zhang, Jian et al. "Accumulation of Heavy Metals in Tea Leaves and Potential Health Risk Assessment: A Case Study from Puan County, Guizhou Province, China." *International journal of environmental research and public health* vol. 15,1 133. 13 Jan. 2018, doi:10.3390/ijerph15010133

6. Hopkins, Allison L et al. "Hibiscus sabdariffa L. in the treatment of hypertension and hyperlipidemia: a comprehensive review of animal and human studies." *Fitoterapia* vol. 85 (2013): 84-94. doi:10.1016/j.fitote.2013.01.003

7. Serban C, Sahebkar A, Ursoniu S, Andrica F, Banach M. "Effect of sour tea (Hibiscus sabdariffa L.) on arterial hypertension: a systematic review and meta-analysis of randomized controlled trials." J Hypertens. 2015 Jun;33(6):1119-27. doi: 10.1097/HJH.0000000000000585. PMID: 25875025.

8. Egert S, Tereszczuk J, Wein S, Müller MJ, Frank J, Rimbach G, Wolffram S. Simultaneous ingestion of dietary proteins reduces the bioavailability of galloylated catechins from green tea in humans. Eur J Nutr. 2013 Feb;52(1):281-8. doi: 10.1007/s00394-012-0330-8. Epub 2012 Feb 25. PMID: 22366739.

9. Blahová, Jana, and Zdeňka Svobodová. "Assessment of coumarin levels in ground cinnamon available in the Czech retail market." *TheScientificWorldJournal* vol. 2012 (2012): 263851. doi:10.1100/2012/263851

10. Zhang, Yuesheng. "Allyl isothiocyanate as a cancer chemopreventive phytochemical." *Molecular nutrition & food research* vol. 54,1 (2010): 127-35. doi:10.1002/mnfr.200900323

11. Bolling, Bradley. "Almond Polyphenols: Methods of Analysis, Contribution to Food Quality, and Health Promotion." *Comprehensive Reviews in Food Science and Food Safety* vol. 16. 2017, doi: 10.1111/1541-4337.12260

12. Chen, C-Y Oliver et al. "Polyphenols in Almond Skins after Blanching Modulate Plasma Biomarkers of Oxidative Stress in Healthy Humans." *Antioxidants (Basel, Switzerland)* vol. 8,4 95. 10 Apr. 2019, doi:10.3390/antiox8040095

13. Almekinder, Elisabeth, "20 Healthy Flours form Lowest to Highest Carbohydrates." TheDiabetesCouncil.com *2020 May.* https://www.thediabetescouncil.com/20-healthy-flours/

14. Kelishadi, Roya et al. "Acute and long term effects of grape and pomegranate juice consumption on endothelial dysfunction in pediatric metabolic syndrome." *Journal of research in medical sciences : the official journal of Isfahan University of Medical Sciences* vol. 16,3 (2011): 245-53.

15. Lentza-Rizos C, Avramides EJ. Pesticide residues in olive oil. Rev Environ Contam Toxicol. 1995;141:111-34. doi: 10.1007/978-1-4612-2530-0_4. PMID: 7886254.

Play 29: Real Food Recipes for Longevity Jocks

1. Yang, Tianxi, et al. "Effectiveness of Commercial and Homemade Washing Agents in Removing Pesticide Residues on and in Apples." *J. Agric. Food Chem.* 2017, 65, 44, 9744–9752. Publication Date:October 25, 2017, doi.org/10.1021/acs.jafc.7b03118

2. Yadav BS, Sharma A, Yadav RB. "Studies on effect of multiple heating/cooling cycles on the resistant starch formation in cereals, legumes and tubers." *Int J Food Sci Nutr.* 2009;60 Suppl 4:258-72. doi: 10.1080/09637480902970975. PMID: 19562607.

3. Mozaffari-Khosravi H, Jalali-Khanabadi BA, Afkhami-Ardekani M, Fatehi F. Effects of sour tea (Hibiscus sabdariffa) on lipid profile and lipoproteins in patients with type II diabetes. J Altern Complement Med. 2009 Aug;15(8):899-903. doi: 10.1089/acm.2008.0540. PMID: 19678781.

4. Serban C, Sahebkar A, Ursoniu S, Andrica F, Banach M. "Effect of sour tea (Hibiscus sabdariffa L.) on arterial hypertension: a systematic review and meta-analysis of randomized controlled trials." J Hypertens. 2015 Jun;33(6):1119-27. doi: 10.1097/HJH.0000000000000585. PMID: 25875025.

5. Da-Costa-Rocha I, Bonnlaender B, Sievers H, Pischel I, Heinrich M. Hibiscus sabdariffa L. - a phytochemical and pharmacological review. Food Chem. 2014 Dec 15;165:424-43. doi: 10.1016/j.foodchem.2014.05.002. Epub 2014 May 27. PMID: 25038696.

6. Lucy N Lewis, Richard P G Hayhoe, Angela A Mulligan, Robert N Luben, Kay-Tee Khaw, Ailsa A Welch. "Lower Dietary and Circulating Vitamin C in Middle- and Older-Aged Men and Women Are Associated with Lower Estimated Skeletal Muscle Mass." *The Journal of Nutrition,* Volume 150, Issue 10, October 2020, Pages 2789–2798, doi.org/10.1093/jn/nxaa221

7. Grussu D, Stewart D, McDougall GJ. "Berry polyphenols inhibit α-amylase in vitro: identifying active components in rowanberry and raspberry." *J Agric Food Chem.* 2011 Mar 23;59(6):2324-31. doi: 10.1021/jf1045359. Epub 2011 Feb 17. PMID: 21329358

8. "Arsenic in Your Food." *Consumer Reports* Nov 2012. https://www.fda.gov/files/food/published/Arsenic-in-Rice-and-Rice-Products-Risk-Assessment-Report-PDF.pdf

9. Raab, Andrea & Baskaran, Christina & Feldmann, Jörg & Meharg, Andrew. (2009). Cooking rice in a high water to rice ratio reduces inorganic arsenic content. Journal of environmental monitoring : JEM. 11. 41-4. 10.1039/b816906c.

10. Roher, Alex E et al. "Cerebral blood flow in Alzheimer's disease." *Vascular health and risk management* vol. 8 (2012): 599-611. doi:10.2147/VHRM.S34874

11. Presley, Tennille D et al. "Acute effect of a high nitrate diet on brain perfusion in older adults." *Nitric oxide : biology and chemistry* vol. 24,1 (2011): 34-42. doi:10.1016/j.niox.2010.10.002

12. Oracz, J., Nebesny, E. & Zyzelewicz, D. Changes in the flavan-3-ols, anthocyanins, and flavanols composition of cocoa beans of different *Theobroma cacao* L. groups affected by roasting conditions. *Eur Food Res Technol* 241, 663–681 (2015). https://doi.org/10.1007/s00217-015-2494-y

13. Miller KB, Hurst WJ, Payne MJ, Stuart DA, Apgar J, Sweigart DS, Ou B. Impact of alkalization on the antioxidant and flavanol content of commercial cocoa powders. J Agric Food Chem. 2008 Sep 24;56(18):8527-33. doi: 10.1021/jf801670p. Epub 2008 Aug 19. PMID: 18710243.

14. Lukasik J, Bradley ML, Scott TM, Dea M, Koo A, Hsu WY, Bartz JA, Farrah SR. Reduction of poliovirus 1, bacteriophages, Salmonella montevideo, and Escherichia coli O157:H7 on strawberries by physical and disinfectant washes. J Food Prot. 2003 Feb;66(2):188-93. doi: 10.4315/0362-028x-66.2.188. PMID: 12597475.

INDEX

A

acrylamide, 57-61

AGEs (advanced glycation end products, glycotoxins): aging, 16-21, 23, 54-61; cooking methods, 58-59; foods, 54-55; glycation, 15-16

aging influences, 85

almonds: blood sugar, 21; brain-friendly, 65; chemical fumigation, 214; Cocoa Almond Milkshake, 243; Five-Minute Almond Milk, 244; flour, 21, 121, 222; prebiotics, 23; shopping for, 214

ALA, 95-96

algal oil, 96

Alzheimer's disease: amyloid plaque, 184-185; balance, 186; cardiovascular disease, 70; cholesterol, 184-185; chronic inflammation, 27; damage to mitochondria, 12; memory loss, 184-185; nitrates, 44; smell test 182-183; TMAO, 37, type 2 diabetes, 17; type 3 diabetes, 18; vascular health, 62

antibiotics: gut health, 25; damage to mitochondria, 12

anti-nutrients, 104

antioxidants, 10, 14, 38-49, 62-65, 165-169

arsenic: cooking rice, 257-258; shopping for, 226-227

arterial stiffening: AGEs (glycotoxins), 16-18; triglycerides, 189; sit-and-reach test, 181; sodium, 20; sugar, 15-16,

arthritis: chronic inflammation, 27; weight gain, 128-130; pain, 183-184

Athlete Cheat Sheet, 331

B

ATP (adenosine triphosphate), 9

avocado oil: daily servings, 80; saturated fat, 34; shopping for, 223-227

balance, 186

barley, 102, 104, 108-111; Barley with Fresh Figs, Arugula, and Maple Mustard Vinaigrette, 275; prebiotics, 24

beans: cooking, 88; daily servings, 78; flatulence, 88; phytohaemagglutinin (PHA), 88-89; shelf life, 89

belly fat: fatty liver, 187-189; flour, 21; triglycerides, 188-189; visceral fat, 187

berries: brain-friendly, 63; daily servings, 78; starch blockers, 250; washing, 294

beta-glucans, 108-111

blood vessels: aging, 3; blood sugar, 30; inflammation, 27; sit-and-reach test, 181; sodium, 20, 70

bone broth, 19

bone loss (see osteoporosis)

breakfast: cereal, 106-111; plant-based protein, 152-153; road food, 174-175

buckwheat: fiber, 104; freezing, 210; pseudo-grain, 103; soba, 162

C

caffeine, 242

chia seeds: daily servings, 79; nutrition, 96, 98; protein source, 153, 163; shopping for, 213

ATHLETE CHEAT SHEET

▸ **FIBER RULE**
Carbohydrates
to Fiber Ratio → **5-to-1**

1-to-1 ← **SODIUM RULE** ◂
Calories to
Sodium Ratio

▸ **OMEGA-6 to
OMEGA-3**
No more than
4-to-1 Ratio → **1-to-1**

BREAKFAST CEREAL
(The Big Five)

1
First ingredient is a "whole"
or "sprouted" grain.

2
Meets the 5-to-1 Fiber Rule.

3
Meets the 1-to-1 Sodium Rule.

4
Contains 5+ gm fiber.

5
Less than 5 gm added sugar.
(Better yet, *none*.)

O-BBBOY! SOLUBLE FIBER

Oats Barley Beans Berries Onions Yams

LIMITS PER DAY

SODIUM
Ages 19-50:
1,500 mg
(~2/3 tsp salt)

Ages 51-70:
1,300 mg
(~1/2 tsp salt)

Ages 71+:
1,200 mg
(1/2 tsp salt)

**ADDED
SUGAR***

Men: 9 tsp or
less (36 gm)

Women: 6 tsp
or less (24 gm)

*Ideally 0 gm
added sugar
per day

OIL
1 tsp per
1,000
calories

**SATURATED
FAT**
Less than 5% to
6% of total daily
calories

PROTEIN RECOMMENDATIONS (gm)

50 years old | Weight* × **0.8 gm per kg** OR **0.36 gm per lb**

Weight* × **1.0 to 1.5 gm per kg** OR **0.45 to 0.68 gm per lb** | **50** years old

Athletes Endurance & Strength-trained

 Weight* × **1.2 to 1.7 gm per kg** OR **0.55 to 0.77 gm per lb**

*Use "ideal" body weight for healthy adults

Sample Shopping List

BUILD YOUR PANTRY, FRIDGE, AND FREEZER AROUND THESE COLOR-FUL ANTI-AGING STAPLES

☐ **Fresh fruits** e.g., apples, bananas, cantaloupe, grapefruit, oranges, peaches, plums, strawberries, watermelon

☐ **Fresh vegetables** e.g., artichokes, avocado, bell peppers, broccoli, carrots, celery, cucumbers, Romaine lettuce, tomatoes, zucchini

☐ **Starchy vegetables** corn, orange and purple sweet potatoes (a.k.a. Hawaiian or Okinawa sweet potatoes), peas, taro, winter squash

☐ **Frozen and dried fruits/vegetables** e.g., berries. cherries, green beans, mango, peas, pineapple

☐ **Intact grains and pseudo-grains** e.g., barley, buckwheat, bulgur, farro, oats, quinoa, rice (black, brown, red, or wild)

☐ **Sprouted whole grain products** e.g., Ezekiel 4:9® bread, cereal, English muffins, tortillas

☐ **Legumes** e.g., beans (canned or dried), edamame, lentils (all colors), soybeans, tofu

☐ **Protein pasta** e.g., black bean, edamame, lentil, or soybean pasta

☐ **Plant-based dairy** e.g., soy milk, almond milk Greek yogurt

☐ **Nuts and seeds** e.g., almonds, pistachios, walnuts; flax, chia, hemp seeds, pepitas

☐ **Low-mercury fish rich in omega-3s** SMASH: Salmon, Mackerel, Anchovies, Sardines, Herring (fresh, frozen, or canned)

☐ **Tea** green, black, and hibiscus

THE HUNGER SCALE

DESPERATE

1 You're ravenous, dizzy, weak, shaky. You're so hungry you'll eat year-old Slim Jims you found in your golf bag or lint-covered mints buried at the bottom of your purse or pocket.

Your stomach is growling a lot, your brain demands energy, and your head aches. You're irritable, beyond hungry, and eyeing Benji's peanut butter biscuits.

2 **UNCOMFORTABLY HUNGRY**

CRAZY HUNGRY

3 Your stomach is beginning to growl. You have hunger pangs. The urge to eat is strong. You can't concentrate on simple tasks, such as complaining about your botched two-inch putt.

You're beginning to feel hungry. It's time to think about what to eat. You can wait, but when asked if you want a 6" or footlong sub, you reply, "Both."

4 **A LITTLE HUNGRY**

NEUTRAL
(Neither Full Nor Hungry)

5 You're not preoccupied with eating. "My mind is on my game, not food."

You are pleasantly full, and think, "I could still eat a few more bites…"

6 **SATISFIED & LIGHT**

FULL

7 You feel slightly uncomfortable. You won't be hungry for 3 to 4 hours. You're able to make it most of the way home from a restaurant without digging into your doggie bag.

You feel stuffed, and you're busting out of your pants. You don't want anything else, and declare, "I can't eat another bite… Oh look, pie!"

8 **VERY FULL**

VERY UNCOMFORTABLY FULL
(Thanksgiving Full)

9 You feel heavy. Your stomach aches. This time, you really can't eat another bite!

You are physically miserable. You can't move. You feel so full you may lose your cookies.

10 **PAINFULLY FULL**

Check off all the First-Stringers you eat in one day.
THE POWER PLATE PLAYERS (DAILY ROSTER)

FIRST STRING – GO FOR IT!

BERRIES
- 1/2 cup (fresh or frozen)
- 1/4 cup dried

1 DAILY SERVING
☐

OTHER FRUITS
- 1 medium fruit
- 1 cup cubed
  (fresh or frozen)
- 1/4 cup dried

3 DAILY SERVINGS
☐ ☐ ☐

LEAFY GREENS
- 1 cup raw
- 1/2 cup cooked

2 DAILY SERVINGS
☐ ☐

CRUCIFEROUS VEGETABLES
- 1/2 cup chopped
- 1/4 cup Brussels or broccoli sprouts
- 1 Tbsp horseradish

1 DAILY SERVING
☐

OTHER VEGETABLES
- 1/2 cup raw or cooked
- 1/4 cup dried mushrooms
- 4 oz vegetable juice

2 DAILY SERVINGS
☐ ☐

RED FRUIT OR VEGETABLE
Lycopene
Include 10K mcg, such as:
- 2/3 cup minestrone
- 4 oz. tomato juice
- 1/3 cup spaghetti sauce
- 1-1/2 cups watermelon

BEANS
- 1/2 cup cooked
- 1 cup fresh peas/ sprouted lentils
- 1/4 cup hummus or bean dip
- 1/2 cup cooked lentil/bean pasta

3 DAILY SERVINGS
☐ ☐ ☐

INTACT & SPROUTED GRAINS
- 1/2 cup cooked intact grains
- 1 slice sprouted whole grain bread
- 3 cups popped popcorn

3 DAILY SERVINGS
☐ ☐ ☐

FLAXSEEDS
- 1 to 2 Tbsp ground

1 DAILY SERVING
☐

NUTS & SEEDS
- 1 oz (about 1/4 cup)
- 2 Tbsp nut or seed butter

1 DAILY SERVING
☐

NUTRITIONAL YEAST
- 2 tsp

1 DAILY SERVING
☐

TURMERIC
- 1/4 to 1 tsp

1 DAILY SERVING
☐

HERBS & SPICES
- Eat liberally

1 DAILY SERVING
☐

BEVERAGES
- **Green Tea or Matcha**
  1 cup (1-4 servings)
  ☐ ☐ ☐ ☐
- **Hibiscus Tea**
  1 cup (1 serving)
  ☐
- **Water & Other Beverages**
  1 cup (3-6 servings)
  ☐ ☐ ☐ ☐ ☐ ☐

8 DAILY SERVINGS
☐ ☐ ☐ ☐ ☐ ☐ ☐ ☐

VINEGAR
- 2 tsp with each meal

3 DAILY SERVINGS
☐ ☐ ☐

FIRST STRINGERS ARE:
- Recommended – the healthiest choices
- Naturally rich in water ("water-rich")
- High volume
- High in fiber (requires more chewing)
- Low in calories
- Low in sodium

ABOUT THE COACH

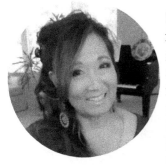

Karen Owoc, ACSM-CEP, ACSM/ACS-CET is a cardiopulmonary rehabilitation physiologist at the Palo Alto VA Medical Center and also a private medical fitness trainer with a focus on functional longevity. She grew up playing and competing in many sports, with skiing being her passion. Karen's unique approach to a healthy mindset and weight loss has been popularized in her e-books: *Why-Can't-I-Lose-Weight Troubleshooting Guide*, *The Happy Brain Blueprint*, and *The Happy Brain Hormone Guide*.

As a medical weight management facilitator and clinical exercise physiologist, Karen has helped hundreds of men and women manage their chronic health conditions and live happier, more functional lives. Weight loss is often a beneficial side effect. She believes the reason most people can't lose weight is because they've been trained to diet, that is, to deprive themselves of food vs use it as medicine.

Karen has extensive experience teaching nutrition and prescribing exercise as a treatment and prevention strategy for high-risk adults challenged with conditions often associated with lifestyle, such as cardiovascular and neurodegenerative diseases, type 2 diabetes, metabolic syndrome, osteoarthritis, osteoporosis, sarcopenia, and cancer. She teaches plant-based nutrition classes and appears on the KRON 4 morning news every weekend in the San Francisco Bay Area as their expert on healthy living. As a frequent health contributor, Karen has appeared on ABC 10 and has been quoted in media outlets, such as CNN Health, FoxNews.com, NBC Bay Area, Livestrong, Newsday, USA Gymnastics, and USA Volleyball.

For more coach's tips and recipes, visit KarenOwoc.com

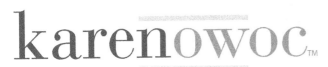

3 1901 10064 6670

CPSIA information can be obtained
at www.ICGtesting.com
Printed in the USA
LVHW061753130322
713348LV00004B/61